Police Custody Healthcare for Nurses and Paramedics

Police Custody Healthcare for Nurses and Paramedics

FIRST EDITION

Edited by

Matthew Peel

Leeds Community Healthcare NHS Trust, Leeds, UK & UK Association of Forensic Nurses and Paramedics

Jennie Smith

Mitie Care and Custody Health Ltd, London, UK & UK Association of Forensic Nurses and Paramedics

Vanessa Webb

Nurture Health and Care Ltd, Norwich, UK

Margaret Bannerman

Nurture Health and Care Ltd, Norwich, UK

WILEY Blackwell

Registered Offices
John Wiley & Sons, Inc., 111 River Street, Hoboken, NJ 07030, USA
John Wiley & Sons Ltd, New Era House, 8 Oldlands Way, Bognor Regis, West Sussex, PO22 9NQ, UK

For details of our global editorial offices, customer services, and more information about Wiley products visit us at www.wiley.com.

Wiley also publishes its books in a variety of electronic formats and by print-on-demand. Some content that appears in standard print versions of this book may not be available in other formats.

Library of Congress Cataloging-in-Publication Data Applied for:

Paperback ISBN: 9781394204892

Cover Design: Wiley
Cover Images: © New Africa/Adobe Stock Photos, © Wasan/Adobe Stock Photos

Set in 9.5/12pt STIXTwoText by Straive, Pondicherry, India

Printed and bound by CPI Group (UK) Ltd, Croydon, CR0 4YY

C9781394204892_030225

The manufacturer's authorized representative according to the EU General Product Safety Regulation is Wiley-VCH GmbH, Boschstr. 12, 69469 Weinheim, Germany, e-mail: Product_Safety@wiley.com.

Contents

4 Vulnerability and Appropriate Adults   31

Chris Bath and Roxanna Dehaghani

5 Managing Long-Term Conditions   41

Vanessa Webb

10   Substance Use and Misuse   105

11   Use of Force   120

15 Writing Statements and Giving Evidence   180

Matthew Peel

16 Special Circumstances   190

Matthew Peel and Thomas Bird

17 Governance   203

Vanessa Webb

18 Professional Ethics   212

Vanessa Webb

19 Emergencies — 221

Matthew Peel, Nick Hart, and Nick Skinner

List of Contributors

Margaret Bannerman
Nurture Health and Care Ltd, Norwich, UK

Chris Bath
National Appropriate Adult Network, Ashford, UK

Thomas Bird
Mitie Care and Custody Health Ltd, London, UK & UK Association of Forensic Nurses and Paramedics

Roxanna Dehaghani
Cardiff University, Cardiff, Wales

Alex Guymer
Mitie Care and Custody Health Ltd, London, UK

Nick Hart
Leeds Community Healthcare NHS Trust, Leeds, UK

Samantha Holmes
Leeds Community Healthcare NHS Trust, Leeds, UK

Abdulla Kraam
North Lincolnshire CAMHS, Scunthorpe, UK

Amanda McDonough
Mitie Care and Custody Health Ltd, London, UK

Esther McPhail
Mitie Care and Custody Health Ltd, London, UK

Dipti Patel
Mountain Healthcare Ltd, Stevenage, UK

Matthew Peel
Leeds Community Healthcare NHS Trust, Leeds, UK & UK Association of Forensic Nurses and Paramedics

Nicola Sheridan
Mitie Care and Custody Health Ltd, London, UK

Nick Skinner
Leeds Community Healthcare NHS Trust, Leeds, UK

Mandy Smail
Mitie Care and Custody Health Ltd, London, UK

Jennie Smith
Mitie Care and Custody Health Ltd, London, UK & UK Association of Forensic Nurses and Paramedics

Vanessa Webb
Nurture Health and Care Ltd, Norwich, UK

Preface

As a team of editors, each with a rich and diverse background in police custody healthcare and education, we are proud to present this comprehensive text, a culmination of our collective experiences and insights.

Our journey in this field has given us a profound understanding of the complexities and challenges inherent in police custody healthcare. Matthew brings over 12 years of experience in police custody. Jennie Smith, the President of the UK Association of Forensic Nurses and Paramedics, contributes with her 17 years of dedication to this field. Dr Vanessa Webb offers a unique dual perspective with her extensive experience as both a nurse and a doctor in police custody. Margaret, with her 20 years in higher education, has been pivotal in developing advanced standards in education and training for custody healthcare professionals, including the UK's first advanced master's programme in this specialty.

This text is born from our shared desire to create a resource that we wished we had at the outset of our careers. It is designed to guide those new to the setting and to enrich the practice of our seasoned colleagues. Our collective goal has been to create a book that not only educates but also resonates with the realities of working in such a dynamic and challenging environment.

We recognise that the practices in police custody vary greatly and can be inconsistent nationally. In this book, we have endeavoured to address these variations, aiming to bring clarity and a unified approach to the field. Our combined expertise and experiences have allowed us to cover a wide range of topics, offering practical advice, and in-depth knowledge, all while highlighting the best practices and standards necessary for effective and compassionate care in custody.

We hope this book will serve as a resource for those navigating the intricate world of police custody, providing a solid foundation for both the novices and the veterans in the field. It is with great pride and anticipation that we share this work with you, our readers, as you embark on or continue your journey in this vital area of healthcare.

MATTHEW PEEL, JENNIE SMITH,
VANESSA WEBB, AND MARGARET BANNERMAN

Acknowledgements

I extend my heartfelt thanks to those who have mentored and guided me throughout my career. Your mentorship and guidance have been invaluable in shaping my professional journey. Equally, I am grateful to the colleagues I have had the privilege to mentor. Your probing questions and eagerness to learn have in turn deepened my own understanding and perspectives.

I express my sincere appreciation to the editorial team – Jennie, Ness, and Marg. Your dedication, hard work and attention to detail have been pivotal in the creation of this text. A special note of thanks goes to all contributors who have enriched this book with their insights, whether through reviewing chapters, contributing texts, or sharing their expertise. Your collective contributions have been immeasurable.

I am grateful to Ian Peate for his support and advice during the initial stages of this project. His insights and encouragement were crucial in transforming the initial thoughts around this text into reality.

Lastly, but most importantly, I extend a massive thank you to my partner and family. Your unwavering support, understanding and love have been the bedrock upon which this endeavour was built. Without you, none of this would have been possible.

MATTHEW PEEL

When my best friend's father mentioned that Merseyside Police were setting up a forensic nursing team and that I should apply for the manager role, little did I know the amazing journey he would set me upon.

I could not have imagined the all of the amazing, driven, passionate, funny and quirky people I would meet. Not only work colleagues, many of whom have become life-long friends, but also the many hundreds of patients I have assessed that have all added to the rich tapestry my nursing career has been and continues to be. To every single one of those people, I am forever grateful and indebted. You have added the colour and texture to my working life, provided knowledge and experience from which I have been able to draw upon in this work.

I have special personal thanks to my colleagues, Esther, Mandy, Mandy, Nic and Alex who agreed without question to give their time and knowledge to bring this project to life, and to all of the contributors.

Matt, to me you are a visionary and an extraordinary talent, thank you for asking me to be part of this. For Marg and Ness for tolerating my slowness and procrastination, I am always thankful.

And finally, thanks to the person who allow me to be me, and do what makes me happy even if that is work. Who has never once complained about the hours spent at my lap-top, taking from the time we could spend together. My John, I couldn't do it without you.

JENNIE SMITH

As I reflect on my journey as an editor, my heart is filled with immense gratitude for the myriad of friends whose support has made it possible for the magic of unicorns, the sparkle of glitter and the promise of rainbows to align. At the heart of this remarkable adventure stands my family—Pete, Jack, Emma, Sam, Alice, Tommy and Arthur—whose unwavering faith in my endeavours lay the foundation of encouragement and love.

To Matt, Marg and Jennie—my esteemed editors— you have not only honed my thoughts with your profound wisdom but also enabled me to discover a harmony in our collective narrative.

There are a collection of others including Dipti that have been instrumental in weaving the fabric of this work. Thank you all for accompanying me on this journey. Your collective spirit and unwavering support have been the greatest gifts, reminding me that together, we are capable of creating something truly magical

VANNESSA WEBB

I thank my students over the years who have provided me with a wealth of knowledge and understanding of the challenges of working as a Forensic Healthcare practitioner within a Custody setting. You are all amazing individuals, working so hard to provide a quality service for your patients but so rarely appreciated.

However, my most sincere gratitude must go to my husband Neil, whose unwavering love and support mean the world to me. I also want to thank my family, especially my beautiful daughters; Katy and Sarah of whom I am so proud, as well as my parents, George and Betty, who shaped me into the person I am today. Thank you all for being there when I needed you.

MARGARET BANNERMAN

Reviewed from a Scotland and Northern Ireland perspective by:

Northern Ireland
Barry Nevin
RN, BSc (Hons), NMP, DLM
Lead Nurse, Custody Healthcare, Belfast Health and Social Care Trust

Scotland
Jessica Davidson MBE
RN, RNMH, QN, FRCN
Clinical Lead, South East Healthcare & Forensic Medical Services for People in Police Care, NHS Lothian
Nurse Lead for SARCS Network
Programme Lead (Associate) – Advanced Forensic Nursing Practice, Queen Margaret University

About the Companion Website

This book is complemented by a companion website.

www.wiley.com/go/policecustodyhealthcare

The companion website provides colour images of all figures used in the book and 25 multiple-choice questions for readers to test their knowledge and understanding regarding each chapter topic. Additionally, suggested responses to each scenario within the book are provided.

Introduction to Police Custody

Matthew Peel[1], Jennie Smith[2], Vanessa Webb[3], and Margaret Bannerman[3]

[1] Leeds Community Healthcare NHS Trust, Leeds, UK & UK Association of Forensic Nurses and Paramedics
[2] Mitie Care and Custody Health Ltd, London, UK & UK Association of Forensic Nurses and Paramedics
[3] Nurture Health and Care Ltd, Norwich, UK

CHAPTER 1

AIM

The aim of this introductory chapter is to provide a foundational understanding of the multifaceted realm of police custody healthcare in the United Kingdom. This will include the current state of forensic healthcare, the role of the healthcare professional, including training and induction. A broad overview of police custody, including the purpose, standards, individuals working in custody and the relevant legislations, will be provided.

LEARNING OUTCOMES

After reading this chapter, you will be able to:

- Understand the current landscape and varying levels of consensus in forensic healthcare within the United Kingdom

- Describe the structural and operational differences in police custody across the devolved nations

- Identify the key demographics and vulnerabilities of individuals detained in police custody

SELF-ASSESSMENT

1. What are the primary roles and responsibilities of HCPs in police custody?

2. Who are the typical detained individuals in police custody and what are their common demographics and vulnerabilities?

3. What standards of care and professional conduct are expected from HCPs working in police custody?

INTRODUCTION

Forensic science is guided by Locard's principle: *'Every contact leaves a trace'* (Locard 1934). However, this ethos extends beyond physical evidence to the compassionate care that healthcare professionals (HCPs) provide to those detained, often in their most vulnerable moments. HCPs must strive to positively impact individuals through respect, dignity and hope. This approach blends assessment, examination and forensic strategy, along with advice, treatment, brief interventions and signposting, aiming to leave a beneficial impact on those they encounter.

This chapter delves into the unique challenges of police custody healthcare, where HCPs work with limited evidence-based guidance to prioritise patient safety and well-being. It addresses the diversity in practices, the absence of consensus in certain areas and the crucial role of risk assessment.

Police Custody Healthcare for Nurses and Paramedics, First Edition. Edited by Matthew Peel, Jennie Smith, Vanessa Webb, and Margaret Bannerman.
© 2025 John Wiley & Sons Ltd. Published 2025 by John Wiley & Sons Ltd.
Companion website: www.wiley.com/go/policecustodyhealthcare

It emphasises the need to balance healthcare needs and human rights with police procedures; this introduction sets the stage for exploring the dynamic and ethical landscape of police custody healthcare.

CONSENSUS

Within police custody, there is a scarcity of comprehensive, evidence-based guidelines, providing a unique challenge for healthcare providers to navigate this uncertain terrain with the patient's safety and best interests, as their guiding principle. This has given rise to a spectrum of practices, each supported by its own evidence, albeit limited and characterised by distinct advantages and potential risks. The variety in clinical approaches reflects not a shortcoming but rather the complex nature of forensic healthcare, where clinical judgment intertwines intricately with the dynamic interface of police procedures and healthcare provisions. These practices are informed by a multifaceted interplay of factors. Recognising these variations, this text identifies areas where there is no consensus in practice, offering a comprehensive view of the diverse methodologies currently in use. For practitioners keen on delving deeper into the development of standardised practices and understanding how to bridge professional opinions, the National Institute of Clinical Excellence (NICE) provides invaluable resources, particularly its guidelines on managing differences in professional opinion.

FORENSIC HEALTHCARE PRACTITIONERS

Forensic healthcare practitioner (FHP) is the umbrella term for HCPs working in forensic healthcare settings (police custody and sexual assault referral centres), typically doctors, nurses, paramedics and midwives. They are distinct from those working in forensic mental health settings.[1] Within this text, we will refer to FHPs as HCPs; however, both titles should be considered synonymous. In police custody, FHPs are more commonly referred to as:

- Custody healthcare practitioner or professional
- Custody nurse/paramedic
- Custody nurse/paramedic practitioner
- Forensic nurse/paramedic examiner

HCPs work at the front door of the criminal justice system, at an intersection between health, justice and forensics, with a dual patient and medico-legal responsibility. For nurses and paramedics, this involves working at an advanced practice level with a high degree of autonomy and complex decision-making (National Health Service 2017).

They have medico-legal responsibilities, such as advising on fitness to interview. In addition, they are responsible for clinically examining and treating individuals presenting with undifferentiated and undiagnosed injuries or illnesses. They also undertake forensic examinations and sampling, providing written statements and oral testimony in court.

EDUCATION AND TRAINING

While HCPs bring with them several years of post-registration clinical experience, knowledge and skills, they still require thorough induction, supervision and support. Figure 1.1 demonstrates a path from novice to expert[2] (Benner 1984). As HCPs come from a wide range of clinical backgrounds and specialities, induction training programmes should be flexible to meet individual needs.

Induction

The UK Association of Forensic Nurse and Paramedics (UKAFNP) has developed standards for induction for healthcare providers to deliver locally, see Box 1.1.

Ongoing Training

Ongoing training and development are essential following induction across all healthcare settings and forensic healthcare is no different. Ongoing training should include both in-house training and external training.

Post-graduate Education (and Exams)

Several stand-alone master's level post-graduate modules will be of interest to HCPs; these include:

- Independent prescribing
- Minor illness
- Minor injuries
- Mental health
- Substance misuse
- Human rights
- Law

Alternatively, HCPs may undertake a master's level post-graduate qualification.

Advanced forensic practice (PgCert, PgDip, MSc) An advanced forensic practice programme,[3] aligned to the UKAFNP ASET award (advanced standards in education and training), is available, including a taught and assessed clinical aspect evidenced by completing a competency document and taught and practical assessments of forensic science knowledge,

---

[1] Forensic mental health service provides long-term treatment, rehabilitation and aftercare for people who are mentally unwell or learning disabled and who are in the criminal justice system (courts or prisons).

[2] Expert in the sense of Benner's clinical expertise, this does not automatically confer expert witness status.
[3] Programme titles may differ.

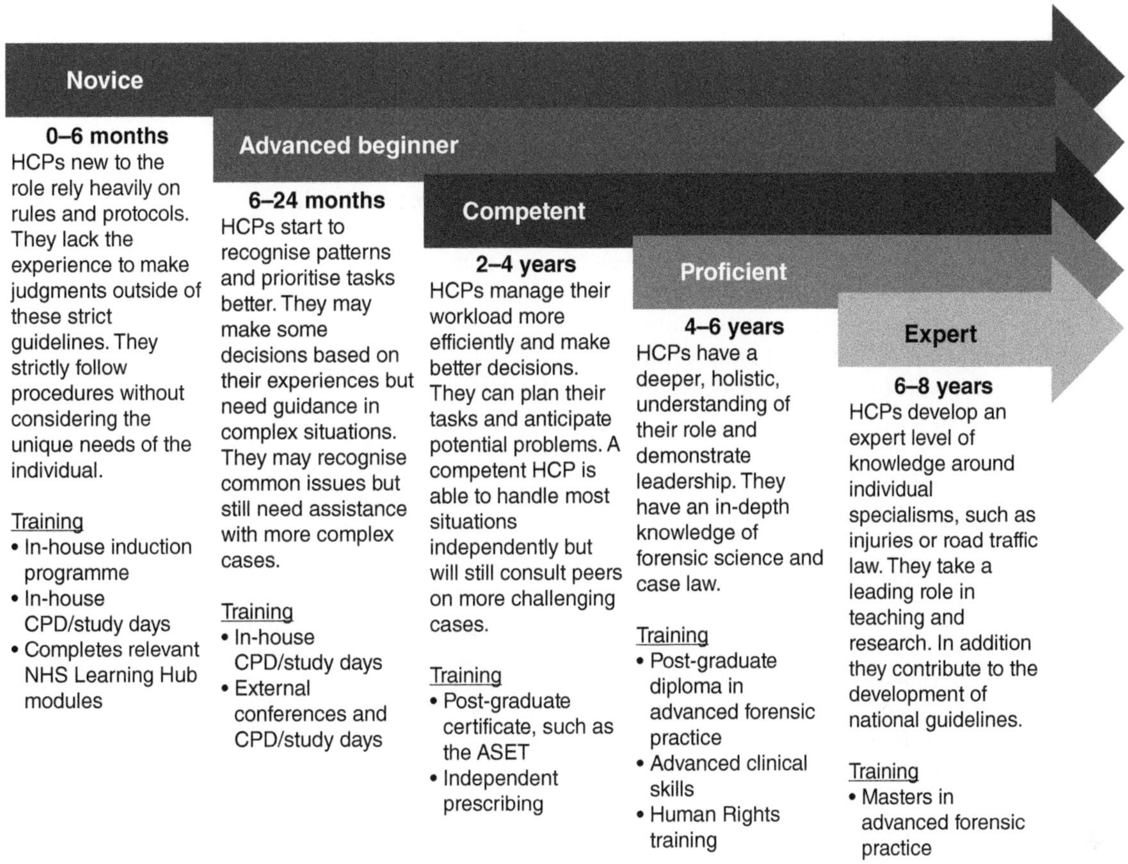

Novice

0–6 months
HCPs new to the role rely heavily on rules and protocols. They lack the experience to make judgments outside of these strict guidelines. They strictly follow procedures without considering the unique needs of the individual.

Training
• In-house induction programme
• In-house CPD/study days
• Completes relevant NHS Learning Hub modules

Advanced beginner

6–24 months
HCPs start to recognise patterns and prioritise tasks better. They may make some decisions based on their experiences but need guidance in complex situations. They may recognise common issues but still need assistance with more complex cases.

Training
• In-house CPD/study days
• External conferences and CPD/study days

Competent

2–4 years
HCPs manage their workload more efficiently and make better decisions. They can plan their tasks and anticipate potential problems. A competent HCP is able to handle most situations independently but will still consult peers on more challenging cases.

Training
• Post-graduate certificate, such as the ASET
• Independent prescribing

Proficient

4–6 years
HCPs have a deeper, holistic, understanding of their role and demonstrate leadership. They have an in-depth knowledge of forensic science and case law.

Training
• Post-graduate diploma in advanced forensic practice
• Advanced clinical skills
• Human Rights training

Expert

6–8 years
HCPs develop an expert level of knowledge around individual specialisms, such as injuries or road traffic law. They take a leading role in teaching and research. In addition they contribute to the development of national guidelines.

Training
• Masters in advanced forensic practice

FIGURE 1.1   Novice to expert.

| BOX 1.1 | STANDARD FOR INDUCTION |

• Overview of organisation, including local mandatory and statutory training

• Governance, patient safety, the duty of candour, reflection and equality, diversity and inclusion

• Resuscitation

• Medicines management, including patient group directions or non-medical prescribing

• Children's Act, Mental Capacity Act and consent

• Mental Health Act, mental state examinations, including risk to self and others

• Level 3 safeguarding children and adults; in addition to PREVENT and female genital mutilation

• GDPR, confidentiality and records management

• Forensic strategy, forensic sampling (including toxicology), chain of evidence

• Ongoing continuity of care

Source: Adapted from UKAFNP (2023).

practice and legal skills, including statement writing and providing oral evidence. These courses are a blend of forensics and advanced clinical practice. It is important to note that the requirements for 'advanced practice' differ across the different countries.

Advanced clinical practice (PgCert, PgDip, MSc) Most universities offer advanced clinical practice programmes. Most programmes are generic, including a taught element and practical examination.

Licentiate of the Faculty of Forensic & Legal Medicine (FFLM) The licentiate is an examination and competency assessment:

• **Part 1:** A three-hour theoretical examination of medico-legal and clinical practice, tested by a single best-answer paper

• **Part 2**: Clinical competency assessment, tested by a 14-station Objective Structured Clinical Examination (OSCE) and a short answer question paper

Completing all the elements may entitle the use of the post-nominals LFFLM.[4]

---

[4] Requires annual membership to use postnominals.

Diploma of Legal Medicine The Diploma of Legal Medicine (DLM) is a stand-alone examination offered by the FFLM consisting of a three-hour examination with 150 best-of-five multiple-choice questions.

ABOUT POLICE CUSTODY HEALTHCARE

The healthcare provided in custody settings is a critical welfare component, ensuring individuals have timely access to physical and mental health assessments and treatments. This care must be patient-centred, with HCPs advocating for individuals' health needs, whilst remaining objective in the participation of the criminal justice system.

Substance misuse is a prevalent issue amongst the population. Providing appropriate services and managing medicines within custody suites is a complex task that requires specialised knowledge and skills. HCPs must be adept at handling these challenges, providing necessary interventions and referring to external services when appropriate.

The safeguarding of vulnerable individuals, including those with mental health issues or those who are intoxicated, is paramount. Police custody HCPs must work closely with custody officers to ensure individuals are monitored, ensuring signs of distress or deterioration are acted upon swiftly.

The responsibility also extends to the release process, where HCPs should ensure continuity of care and facilitate connections with community health services if necessary. This transition is a critical juncture where effective communication and planning can significantly impact the ongoing well-being of the individual after release from custody.

In essence, the healthcare provision in police custody is not merely about treating illness or injury but is an integral part of the broader custodial care system. It requires a holistic approach, addressing physical, mental and social health determinants, contributing to the overall aim of the custodial system to ensure safety, security and preparation for release or transfer.

COMMISSIONING

The commissioning of police custody healthcare differs across the United Kingdom. In England and Wales, the commissioning of police custody healthcare rests with the local force and their Police and Crime Commissioner (or equivalent). However, they are supported by NHS England. Most forces outsource their healthcare to private healthcare organisations (most specialising in forensic healthcare) and some NHS Trusts. A very small number of forces deliver healthcare in-house. In Scotland, commissioning sits with NHS Scotland and in Northern Ireland, the Police Service Northern Ireland works collaboratively with the Department of Health, the Public Health Agency and the Health and Social Care Trust.

DETAINED INDIVIDUALS

Individuals detained in police custody are often referred to as a 'detained person' or reduced to 'DP'. The editors have purposefully chosen to avoid both 'detained person' and 'DP'. Such language groups all those in custody as a single homogenous group, which fails to acknowledge or appreciate their individual histories, needs and vulnerabilities. Mostly, we refer to those in custody as 'individuals'. However, other terms used are 'suspect' and 'patient', see Box 1.2.

CONDITIONS OF DETENTION

Individuals brought into police custody are forced into an environment where their freedoms are significantly restricted. Yet, it is a fundamental expectation their treatment is grounded in respect, dignity and upholding their human rights. This begins with the initial interaction and continues throughout the entire custody period. Police custody staff, including HCPs, play a pivotal role in this process.

Individuals are entitled to conditions respecting their dignity and basic human needs. Individuals should be housed alone in well-ventilated, clean and properly heated cells, with access to bedding, toilet and washing facilities. Suitable clothing must be provided if necessary. Individuals are entitled to at least three meals daily with additional drinks, time outdoors for fresh air, and specific health, hygiene and welfare provisions, such as menstrual products. Faith-related items should be made available as required. Additionally, they have the right to an uninterrupted rest period of 8 hours within a 24-hour time frame.

Individuals' diverse needs must be recognised and met. This involves a thorough risk assessment to manage any health, welfare or security concerns effectively. The assessment must be competent, and individuals must be informed of their rights and entitlements promptly and clearly (see Box 1.3). The custody environment itself must be safe and clean, and any use of force must be lawful, necessary and proportionate.

BOX 1.2	DESCRIPTIVE TERMS USED
Individual	For the most part, the text uses the term individual, recognising their own unique experiences, beliefs, vulnerabilities and needs.
Suspect	Used where a person is under investigation or arrest and, is going to be interviewed or have forensic samples taken (including road traffic procedures). Not all those detained in custody are suspects.
Patient	An individual who requires clinical attention or treatment.

SCENARIO 1.1   Conditions of detention

A 45-year-old male with known arthritis was brought into custody on a wet, chilly winter night. In the morning, he complains of not feeling well and he is booked to see the HCP, where he states he is stressed from the arrest and feels increasingly uncomfortable as the cell temperature dropped during the night. He reports he was left in wet clothing in a cold cell without a blanket overnight. He appears distressed and upset, his heart rate and blood pressure are raised and his temperature is 35.2°C.

1. *Outline your approach and clinical management of this individual*

2. *How do you respond to his complaints about detention?*

3. *What is the mechanism or structure for reporting concerns about an individual's conditions of detention?*

The expectations and conditions outlined are comprehensive and demanding. Yet, they are crucial for safeguarding the health and well-being of individuals, ensuring legal compliance, and fostering public trust in the police. HCPs working in this environment are not only caregivers but also custodians of human rights and their role is vital in upholding the standards in police custody.

THOSE WORKING IN CUSTODY

Various roles work in custody, including numerous police staff and outside agencies. Each has its own defined role and scope. There may be some regional differences.

POLICE STAFF

There are several ranks of police staff working in police custody, identifiable by the insignia on their epaulettes, see Figure 1.2.

Custody Officer (Custody Sergeant)

The Custody Officer is an officer at least a rank of Sergeant. Their role involves managing and leading the custody suite, including the care and welfare of detainees. The Custody Sergeant is responsible for authorising or refusing detention of persons presented to them and ensuring adherence to the Police and Criminal Evidence Act 1984 (PACE) Codes of Practice (or equivalent). They also direct resources to ensure safe detention and delegate tasks to assist them in the suite's safe and lawful operation. In England, Wales and Northern Ireland, a Custody Sergeant can authorise non-intimate samples.

Detention Officer

A Detention Officer, sometimes called a Civilian Detention Officer, assists Custody Sergeants in processing individuals arrested and detained. This includes undertaking regular observations and providing food and drinks. They also assist by taking fingerprints, photographs and deoxyribonucleic acid (DNA) samples. If needed, they are involved in restraints. Detention Officers are civilian employees; Police Constable Gaolers are police constables who perform the same role in custody.

Inspector

In England, Wales and Northern Ireland, before charge, Inspectors review each detention six hours post-detention and then every nine hours following to ensure detention remains necessary. Inspectors can authorise intimate samples. In England and Wales, individuals arrested and detained under Section 136 of The Mental Health Act 1983, an Inspector (or above) must authorise their detention in custody.

In Scotland, Inspectors must review the detention of any child likely to be detained over four hours. Inspectors review each detention following 6 hours of detention, then review at 12 hours and authorise (if necessary) a 12-hour investigative extension, which is then reviewed after 6 hours (or 18 hours of detention). Inspectors can authorise non-intimate samples only.

Superintendent

In PACE (and PACENI) a Superintendent has the authority to extend the maximum period a person may be detained without charge. After an initial detention period and the first review, if further detention is deemed necessary, a Superintendent can authorise an extension by up to 12 hours. The Superintendent's role is critical in ensuring the extension of detention is justified, documented and in accordance with the legal framework provided by PACE or PACENI.

APPROPRIATE ADULTS

Appropriate Adults (AA) help safeguard the rights and welfare of juveniles (under 18) and vulnerable adults detained or questioned by the police. Their duties include ensuring individuals

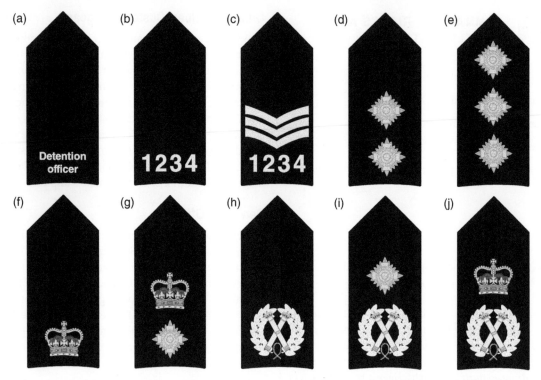

FIGURE 1.2 Police insignia. (a) Detention officer. (b) Constable. (c) Sergeant. (d) Inspector. (e) Chief inspector. (f) Superintendent. (g) Chief superintendent. (h) Assistant chief constable. (i) Deputy chief constable. (j) Chief constable (regional variations exist).

understand their rights, their reason for detention and the police. Additionally, they can ensure legal rights are exercised, such as consulting with a solicitor. For further information, see Chapter 3 – Vulnerability and Appropriate Adults.

LIAISON AND DIVERSION PRACTITIONERS

Liaison and Diversion (L&D) services differ across the United Kingdom. In Wales, it is known as the Criminal Justice Liaison Service and Northern Ireland currently has no such service. NHS Scotland has most recently introduced L&D practitioners in response to Scotland's Mental Health Strategy (2017–2027). L&D practitioners serve as a bridge between the criminal justice and mental health services. They screen for vulnerabilities, such as mental health issues, learning disabilities and substance misuse. Their role includes early intervention, diverting people to appropriate health, social care or other supportive services, reducing the likelihood of reoffending. L&D is commissioned by the NHS. L&D practitioners include registered professionals (i.e. nurses and social workers) and may include unregistered mental health professionals. It is important to be familiar with your local service and the referral mechanisms.

SOLICITOR AND LEGAL REPRESENTATIVES

A solicitor or legal representative plays a crucial role in the criminal justice process in police custody. They provide legal advice, guiding their clients and advocating for their interests.

This involves explaining legal rights, the implications of different choices, such as whether to provide responses during a police interview and potential legal strategies. Across the United Kingdom, individuals detained in police custody are entitled to free, independent, legal advice at any time. This can include a named solicitor (or firm) or can be provided through the duty scheme. The scheme provides legal representation to individuals in police custody and is available 24 hours a day, 365 days a year.

DRUG INTERVENTION PROGRAMME WORKERS

Drug intervention programme (DIP) workers are a critical part of the UK's strategy to address drug abuse, particularly within the criminal justice system. The program aims to engage drug-misusing offenders by involving them in formal addiction treatment and support, thereby aiming to reduce drug-related harm and criminal behaviour. Individuals are typically identified through the criminal justice system at key points, such as after a positive drug test in police custody, and are then directed towards treatment and comprehensive support.

LEGISLATION

HCPs working within police custody must navigate a complex interplay of healthcare ethics, patient care and legal mandates. A deep understanding of relevant legislation such as PACE,

PACENI and the Criminal Justice Act (Scotland) 2016 is vital for ensuring legal compliance in their professional activities. This knowledge base assists HCPs in upholding the rights of individuals, guaranteeing those in custody receive their entitled medical care and legal representation.

Furthermore, a firm grasp of these laws underpins the ethical practice of healthcare within the custodial setting. It allows HCPs to advocate effectively for the health needs of individuals, particularly those who are most vulnerable, such as those experiencing mental health crises or substance misuse issues. By understanding the legal framework, HCPs are better equipped to manage the risks associated with custodial care, ensuring the welfare of individuals and mitigating potential harm.

Effective communication between HCPs and police is critical, and being knowledgeable with custody-related legislation facilitates clearer dialogue and understanding. For HCPs involved in forensic evidence collection, legal literacy is essential to ensure evidence is managed in a manner that maintains its integrity for potential court proceedings.

Additionally, the professional accountability of HCPs extends beyond immediate patient care. They may be called upon to provide testimony or input during legal proceedings or inquiries. In such scenarios, their insight into the legislative context is indispensable for contributing objective, accurate and authoritative information.

Lastly, HCPs with a sound understanding of the legalities surrounding police custody are well-positioned to influence policy development. They can offer informed opinions on the creation and refinement of protocols and guidelines that directly impact the health and well-being of individuals. Through this, HCPs not only fulfil their role as caregivers but also as crucial advocates for health in the justice system.

POLICE AND CRIMINAL EVIDENCE ACT 1984

The Police and Criminal Evidence Act 1984 (PACE) is a significant piece of legislation in England and Wales that sets out the powers and responsibilities of the police concerning the prevention and investigation of crimes. PACE and its accompanying Codes of Practice aim to balance the needs of the police to gather evidence with the rights and freedoms of the public. See Box 1.4 for an overview of the main provisions.

BOX 1.4	OVERVIEW OF PACE
Police powers	PACE defines the powers of the police to stop and search individuals, enter and search premises, seizing property found during searches. It also outlines the conditions under which the police can arrest and detain individuals.
Detention and treatment	PACE stipulates how long a person can be held in police custody before they are charged or released, and it sets standards for the treatment and welfare of detainees to ensure their rights are protected while in custody.
Evidence	PACE provides a framework for the gathering, handling, and admissibility of evidence. This includes rules on the conduct of searches, the seizure of items, and the handling of confessions and statements.
Codes of practice	The Act is accompanied by Codes of Practice (Codes A to H) that provide detailed guidance on various aspects of police procedures:
	• **Code A**: Governs the practice of stop and search
	• **Code B**: Deals with searching of premises and seizure of property
	• **Code C**: Concerns the detention, treatment, and questioning of persons by police officers
	• **Code D**: Relates to the identification of persons by police officers
	• **Code E**: Cover the audio recording of interviews with suspects
	• **Code F**: Cover the visual recording of interviews with suspects
	• **Code G**: Relates to the powers of arrest
	• **Code H**: Involves the detention, treatment and questioning of terrorism suspects
	• **Code I**: Involves the detention, treatment and questioning of persons in relation to the National Security Act 2023
Safeguards	PACE introduced several safeguards to prevent the misuse of these powers, including the requirement for the police to maintain detailed records of searches, arrests, and detentions, and the provision of legal advice and appropriate adults.
Independent oversight	The Act also established the Police Complaints Authority (which has since been replaced by the Independent Police Complaints Commission and then the Independent Office for Police Conduct) to provide independent oversight of complaints against the police.

PACE was designed to standardise police practices across England and Wales to ensure fair treatment for individuals who encounter the police. It is often updated and amended to adapt to new legal decisions and changes in society, so it is crucial for HCPs to stay current with these updates. For HCPs working in police custody, understanding PACE, in particular Code C, is essential to ensure the rights and well-being of individuals are upheld.

POLICE AND CRIMINAL EVIDENCE (NORTHERN IRELAND) ORDER 1989

The Police and Criminal Evidence (Northern Ireland) Order 1989 (PACENI) is the PACE equivalent legislation for Northern Ireland. While it is broadly similar to PACE and was based on the same principles, it has been tailored to fit the specific legal and policing context of Northern Ireland. PACENI also has its own set of Codes of Practice, which broadly mirror those in PACE, addressing similar areas such as stop and search, arrest, detention and the treatment of detainees, but with adjustments for local requirements.

CRIMINAL JUSTICE ACT (SCOTLAND) 2016

The Criminal Justice Act (Scotland) 2016 is a legislative measure enacted by the Scottish Parliament that brought about key changes to criminal practices and procedures within Scotland. Aimed at modernising and streamlining the Scottish criminal justice system, the Act sought to improve its overall efficiency.

The legislation was approved by the Scottish Parliament on 8 December 2015 and granted royal assent on 6 April 2016. The provisions of the Act were implemented in stages from 2016 to 2019 and have been subject to further modifications since then. Unlike PACE and PACENI, there are no Codes of Practice. Rather, Police Scotland has developed several standard operating procedures.

The initial part of the Act overhauled the police's authority concerning the arrest and holding of individuals. It replaced the pre-existing common law powers and various statutory detention powers with a unified statutory power of arrest, akin to the one outlined in section 24 of PACE applicable in England and Wales. According to section 3 of the Act, individuals arrested under this new power must be cautioned and informed about the grounds for their arrest. Additionally, the Act enshrines the right of those in police custody to legal counsel, a move influenced by the Cadder v HM Advocate case and the subsequent Carloway Review. Section 50 obligates the police to avoid holding individuals in custody without reasonable or necessary cause.

CONSENT

Consent is a fundamental principle that guides the ethical and legal practice of HCPs. Consent may be complicated in custody; individuals may be under significant stress or influenced by substances, mental health issues, or the intimidating environment of custody. Consent, at its core, is the voluntary agreement to an intervention by a competent and informed individual. It must be given freely, without coercion and with an adequate understanding of the nature and consequences of the procedure or treatment.

Consent may be implied and explicit. Implied consent occurs when an individual's actions indicate consent, such as presenting an arm for a blood pressure check. Alternatively, express consent is given either verbally or in writing and is necessary for more significant interventions. While practice varies, there is often a preference for written consent before undertaking forensic examinations.

CONFIDENTIALITY AND INFORMATION SHARING

In police custody healthcare, maintaining confidentiality while effectively sharing information with the police is a delicate balance. This is discussed further in Chapter 18 – Professional ethic; however key principles are identified as follows.

CONFIDENTIALITY AND LEGAL OBLIGATIONS

Confidentiality is a cornerstone of healthcare, embedded deeply in the individual codes of practice for nurses and paramedics. In the United Kingdom, this is further reinforced by legislation such as the Data Protection Act and the Human Rights Act.[5] These laws provide a legal framework that protects personal information, requiring HCPs to handle it with the utmost care and discretion.

BALANCING CONFIDENTIALITY WITH INFORMATION SHARING

In police custody, HCPs often find themselves in situations where they need to share information with the police. This is crucial for ensuring proper care and preventing harm. However, this need must be balanced against the individual's right to confidentiality. The decision to share information should be guided by professional judgment, considering the potential benefits and risks. Information should only be shared if doing so reduces the risk of harm to the individual. Police asking for speculative searches of an individuals' health or medication records should be refused.

LIMITS OF CONFIDENTIALITY

When interacting with individuals in custody, it is important to inform them about the limits of confidentiality. Such disclosure would typically be in situations where there is a significant

---

[5] Article 8 – Right to privacy.

risk of harm to the individual or others, including self-harm or safeguarding concerns. Individuals should understand that conversations with HCPs are not subject to legal privilege and in certain circumstances, a court may require HCPs to disclose confidential information. Therefore, they should avoid discussing the allegation against them.

COMPLEX SITUATIONS

There are instances where an individual might expressly forbid the sharing of certain information with the police. In such cases, HCPs should consult their colleagues or superiors to weigh the ethical implications and legal requirements. This consultation process is essential for making informed decisions about whether to breach confidentiality, especially when the individual's or public's safety is at stake. HCPs may wish to seek advice from their Caldicott Guardian, who are experts in confidentiality and information-sharing issues within healthcare settings. They can provide guidance on the legal and ethical implications of sharing patient information, helping HCPs navigate the complexities of such situations.

TRAUMA-INFORMED CARE

Trauma-informed care is an approach in healthcare that assumes an understanding of the prevalence of trauma and recognises the widespread impact of trauma on individuals, including patients, staff and others involved in the healthcare system. It is an approach particularly relevant in settings such as police custody healthcare, where individuals may have experienced various forms of trauma. There are six key principles of trauma-informed care, see Box 1.5.

For HCPs working in police custody, these principles should be integrated into all levels of organisational operation, influencing policy, physical space design, staff training and treatment to ensure services are delivered in a way that is respectful and appropriate for individuals who have experienced trauma.

Implementing trauma-informed care can also involve specific strategies, such as training staff on recognising the signs of trauma, creating environments that avoid re-traumatisation and developing policies that support recovery from trauma. This approach can be particularly critical when dealing with distressed individuals, mental health crises, substance misuse and the vulnerable.

Incorporating trauma-informed principles could be beneficial, not only for the patients but also for the practitioners, as it can help in managing their own stress and preventing burnout.

SECURITY

HCPs working in custody must have an awareness of security measures to adhere to.

BOX 1.5	PRINCIPLES OF TRAUMA-INFORMED CARE
Safety	Ensuring physical and emotional safety for patients and staff.
Trustworthiness and transparency	Assessments and decisions are conducted with transparency with the goal of building and maintaining trust among HCPs and patients.
Peer support	Peer support and mutual self-help are key vehicles for establishing safety and hope, building trust and enhancing collaboration.
Collaboration and mutuality	There is recognition that healing happens in the meaningful sharing of power and decision-making. The organisation recognises everyone has a role to play in a trauma-informed approach.
Empowerment, voice and choice	Individuals' strengths are recognised, built on, and validated and new skills are developed as necessary. HCPs are facilitated to work collaboratively with patients in a way that is empowering and supportive.
Cultural, historical and gender issues	The organisation actively moves past cultural stereotypes and biases, offers gender-responsive services, leverages the healing value of traditional cultural connections, and recognises and addresses historical trauma.

AWARENESS OF THE NATIONAL THREAT LEVEL

Awareness of the national threat level is paramount for HCPs working in police custody. This awareness becomes even more crucial in Northern Ireland, considering its unique history. HCPs must remain vigilant, especially in areas such as secure police car parks or secure entrances. The use of police ID for accessing restricted areas is a key protocol in ensuring only authorised personnel gain entry, thereby maintaining a secure environment. Therefore, HCPs should ask for the ID of anyone tailgating them entering (or leaving).

ESCORTING INDIVIDUALS

When escorting detained individuals, it is advised they walk a step or two ahead of the HCP. This practice allows the HCP to always keep the individual within sight, mitigating the risk of an attack from behind. This simple yet effective measure is vital for the safety of the HCP. Additionally, HCPs should be familiar with the panic alarms available on their route between the medical room and the custody desk.

MEDICAL ROOM SECURITY

Ideally, individuals will be seen in the medical room privately.[6] However, in practice, there is no consensus and will vary between local services, practices and risk assessments. Custody is a relatively controlled environment with individuals searched and risk assessed. However, some may have a propensity for violence or aggression. Therefore, HCPs should take reasonable steps to protect themselves.

Sharp Objects

Sharp objects, such as scissors and sharps bins, must be kept securely and out of reach. Storing these items in cupboards or drawers reduces the risk of them being used inappropriately by individuals in custody.

Tidy Desk Policy

A tidy desk policy in medical rooms is essential. This involves ensuring only necessary items are on the desk, out of reach, reducing the risk of objects being taken into cells and used as weapons or for self-harm. Desks should be checked after each assessment to ensure nothing is missing.

Data Security

Data security is a critical component of maintaining confidentiality and trust in the healthcare environment, especially in the sensitive setting of police custody. All HCPs must protect their passwords. Lock computers when not in use to prevent unauthorised access to sensitive information. This simple action can significantly reduce the risk of data breaches. Although much of today's documentation is digital, paper records must be stored securely. This involves locking file cabinets and ensuring that sensitive information is not left unattended. In addition to these measures, HCPs must also be cognisant of the General Data Protection Regulation (GDPR). GDPR requires the safeguarding of personal data and privacy for individuals within the European Union and the United Kingdom

Medication Security

The security of medication is of utmost importance. Medication cupboards should always be locked, and keys should be kept secure. Opening medication cupboards in the presence of detained individuals should be avoided to reduce risks.

SCENARIO 1.2 Security

You are asked to see a very angry male who has recently just come into custody. The custody risk assessment was not completed because of his level of aggression. He has requested to speak to the HCP because of his mental health.

1. *Outline the risks associated with seeing this man in the medical room*
   - *What (if anything) can be done to mitigate the risks*
2. *Outline the risks associated with seeing this man at the cell*
   - *What (if anything) can be done to mitigate the risks*
3. *How would you respond to this request?*

RISK ASSESSMENT AND COMMUNICATION

If possible, before any interaction with the individual, review the police risk assessment. This review, coupled with discussions with police and an examination of recent detention logs, helps HCPs understand their behaviour and potential risks.

CONCLUSION

This chapter has introduced the intricate landscape of police custody healthcare, a field where evidence is scarce and practices vary. In this complex environment, HCPs face the challenge of making decisions that prioritise the safety and well-being of individuals, often in the absence of clear, evidence-based guidelines. The diversity in approaches, as we have seen, is not a shortfall but a reflection of the multifaceted nature of forensic healthcare. It is a domain where clinical judgement must balance the scales between police procedures, healthcare needs, risk mitigation and human rights considerations.

As practitioners in this field, it is imperative to stay informed and adaptable, recognising the landscape of police custody healthcare is continuously evolving. Ultimately, the commitment to the welfare of those in custody remains the cornerstone of our practice, guiding us through the challenges and informing our decisions, ensuring every contact leaves a positive, lasting trace.

Throughout this text, readers will find various scenarios with probing questions. These are designed to expand the reader's understanding of specific topics or subject areas. Readers are encouraged to work through and explore these scenarios alone or with their colleagues and peers, using them to generate discussions and appropriate approaches or responses. Example responses to each scenario can be found on the accompanying website.

---

[6] HCPs should consider the need for a chaperone, not just for security reasons. Male HCPs should consider a female chaperone when seeing females.

LEARNING ACTIVITIES

1. Write a reflection relating to a confidentiality dilemma. Consider your attitude, values and beliefs along with the impact of any external pressure or influence from the police or detained individual. What were the tensions with your professional code of practice, if any?

2. Engage in role-playing exercises to simulate interactions between HCPs, detained individuals and police staff, focusing on communication skills, confidentiality and handling complex scenarios.

3. Review and critique your current policies, consider the language used and if there is evidence, they are trauma-informed. Identify areas for improvement or further research.

RESOURCES

Online

- NHS England | About liaison and diversion | https://www.england.nhs.uk/commissioning/health-just/liaison-and-diversion/about/

- Home Office & National Appropriate Adult Network | Guide for appropriate adults https://assets.publishing.service.gov.uk/government/uploads/system/uploads/attachment_data/file/117682/appropriate-adults-guide.pdf

- Police Scotland | Standard operating procedures | https://www.scotland.police.uk/access-to-information/policies-and-procedures/standard-operating-procedures/standard-operating-procedures-a-b/

Organisations

- Faculty of Forensic & Legal Medicine | https://fflm.ac.uk/

- National Police Chief's Council | https://www.npcc.police.uk/

- Police Scotland | https://www.scotland.police.uk/

- Police Service Northern Ireland | https://www.psni.police.uk/

- UK Association of Forensic Nurses and Paramedics | https://ukafnp.org/

REFERENCES

Benner, P. (1984). *From Novice to Expert: Excellence and Power in Clinical Nursing Practice*. Menlo Park, CA: Addison-Wesley Publishing Company.

Locard, E. (1934). *La police et les méthodes scientifiques*. Paris: Editions Rieder.

National Health Service (2017). Multi-professional framework for advanced clinical practice in England. https://www.hee.nhs.uk/sites/default/files/documents/multi-professionalframeworkforadvancedclinicalpracticeinengland.pdf (accessed 4 November 2022).

UK Association of Forensic Nurses and Paramedics (2023). Standards for induction. LINK: https://irp.cdn-website.com/552775eb/files/uploaded/Standards_for_Induction_Final.xlsx

FURTHER READING

National Institute for Health and Care Excellence | Developing NICE guidelines: the manual | https://www.nice.org.uk/process/pmg20/resources/developing-nice-guidelines-the-manual-pdf-72286708700869

History of Forensic Science

CHAPTER 2

Esther McPhail

Mitie Care and Custody Health Ltd, London, UK

AIM

The aim of this chapter is to provide readers with a comprehensive overview of the evolution and development of forensic science from its earliest inception to the present day. This exploration seeks to elucidate the significant milestones and key figures that have shaped the field, highlighting how these advancements have influenced and enhanced criminal investigations.

LEARNING OUTCOMES

After reading this chapter, you will be able to:

- Identify key historical milestones

- Recognise pioneering figures

- Comprehend the evolution of forensic science techniques

SELF-ASSESSMENT

1. Explain the principle of *'every contact leaves a trace'* as formulated by Dr Edmond Locard. How is this principle relevant in modern forensic science?

2. What was the purpose of establishing the Forensic Science Regulator, and how does it impact forensic practices in the United Kingdom?

INTRODUCTION

Forensic science is the application of scientific methods and techniques to matters under criminal investigation or court proceedings (Home Office 2016). Its intricate mosaic of methods and applications has evolved dramatically from its earliest days. This chapter embarks on a journey through time, tracing the evolution of this fascinating field. Beginning with the ancient civilisations, we explore the seminal developments in forensic science that have shaped our understanding of crime investigation. This chapter is a chronicle of breakthroughs, from the pioneering works of Sung Tz'u in medieval China to the innovative contributions of Mathieu Orfila and Alphonse Bertillon. It highlights the pivotal moments that have marked the transition from rudimentary practices to the sophisticated techniques employed in modern forensics. Through this historical lens, healthcare professionals in police custody will gain a profound appreciation for the science that underpins their vital role in the criminal justice system.

EARLY EVIDENCE OF FORENSIC SCIENCE

The origins of forensic science can be dated back to ancient Greek and Roman societies. In a book written in 1247 AD by Sung Tz'u titled The Washing Away of Wrongs, we can read about the first documented account of the use of forensic medicine. It is in this book we learn of an account of a forensic investigation into a murder victim in Medieval China in 1235. The village lawman questioned the farmers who worked in

Police Custody Healthcare for Nurses and Paramedics, First Edition. Edited by Matthew Peel, Jennie Smith, Vanessa Webb, and Margaret Bannerman.
© 2025 John Wiley & Sons Ltd. Published 2025 by John Wiley & Sons Ltd.
Companion website: www.wiley.com/go/policecustodyhealthcare

the fields closest to the murder site. While their sickles lay on the ground before them during their questioning, over the course of a few hours, the flies were attracted to one particular sickle as, although it had been wiped clean, there were traces of blood left behind that attracted the insects. As a result, the owner of the sickle confessed to the murder.

Although inadmissible as hard evidence in a court today, this account documented the foundation of forensic entomology.

1700S – ADVANCEMENTS IN FORENSIC SCIENCE

It was not until the early 1700s that forensic science was driven forward with developments in techniques such as identification of the victim by their false teeth, securing a murder conviction by matching the torn edge of newspaper in a pistol with the remaining piece of the paper found in the person's pocket, toxicology used to detect poisoning in the victim and bullet comparison techniques to catch a murderer. Criminal investigations became more evidence based and rational. Practices in obtaining confessions by torture were scaled down and the use of torture altogether was gradually diminished in favour of physical evidence.

One example of the early, rudimentary application of forensic science to physical evidence was in 1784 when John Toms, an Englishman of Lancaster, UK, was tried and convicted of murdering his victim Edward Wilshaw by shooting him in the head with a pistol. A pistol wad (a crushed ball of paper used to secure the gunpowder and ball in the muzzle of the pistol), was found in the victim's head wound. This torn piece of paper was matched to a piece of newspaper found in John Tom's pocket, which secured his conviction. On the strength of this physical evidence, he was sentenced to be executed by hanging on 29 March 1784. This was the first documented use of physical evidence to secure a conviction in the legal system.

1813 – THE FORENSIC DETECTION OF ARSENIC

Mathieu Orfila (24 April 1787–12 March 1853), a Spanish Toxicologist and chemist, was regarded as the founder of the science of toxicology. As arsenic was the most common form of poisoning of his time, its effects became the basis of much of his work. His research into the effects of arsenic poisoning, branded him as a pioneer in the effects of toxins and antidotes. Throughout his life, he continuously worked to develop a reliable and systematic method to detect the presence of poisonous substances in the human body.

A murder case in 1840, investigating the death of Charles Lafarge, summoned Orfila to look at the forensic evidence of the case. Marie Lafarge was on trial, accused of murdering her husband with arsenic. Due to a lack of a trustworthy process, no evidence of arsenic could be found in the victim's body.

Considered a forensic toxicology specialist, Orfila conducted a meticulous study of the evidence, including the methodology of testing and concluded the tests were not being conducted correctly. His study of the evidence revealed the presence of arsenic in the body of the victim and as such, the court declared the victim's wife, Marie Lafarge, guilty of his murder.

His four-volume Traité des Poisons (1813) are regarded as the first reference books in forensic science. In these books, Orfila documented his findings, from his clinical research into the effects of arsenic and other poisonous substances, along with refining new procedures to determine a predictable and reliable way to check for poison in the body.

1835 – THE FIRST USE OF BULLET COMPARISON

Before guns were mass produced, the barrels and bullet moulds were handmade by gunsmiths. Bullets fired from a barrel always bore the same distinctive markings, or exclusive impressions unique to that specific firearm. The first case of this being used in an investigation was documented in 1835 by Henry Goddard.

Henry Goddard was a member of the Bow Street Runners from 1824 until 1839. They were known as the first British police force and were eventually disbanded in 1839, following the establishment of the Metropolitan Police Force by Sir Robert Peel. During this time, Goddard earned himself an exceptional reputation for his participation in major crime investigations such as murder and arson. It was his participation in a murder investigation in 1835 that led Henry Goddard to use bullet comparison during an active murder investigation, to establish the murder weapon by tracing the bullet back to its mould.

The victim, Mrs Maxwell, had been shot dead at her home in Southampton, UK. Her butler, Joseph Randall, claimed at the time, a gunfight with burglars had taken place. Examining both Randall's weapon and the bullets found at the scene, including those that had killed Mrs Maxwell and the bullets Randall claimed had been shot at him, Goddard identified an identical defect on the surface of all the bullets. During the course of the investigation, Goddard found a bullet mould at Randall's home and when he examined the mould, the distinctive marks matched those found on the bullets. Goddard was able to confidently conclude that, based on the physical evidence, Randall had carried out the murder himself. This became known as forensic ballistics.

1850S – THE USE OF ANTHROPOMETRIC DATA

Alphonse Bertillon, a French Police Officer and biometrics researcher, created a system of identification based on physical measurements, Figure 2.1. As a records clerk for the Parisian police, he was dissatisfied at the disorderly methods adopted at the time, to identify and process the captured criminals. Prior to the application of Bertillon's anthropometry, criminals

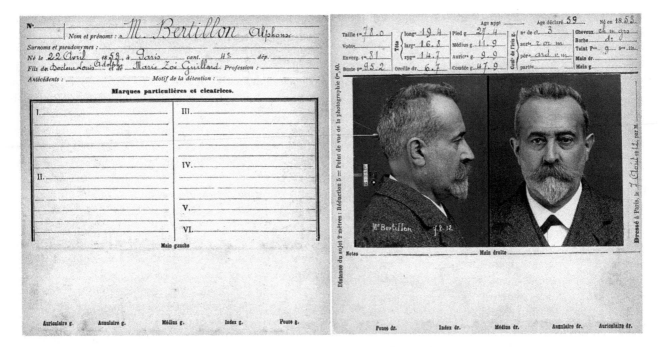

FIGURE 2.1 Anthropometric data sheet of Alphonse Bertillon. *Source:* Jebulon / Wikimedia Commons / CC0 1.0.

could only be identified by eyewitness account, name or photograph. The introduction of anthropometry was considered to be the first scientific system used by the police to identify criminals.

Bertillon's systematic approach to documenting the various measurements of an individual, recorded various physical characteristics such as head length, length of middle finger, length of the left foot, shape formations of the facial features and distinguishable features such as scars or tattoos. Recorded on a card with a photo, known as a mug shot, it was systematically filed. It could be easily retrieved and cross-indexed. In 1884, Bertillon used his method to identify 241 offenders, which was sufficient evidence for police forces in the United Kingdom, Europe and America to adopt bertillonage – the anthropometric identification system.

His system, although based in scientific measures had its flaws. It was difficult to implement due to human error, the measuring equipment requiring frequent recalibration and it was labour intensive, requiring highly trained and skilled technicians, which proved expensive. Eventually, bertillonage was abandoned by many police forces in favour of fingerprint identification. However, a number of features of his work are retained to this day, such as the mug shot and distinguishing features.

DR EDMOND LOCARD

Dr Edmond Locard, born in 1877, was a French criminologist who became renowned as the father of modern science and criminology and was often referred to as the 'Sherlock Holmes of France'.

A pioneer in forensic science, he formulated what has become known as the essential pillar of forensic science: that *'every contact leaves a trace'*.

LOCARD'S EXCHANGE PRINCIPLE

During his life, Locard published many pieces of work, the most famous of which was his seven-volume series Traité de Criminalistique (Treaty of Criminalistics). It is here he wrote about his most famous forensic work the 'Locard Exchange Principle', see Figure 2.2. He wrote the action of a criminal or

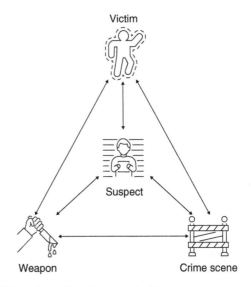

FIGURE 2.2 Locard's exchange principle.

any activity or violation cannot take place without leaving a trace. The indication that when a crime is committed, a trace is left behind by the perpetrator but they also take trace evidence from the scene with them, forms the basis of the principle. The more violent and intense the crime, the more trace evidence is exchanged.

It is this methodological study and forensic analysis of the trace evidence that assisted investigators to compile evidence and find answers to questions that arise during the course of the investigation, in order to impact the outcome of the trial.

After studying medicine and law in Lyon, France, Locard worked as an assistant to a criminologist and Professor Alexandre Lacassagne and remained until 1910, when Locard was offered the opportunity by Lyon police to start the first ever police crime investigation laboratory, where he could analyse evidence gathered from crime scenes and examine them scientifically.

His work as a medical examiner for the French Secret Service during the First World War was mostly dependent on science and physical evidence, attempting to identify cause and location of death through the examination of the stains and damage to the uniforms of soldiers and prisoners. This laboratory became recognised as the first police crime laboratory.

FINGERPRINTS

It was during this time at his laboratory, Locard developed his knowledge in the field of fingerprints and the science of poroscopy – the study of fingerprint pores. His work on the study of fingerprints underpins current-day practices in the area of dactylography – the study of fingerprints. His work surmised if 12 specific points known as 'minutiae points' could be identified between two fingerprints, it was sufficient evidence to be considered a positive identification. Locard's work in this field went on to replace the earlier techniques of Bertillon's anthropometry in this area. The 12-point fingerprint identification is still widely used today.

1900 – HUMAN BLOOD GROUPS IDENTIFIED

In the year 1900, Karl Landsteiner, an Austrian Scientist at the University of Vienna discovered the ABO blood group system through his research, mixing different red blood cell and serums and documenting the results.

His results demonstrated why some blood transfusions at the time were successful and others could be deadly, based on the interactions between the serum and the red cells and the presence of markers known as antigens. These foundational antigens became known as A and B, dependent on which antigen was expressed by the red blood cells in reaction to the antibodies in the serum. He later discovered the O group, which lacked the properties of A and B. The following year, he discovered the group AB as it expressed both the A

and B antigens. Whilst the subject matter of the biochemistry of blood groups is vast and detailed, for the purposes of this section, I will assume the reader understands the basics.

In the application to forensic science, where blood has been spilled at a crime scene, the sample would be collected by the crime scene officers and transported to the lab to be processed by a serologist. The 'ABO System' would allow the serologist to identify whose blood belongs to whom and definitively compare blood evidence from a crime scene and compare to the blood of a suspect.

By the 1960s, scientists used blood typing as a means to exclude individuals from the course of an investigation and as such, use blood typing to prove innocence, but it was not exact enough to prove a crime beyond a reasonable doubt on its own. Therefore, it was used to corroborate other evidence gathered during the course of an investigation such as DNA evidence, witness accounts and trace evidence, for use by the prosecution.

1937 – THE DISCOVERY AND USE OF LUMINOL

Luminol was initially discovered in the late part of the nineteenth century but was of little use to the scientists at the time. It was not until 1928 that German chemist H. O. Albrecht discovered that with the addition of an alkaline solution of hydrogen peroxide, luminol would produce a blue glow, known as chemiluminescence. In the presence of a catalyst that contained a small amount of copper or iron, it was found the mixture of luminol and hydrogen peroxide would glow brightly under ultraviolet light, or by a long-exposure photograph in a fairly dark room.

In 1937, during extensive studies carried out by German forensic scientist Walter Specht into the use of luminol, it was discovered blood itself could act as a catalyst, which meant luminol could be used for the forensic detection of blood at a crime scene. To date, crime scene investigators use luminol to reveal blood residue, even if the blood has been cleaned up due to the amount of iron required to cause a reaction is very small, it allows detection of even a small trace amount of blood at a scene. It can also be used to detect blood stains that are a number of years old. It is used mainly as an indicator of the presence of blood, in order to prompt further forensic investigation of the blood sample, to formally link the forensic relevance of the evidence to the case.

PRESENT DAY FORENSIC SCIENCE

Described as the application of science to civil and criminal law, forensic science specifically relates to the collection, preservation and analysis of evidence gathered, during the course of an investigation. Although during the early years of criminal investigations, a distinct lack of standardisation in forensic practices resulted in a number of criminals escaping conviction for their crimes, built on the foundations of years of development, discoveries and research. From its early formation to the present day, forensic science has become a key part of today's criminal justice system in England and Wales by applying science and technology to criminal investigations and court proceedings.

Today, forensic science still consists of many of the early disciplines including fingerprints, toxicology, trace evidence, handwriting analysis, DNA and forensic medical examinations. However, with the development of technology, digital forensics, the interpretation of evidence contained within mobile devices and CCTV footage, is becoming increasingly relevant.

MOVING TO THE FUTURE – DIGITAL FORENSICS

A Home Office publication in 2016 titled 'Forensic Science Strategy', describes how the field of forensic science is evolving to adapt to the socio-environmental changes that influence changes in criminal behaviour.

As the world becomes more digital, crime is rapidly evolving and there is a notable shift towards an increase in cybercrime being committed, as digital technology facilitates new ways to commit old crimes. Digital crime can now enable criminals to commit crimes in greater volume; crimes such as vehicle theft can be committed on a greater scale and offer a greater prospect of profitability to the criminal. Due to the vast quantity of digital data now available, crimes such as phishing emails and cyberattacks to name but a few, can prove to be devastating to the victim.

Police recorded crimes show a long-term shift from traditional crimes such as burglary and theft, towards crimes with a digital element, online sharing of images and fraudulent online purchases. It noted in 2015, 93% of UK adults owned a smart phone and used this as their preferred method to access online content.

With the shift away from traditional crimes, there is a steady decline in the demand for traditional forensic science such as DNA and fingerprints, leading the way to an increasing demand for digital forensic services to evolve, in order to address the digital as well as the physical evidence.

Real-time forensics is considered an area of ongoing research and development for the future of forensic science, as there is now the demand to develop technology in order to deliver forensic results faster and produce a swifter criminal justice outcome. This indicates a move away from the traditional laboratory and towards real-time analysis at the scene, using tools and techniques to enable rapid analysis of evidence from the crime scene to the court.

Due to the expansion of forensic science provision in England and Wales throughout the twentieth century, the field of forensic science was subject to a number of highly critical reports that documented the overall quality of the service provision as poor. The provision of forensic services was and is subject to ongoing scrutiny, therefore in 2007, to ensure uniform provision of high-quality forensic scientific services, the Forensic Science Regulator was established.

FORENSIC SCIENCE REGULATOR

The forensic science regulator was first appointed in 2007 by the Government to ensure forensic science services in the criminal justice system are carried out with objectivity and impartiality, while also complying with scientific standards. The successful candidate for the position of the forensic science regulator is in post for three years and their numerous responsibilities include:

- To establish and monitor the standards in the field of forensic science services

- To ensure that forensic science service providers are accredited

- To provide advice on the standards in forensic science

Following the Forensic Science Regulator Act of 2021, the role of the regulator was given statutory footing, which meant they were given the powers to enforce compliance with the statutory codes of practice within the forensic science activities in the England and Wales criminal justice system.

FORENSIC CAPABILITY NETWORK

Policing in the United Kingdom faces a series of challenges as it seeks to modernise and improve its efficiency in facing the current and future demands of its service. Forensic science is integral to policing the modern world and as such, faces the same demands and challenges. The Forensic Capability Network (FCN), a national network for forensic science in policing in England and Wales, started in April 2020 and is funded by the Home Office. Hosted by Dorset Police, The FCN reports directly to the National Police Chiefs Council (NPCC).

The FCN works to enable collaborative working between the 43 police forces, private forensic science providers and academic establishments in order to share resources in the field of forensic science. They promote innovation by leading improvement in quality standards and accreditation for facilities and work to strengthen the provision of services nationally and are driven to achieve sustainable forensic services across all forensic disciplines. They work nationally to provide advice on quality and science-related issues, to streamline forensic services by managing crises in the private marketplace and to reduce the backlogs in the processing of samples.

FACULTY OF FORENSIC AND LEGAL MEDICINE

The Faculty of Forensic and Legal Medicine (FFLM) founded in September 2005, was set up in order to maintain high standards of competence and professional integrity in the field of forensic and legal medicine. Originally set up by the Royal College of Physicians in London, it set about establishing training pathways for forensic practitioners and became recognised as an authoritative body for consultation in all matters of forensic and legal medicine.

The FFLM, working in conjunction with several organisations, including the UK Association of Forensic Nurses and Paramedics (UKAFNP), publishes the standards of practice for the collection of forensic samples in police custody. Their 'Recommendations for the Collection of Forensic Specimens from Complainants and Suspects' are updated biannually and provide the latest updated guidelines for evidence-based practice.

The recommendations outline the reason for analysis, the methodology for obtaining the samples and the packaging and storage guidance for each sample.

CONCLUSION

As we conclude our exploration of the history of forensic science, it becomes evident that this field is much more than a collection of techniques and methodologies. It is a testament to human ingenuity and the relentless pursuit of truth. The journey from early forensic practices to the cutting-edge technologies of today illustrates a remarkable evolution. This chapter has navigated through centuries of advancements, each step contributing to the intricate tapestry of forensic science. For professionals in police custody healthcare, understanding this history is not merely academic; it is a foundation for appreciating the profound impact of forensic science on our work. As we look to the future, with emerging fields like digital forensics and real-time analysis, the lessons from the past guide us. They remind us that at the heart of forensic science lies a steadfast commitment to justice, a pursuit that continues to shape and redefine the boundaries of what is possible in the quest to unravel the mysteries of crime.

RESOURCES

Online

- History of Forensic Science | Earliest documented case of forensic science | https://en.wikipedia.org/wiki/Collected_Cases_of_Injustice_Rectified
- John Toms 1784 | conviction secured through forensic evidence | https://www.guinnessworldrecords.com/world-records/118957-first-person-convicted-using-forensic-material-matching
- Mathieu Orfila | Toxicology | https://forensicfield.blog/mathieu-orfila/#google_vignette
- Alfonse Bertillon | The Anthropometric System of documenting criminals | https://en.wikipedia.org/wiki/Alphonse_Bertillon
- Dr Edmond Locard | The Locard Exchange Principle | http://aboutforensics.co.uk/edmond-locard/

Organisations

- Chartered Society of Forensic Sciences | https://www.csofs.org/
- Forensic Capability Network | https://www.fcn.police.uk/
- Forensic Science Regulator | https://www.gov.uk/government/organisations/forensic-science-regulator

REFERENCE

Home Office (2016). Forensic science strategy. https://assets.publishing.service.gov.uk/media/5a800bafe5274a2e8ab4ddc4/54493_Cm_9217_Forensic_Science_Strategy_Print_ready.pdf (accessed 16 January 2024).

FURTHER READING

UK Parliament | Forensic science services and the criminal justice system | https://lordslibrary.parliament.uk/forensic-science-services-and-the-criminal-justice-system/#:~:text=Who%20is%20the%20Forensic%20Science,regulator)%20on%2017%20May%20202

Fitness Assessments

Matthew Peel

Leeds Community Healthcare NHS Trust, Leeds, UK & UK Association of Forensic Nurses and Paramedics

---

AIM

This chapter explores fitness assessments in police custody, including fitness to detain, interview, charge, release and travel. It will outline an approach to holistic assessments to help readers effectively perform assessments, ensuring safety and adherence to legal and ethical standards.

LEARNING OUTCOMES

Upon completion of this chapter, readers should be able to:

- Understand the importance and purpose of fitness assessments in custody, including the roles and responsibilities of custody healthcare professionals

- Identify the key components of holistic fitness assessments, considering the physical, mental and emotional well-being of individuals

- Differentiate between the various types of fitness assessments, such as fitness to detain, interview, charge, release and travel, recognising the specific factors that must be considered for each assessment

SELF-ASSESSMENT

1. What are the key factors to consider when assessing fitness to detain?

2. List three physical and mental health conditions and outline how they may impact an individual's fitness to be interviewed.

3. Outline the legal guidelines and frameworks healthcare professionals (HCPs) must be familiar with when assessing fitness to release.

INTRODUCTION

Fitness assessments are the bedrock of custody work, particularly fitness to detain and interview. Typically, custody officers make a referral where a concern has been identified. However, whenever seeing an individual for whatever reason, always consider their fitness to detain and interview. For example, when assessing drug withdrawal, consider its impact on fitness to detain and interview. Fitness assessments are date and time specific, with opinions based on the available history and examination at that time. Healthcare professionals (HCPs)

must have an understanding of the relevant legislation relating to custody:

- Police and Criminal Evidence Act 1984 (PACE)

- Police and Criminal Evidence (Northern Ireland) Order 1989 (PACENI)

- Criminal Justice (Scotland) Act 2016 (CJA)

Assessments must be thorough and well documented. Fitness assessments are relied upon in much the same way as in-patient clerking's, noting information that may not be

Police Custody Healthcare for Nurses and Paramedics, First Edition. Edited by Matthew Peel, Jennie Smith, Vanessa Webb, and Margaret Bannerman.
© 2025 John Wiley & Sons Ltd. Published 2025 by John Wiley & Sons Ltd.
Companion website: www.wiley.com/go/policecustodyhealthcare

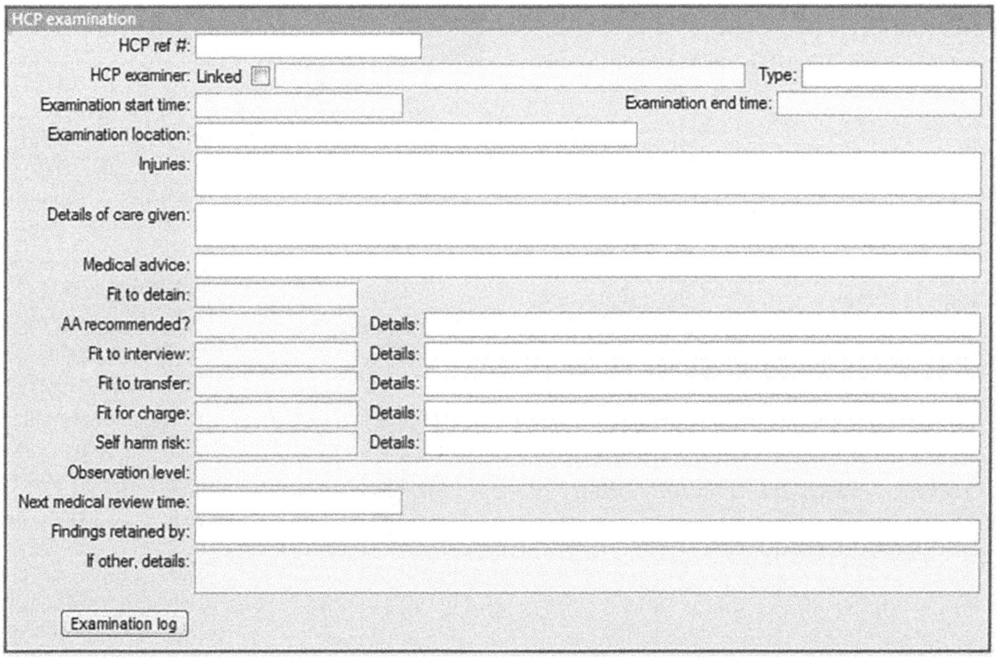
HCP examination
HCP ref #:
HCP examiner: Linked Type:
Examination start time: Examination end time:
Examination location:
Injuries:
Details of care given:
Medical advice:
Fit to detain:
AA recommended? Details:
Fit to interview: Details:
Fit to transfer: Details:
Fit for charge: Details:
Self harm risk: Details:
Observation level:
Next medical review time:
Findings retained by:
If other, details:
Examination log

FIGURE 3.1 Custody record healthcare form. *Source:* Adapted from Matthew Peel.

available later, along with relevant positive and negative findings. For example, it is important to routinely document the presence or absence of intoxication or withdrawal and the presence, or absence of self-harm thoughts. A summary of each assessment should be made in the custody record using a 'Detained Person Medical Form' or similar (see Figure 3.1). Summarising the important and relevant details, advising police on how they should care for the individual.

APPROACH TO FITNESS ASSESSMENTS

All fitness assessments involve a history followed by an examination. The focus depends on the concern raised. Individuals should, wherever possible, be seen in the medical room in private. Providing a degree of separation between the HCP and the police and framing the interaction as therapeutic.

HISTORY

Obtain a collateral history from the police and review the police risk assessment, noting the arrest, arrival times, offence, expected detention duration, likelihood of remand and any previous custody-related issues. Note any evidence of drug or alcohol intoxication, withdrawal, agitation, confusion or bizarre behaviours. Individuals taken straight to a cell without completing a risk assessment should be considered a high clinical risk due to:

- Likely use of force or restraint
- High-risk behaviours prior to arrest
- Risk of acute medical condition (physical or mental health) presenting as aggression or intoxication
- Risk of long-term condition being missed or not effectively assessed or managed

The reason for the arrest is important, as some offences are associated with prolonged detention and intensive interviews. Additionally, some offences are more commonly linked to mental illness, for example arson, possession of weapons, public order may be linked to psychosis or indecent exposure and some sexual assaults to mania. Equally, the circumstances around the offence may suggest a mental health concern, for example an unprovoked attack on a stranger in public. Be sure to review any available records, such as:

- Hospital discharge letters
- Ambulance forms
- Person escort records
- Custody record

Medical and Surgical

Identify conditions that may present a risk during detention, as well as any care (i.e. regular blood sugar checks) or medication needs. Specifically enquire about:

- Asthma/chronic obstructive pulmonary disease
- Diabetes
- Epilepsy

- Heart conditions
- Strokes or neurological conditions (including acquired or traumatic brain injuries)
- Fits or blackouts
- Liver or renal disease

Mental Health

Identify any condition that may negatively impact detention, interview or release. For example, a history of self-harm is a risk factor for repeated self-harm. Ascertain any history of mental illness, who and where a diagnosis was made. Any previous in-patient admissions, duration and status (i.e. voluntary or involuntary). Note any current treatment or engagement with services. Always ask about any history of self-harm or suicide attempts, as well as any current thoughts. For more detail, see Chapter 6 – Mental Health.

Medication

The medication history is essential to meet ongoing medication needs and may highlight undisclosed conditions. Note the medication, dose, frequency, last taken and current whereabouts. It is helpful to understand how individuals use their medication, especially if not as directed. Histories may be confirmed by accessing their National Care Record (formerly Summary Care Record), or similar.[1] In addition, enquire about over-the-counter, herbal, borrowed and any street-bought medications. Street-bought medications are diverted prescription medicines and typically include opioids, benzodiazepines, stimulants and GABA agonists. For more detail, see Chapter 7 – Medicine Management.

Social History

Box 3.1 outlines an approach that provides insight into the individual's support network and protective factors. Identifying opportunities for liaison and diversion, brief interventions or signposting. Additionally, it may identify safeguarding concerns, see Chapter 15 – Safeguarding. Enquiries about occupation, benefits, education and support workers are especially helpful when assessing fitness to interview and identifying vulnerability. Occupation is additionally important, as those regarding themselves with high standing in the community may be at increased risk of suicide post-release, particularly if the offence is associated with shame (i.e. child sex offences).

Finally, enquiries about previous arrests are useful as those not detained before are an unknown risk and may be at increased risk of self-harming. They may also require further explanation of the processes. Enquiries about prison can provide insight into previous court proceedings and convictions. Additionally, those recently released may be less likely to have re-developed alcohol or drug dependency.

---

[1] Welsh GP Record; Emergency Care Record (Scotland); Northern Ireland Electronic Care Record.

BOX 3.1	SOCIAL HISTORY
Partner	• Current partner, recently separated, is the partner the victim?
Children	• How many? Do they live with them? Do they have contact?
Dependents	• Do they care for someone? Are they the victim?
Accommodation	• Who do they live with? Sofa surfing? Homeless? • Are they a care leaver?[a]
Occupation or trade	• Occupation or trade? • Current/previous employment?
Benefits	• Receiving benefits? Which?
Education	• Able to read and write? • Level of education (school, college, university)? • Special educational needs? • Do they identify as being neurodiverse? That is, Autistic Spectrum Disorder (ASD), Attention Deficit Hyperactivity Disorder (ADHD) etc.
Support workers	• Do they have support workers?
Smoking	• Do they smoke?
Previous arrests	• Arrested before? • Previous issues?
Prison or other detention setting	• Have they ever been in prison, Young Offenders Institute or Immigration Removal Centre? • When?

[a] A young person aged 16–25 years old who has been 'looked after' at some point since they were 14 years old and were in care on or after their 16th birthday.

Alcohol History

Because of the close relationship between alcohol and custody, the over-representation of alcohol dependency and deaths from intoxication and withdrawal, it is essential to obtain an alcohol history, see Box 3.2. Determine alcohol use in the previous 24 hours, the amount and over what period. Then determine their typical pattern of use, paying particular attention to those at risk of alcohol withdrawal, see Chapter 10 – Substance Use and Misuse.

Drug Use

As with alcohol, drug use is over-represented amongst the custody population. Drug intoxication is linked to several deaths in custody each year, particularly cocaine. Making the drug use history an essential element, see Box 3.3. All drug use should be explored, including street-bought prescription medications, novel psychoactive substances, so-called 'soft drugs' like cannabis and 'hard drugs' like heroin. Specifically,

BOX 3.2	ALCOHOL HISTORY

Last 24 hours	• Amount?
	• Consumed between (time)?
Pattern of alcohol use	• Social, binge or dependent?
	• How many times a week? Month? Year?
If alcohol dependent	• 'Normal' daily amount?
	• Typical drinking pattern?
	• Previous alcohol withdrawal? Shakes? Sweats?
	• Fits or seizures?
	• Blackouts?

BOX 3.3	DRUG USE HISTORY

Drug	• Clarify if needed
Frequency	• How often?
Amount	• Weight or cost
Route	• Oral, rectal, injected, sniffed (insufflation), other
Last used	• Time?
Length used	• Duration of use?

BOX 3.4	GENERAL SURVEY

• Gait; normal, ataxic, unsteady, antalgic

• Alertness; alert, drowsy, somnolent, obtunded, stupor

• Orientation; orientated or confused

• Behaviour; calm, cooperative, hostile, uncooperative

• Presentation; the presence of any intoxication (toxidrome) or withdrawal

• Speech; normal, rapid, slow, slurred, loud, quiet

• General state of health; good, reasonable, poor

• Dress; appropriate, inappropriate, clean, tidy, unkempt

• Odour; alcohol, tobacco, cannabis, malodorous

• Injuries; presence or absence

BOX 3.5	VITAL SIGNS

• Heart rate

• Respiratory rate

• Blood pressure

• Oxygen saturation

• Temperature

• Blood glucose level

• Pupillary size and response to light

• Glasgow coma score/ACVPU

• NEWS2

enquire about cannabis and prescription drugs, as many do not consider these drugs. Several names can be used for a drug, so clarify if needed. People who inject drugs should be asked about the condition of injection sites.

EXAMINATION

The examination typically begins when you meet the individual, although you may gather useful information by observing them completing the initial risk assessment, or in their cell via CCTV. The focus of the examination will depend on the presenting complaint or concern raised. However, all should have a general survey (see Box 3.4). Note their gait; a steady gait may be reassuring however an unsteady, wide-based, ataxic gait may indicate intoxication, head injury or Wernicke's encephalopathy. Additionally, an antalgic gait (i.e. a limp) may indicate a leg injury. The individual's alertness and level of orientation should be tested and noted. However, be cautious attributing too much significance to minor disorientation to time; cells typically have no clocks.

Vital Signs

Appropriate vital signs should be recorded (see Box 3.5).

FITNESS TO DETAIN

The purpose of the assessment is to ascertain if an individual's health is compatible with detention, highlight any reasonably foreseeable risks and mitigate where possible, see Box 3.6. Where health is compatible with detention, any healthcare needs should be planned for with consideration for the expected duration of detention.

DETERMINING FITNESS TO DETAIN

When assessing fitness to detain, a useful threshold to consider is, in another setting would you discharge the individual home to their family? If someone is unsuitable to be cared for at home by family, they are likely unsuitable for custody. It is essential

---

BOX 3.6   FITNESS TO DETAIN

- Manage minor illness or injury
- Manage drug/alcohol intoxication/withdrawal
- Assess mental health and self-harm risk
- Medication needs
- Referrals (i.e. hospital, liaison and diversion, mental health)
- Consider a medical rest period
- Recommend level and frequency of observation

---

hospitals are aware that custody offers no higher standard of observations than can be provided by family members.

Once the assessment is complete, the outcome should be explained to the individual. The outcome is a 'Yes' or 'No' decision. Yes, they are fit to detain or no, they are not. However, HCPs may impose time limits after which an individual would no longer be fit to detain, or require a further review. For example, someone requiring haemodialysis may be fit to detain until they are due for their dialysis session.

Fit to Detain

If fit to detain, provide a care plan for the custody staff, including any worsening advice and when to refer back to the HCP or call an ambulance. Clearly document a recommended level and frequency of observation, along with any welfare needs, such as clothing, blankets, food, drink, exercise, a glass door or a low-level bench. If necessary, recommend a medical rest period, for example when someone is intoxicated. Medical rest offers a period where the individual cannot be interviewed or undergo other police processes.

Not Fit to Detain

Most individuals are fit to detain, with only 2–3% sent to the emergency department, most commonly with fractures, diabetes, epileptic or neurological emergencies (Dorn et al. 2018; Miles et al. 2020). When unfit to detain, arrange an onward referral to the most appropriate service. A very small proportion may present with healthcare needs that cannot be met in custody and are therefore unfit to detain but do not require a referral to hospital. For example, someone who is particularly frail with major comorbidities and requiring intensive medication, or care needs which cannot be reasonably met while in custody.

As with all fitness assessments, the HCP's role is to advise the custody officer, but it is the custody officer who ultimately decides. HCPs may find situations where they recommend someone is unfit to detain, but the custody officer disagrees. This is less likely to occur when the HCP recommends someone is unfit to be detained due to acute illness or injury

and requires transferring to hospital. However, HCPs should clearly highlight their concerns and the risks involved in continued detention, to the custody officer and an inspector. Discussion and risks should be clearly documented both on the custody record and the healthcare notes. HCPs still have a duty to provide care to those they deem unfit within the limitations of the custody setting.

Referrals to hospital Most individuals will be referred to the Emergency Department. However, pathways may exist enabling direct speciality referrals. For example, suspected deep vein thrombosis may be referred directly to acute medicine, or maternity complications may be referred directly to the maternity assessment unit. Regardless, all referrals should be accompanied by a documented letter outlining the concerns and any treatment provided.

Not all referrals will require an ambulance and many will be safe to be transported by police. This will depend on the nature of their condition, presentation, current treatment and the distance to hospital. Decisions may also be influenced by ambulance delays. Where delays exist, HCPs should consider the risk of delayed hospital treatment against a clinically unsupervised transfer to hospital by the police.

LEVEL OF OBSERVATIONS

Every individual is assigned a level of observation by the custody officer based on their risk assessment. The levels vary slightly between the nations (see Boxes 3.7 and 3.9), but outline how frequently individuals are visited and the level of interaction. Level one is suitable for those with little risk, while level four is reserved for those with the greatest risk. Ultimately, it is the custody officer's responsibility to set the

---

SCENARIO 3.1   Fitness to detain

You are asked to assess fitness to detain for a 38-year-old female with type 1 diabetes who is intoxicated through alcohol. Her blood glucose level is 12.1 mmol/l. She is prescribed a combination of Lantus at night and Novorapid with meals. She has no medication with her; it is currently 02:37 hours.

1. *Describe your approach to the fitness to detain assessment.*

2. *Are they fit to be detained?*
   a. *What are the foreseeable risks?*
   b. *Provide a care plan for the police including a recommended level and frequency of observations with a rationale.*

3. *Outline any further healthcare interventions or requirements.*

BOX 3.7	LEVELS OF OBSERVATIONS (ENGLAND, WALES AND NORTHERN IRELAND)

Level 1 general observation

- The minimum level of observation. It includes the following actions:
- Visited every 30–60 minutes
- If no reasonably foreseeable risk is recognised, sleeping individuals do not require rousing
- If awake, staff should communicate with them
- If any change presenting a new risk is noted, the individual should be roused

Level 2 intermittent observation

- The minimum acceptable level for those under the influence of alcohol or drugs or whose level of consciousness causes concern
- Physically visited and roused at least every 30 minutes
- The individual is positively communicated at frequent and irregular intervals
- Visits are conducted as per PACE/PACENI Code C Annex H (see Box 3.8)

Level 3 constant observation

- The level of observation for those at heightened risk of self-harm, suicide or other significant mental or physical vulnerability harm
- The individual is always under constant observation and accessible
- Physical visits must be carried out at least every 30 minutes
- CCTV is constantly monitored (other technologies can also be used)
- Possible ligatures are removed
- The individual is positively communicated at frequent and irregular intervals
- Review by the forensic healthcare practitioner

Level 4 close proximity

- The level of observation for those at the highest risk of self-harm
- Physically supervised in close proximity to enable immediate physical intervention if necessary
- Possible ligatures are removed
- The individual is positively communicated at frequent and irregular intervals
- Review by the forensic healthcare practitioner

Source: Adapted from College of Policing (2020).

level of observation; the HCP's role is to advise. Whenever recommending reducing levels, do so incrementally, that is not from level four to level one.

FITNESS TO INTERVIEW

Interviews aim to obtain accurate, reliable and relevant information about an individual's involvement (or otherwise) in a crime, which withstands scrutiny. They are key to successful investigations and crucial in a third of convictions. In England, Wales and Northern Ireland, individuals can be convicted solely on confessional evidence. However, Scotland requires corroborating evidence, except where a confession

contains 'special knowledge'. Interviews should be approached with an investigative mindset following the PEACE model, see Box 3.10, introduced to help prevent miscarriages of justice.

Box 3.11 outlines when a custody officer may query an individual's fitness to be interviewed. The assessment aims to highlight where an interview may harm an individual's health, or the reliability of their statements may be questioned in court, see Box 3.12. Interviews conducted without regard to an individual's vulnerabilities risk obtaining evidence that is inadmissible, inaccurate or unfairly incriminating.

At the start of an interview, individuals are reminded of their right to free and independent legal advice and cautioned. In England and Wales, the caution reads, *'You do not have to say anything. But it may harm your defence if you do not mention*

BOX 3.8	PACE & PACENI CODE C ANNEX H OBSERVATION LIST

- If the individual fails to meet any of the following criteria, an appropriate healthcare professional or an ambulance must be called

- When assessing the level of reusability, consider:

Rousability – can they be woken?

- Go into the cell
- Call their name
- Shake gently

Response to questions – can they give appropriate answers to questions such as:

- *What's your name?*
- Where do you live?
- Where do you think you are?

Response to commands – can they respond appropriately to commands such as:

- *Open your eyes!*
- Life one arm, now the other arm!
- Remember to take into account the possibility or presence of other illnesses, injury or mental condition; a person who is drowsy and smells of alcohol may also have the following:
- Diabetes
- Epilepsy
- Head injury
- Drug intoxication or overdose
- Stroke

Source: Crown, 2019 / Public Domain.

BOX 3.9	LEVELS OF OBSERVATIONS (SCOTLAND)

Level 1 general well-being observations

- The minimum level of observations for low-risk individuals
- For the first 6 hours of detention, they must be roused every hour
- After this, if no reasonably foreseeable risk is recognised, sleeping individuals do not require rousing
- However, a single period of sleep should not exceed three hours
- Any evidence of altered breathing patterns should be roused

Level 2 intermittent (health and rousable) observations

- The minimum level of observations for individuals suspected of drug or alcohol intoxication or where there are other concerns regarding consciousness
- Individuals are visited and roused at least every 15 or 30 minutes

Level 3 constant (harm awareness) observations

- The individual is constantly monitored by:
  - CCTV
  - Glass cell door
  - Window or cell hatch
- Visits are conducted every 15–60 minutes

Level 4 close proximity (harm prevention) observations

- For prisoners at the highest risk of harm who should be constantly observed at very close proximity
- The individual is physically supervised in person, with staff either in the cell or outside with the door open

Source: Adapted from Police Scotland (2019).

when questioned something which you later rely on in Court. *Anything you do say may be given in evidence'* (Home Office 2019, p. 40). While the wording in Northern Ireland slightly differs, it is substantially the same. In England, Wales and Northern Ireland, the courts can sometimes draw adverse inferences from a suspect's silence during interview. Allowing courts to interpret an individual's silence as supporting the prosecution's case. However, in Scotland, the caution reads, *'I am going to ask you some questions about (crime/offence). You are not obliged to answer any questions but anything you say may be noted, may be audio and visually recorded, and may be used as evidence'* (Police Scotland 2016). In Scotland, suspects have a right to silence during interviews and no such adverse inferences can be drawn.

BOX 3.10	PEACE INTERVIEW MODEL

- Planning and preparation
- Engage and explain
- Account clarification and challenge
- Closure
- Evaluation

Source: Adapted from College of Policing (2022).

BOX 3.11   **PACE & PACENI CODE C ANNEX G**

A detainee may be at risk in an interview if it is considered that:

a. Conducting the interview could significantly harm the detainee's physical or mental state;

b. Anything the detainee says in the interview about their involvement or suspected involvement in the offence about which they are being interviewed **might** be considered unreliable in subsequent court proceedings because of their physical or mental state.

Source: Crown, 2019 / Public Domain.

BOX 3.12   **FITNESS TO INTERVIEW ASSESSMENT**

• Capacity to understand and follow the interview process

• Recognise those at risk of unreliable confessions

• Identify the need for appropriate safeguards

• Determine where an interview will have an unacceptable detrimental effect on an individual's health

Source: Adapted from Police Scotland and NHS Scotland (2013).

VOLUNTARY INTERVIEWS

Officers can conduct interviews under caution without arresting an individual and may request their fitness to be interviewed assessed. Voluntary interviews, named because the individual voluntarily agrees to one, may occur in a police station or other setting, such as their home.[2] While individuals can leave at any time, they may be arrested if they attempt to. They are still entitled to free and independent legal advice and representation. The assessment follows the standard scheme for those in custody. In England and Wales, the caution differs slightly from those under arrest, *'You do not have to say anything, but anything you do say may be given in evidence'* (Home Office 2019, p. 77). Meaning courts cannot draw adverse inferences from silence during voluntary interviews. In Scotland and Northern Ireland, the cautions remain unchanged.

DETERMINING FITNESS TO INTERVIEW

The assessment considers their physical and mental health, social, education, employment, alcohol and substance misuse history. The assessment can be broken down into two parts:

• **Part 1**: Harm

• **Part 2**: Reliability

---

[2] In Scotland voluntary interviews must take place in a police station.

Part 1: Physical Health

The first part is typically straightforward, will the interview cause significant harm? Those unfit to detain and referred to the Emergency Department will be unfit to interview as a delay could harm their health. However, someone deemed unfit for detention because of their long-term care needs may still be suitable for a voluntary interview. Individuals who are sleep or food deprived should not be interviewed; therefore make inquiries regarding any recent sleep and diet.

Harm is not just physical and HCPs should consider if the interview will have a significant detrimental effect on their mental health. All interviews are likely to cause some stress and anxiety; the HCP's role is to determine where this goes beyond a 'normal response' and causes significant harm.

Part 2: Reliability

The second part, reliability, can be more complex. PACE and PACENI advise on elements that must be considered (see Box 3.13). The individual must understand the above caution in either the original or a simplified form. If not, the individual will be unfit for an interview. Assessing reliability aims to determine if the individuals' replies are rational, or affected by a physical or mental condition. Rational is defined as 'based on clear thought and reason' (Cambridge Dictionary 2023). To determine if responses are likely to be rational HCPs need to consider the individual's mental state (see Chapter 6 – Mental Health) and the three main elements for unreliability: suggestibility, compliance and acquiescence.

Suggestibility   Suggestibility is the tendency to be influenced by external cues or suggestions. Highly suggestible individuals may be more susceptible to leading questions or other

---

BOX 3.13   **PACE & PACENI CODE C ANNEX G**

In assessing whether the detainee should be interviewed, the following must be considered:

a. How the detainee's physical or mental state might affect their ability to understand the nature and purpose of the interview, to comprehend what is being asked and to appreciate the significance of any answers given and make rational decisions about whether they want to say anything.

b. The extent to which the detainee's replies may be affected by their physical or mental condition, rather than representing a rational and accurate explanation of their involvement in the offence.

c. How the nature of the interview, which could include particularly probing questions, might affect the detainee.

Source: Crown, 2019 / Public Domain.

forms of interviewer influence, which can lead to inaccurate or false statements. Additionally, if an interviewer is perceived as having authority or power over the individual, this can increase their suggestibility.

Compliance Some degree of compliance is necessary. Excessive compliance in this context refers to situations where an individual is overly cooperative and agrees with everything the interviewer says or requests, without questioning or resisting.

Acquiescence Acquiescence refers to a situation where an individual passively or uncritically agrees with the assertions, suggestions or demands made by interviewers, without necessarily believing them to be true.

Substance use or misuse The assessment should examine for the presence or absence of any drug or alcohol intoxication or withdrawal. Individuals should not be interviewed where there is evidence of intoxication or moderate withdrawal

symptoms (drug or alcohol) as both can negatively affect reliability. Officers often consider individuals fit to interview when their alcohol concentration is below the legal limit. However, this arbitrary figure may harm those with an alcohol dependency who may develop alcohol withdrawal syndrome before they reach this level. In such circumstances, alcohol concentration levels are unhelpful, and HCPs should rely on clinical and functional assessments.

Norfolk (2001) developed the acronym 'PHIT' (Personality factors, Health, Interview and Totality of circumstances) to help recognise reliability vulnerabilities. Building on Norfolk's (2001) work, re-framing 'Personality factors' as 'Personal factors', which includes 'personality factors', allows for adding personal risks outside their personality, see Box 3.14. For example, cultural differences, fatigue and age. See Chapter 4 – Appropriate Adults and Vulnerabilities for a Greater Understanding. The presence of reliability vulnerabilities does not preclude an interview, but HCPs should recommend an appropriate adult safeguard as a minimum.

BOX 3.14	**RELIABILITY VULNERABILITIES**
Personal factors	• Children and older adults
	• Personality traits (i.e. low self-esteem and tendency to conform)
	• Suggestibility, compliance and acquiescence
	• Fatigue or lack of sleep
	• Perception of authority figures (i.e. a desire to please others)
	• Language barriers
	• Cultural differences
Health	*Physical*
	• Acute illness
	• Moderate-severe pain
	• Hypoglycaemia
	Mental
	• Stress and anxiety
	• Intellectual disabilities or cognitive impairments
	• Mental illness (psychotic, mood or depressive disorders)
	• ADHD, Autism, acquire or traumatic brain injuries
	Substance use and misuse
	• Drug or alcohol intoxication or withdrawal
Interview	• Interview characteristics (i.e. coercive and leading questions)
	• Interview demands (i.e. the number and length of interviews will be much higher for serious offences like murder than less serious offences like theft)
Totality of circumstances	• Consider all the available information, including social distractions (i.e. childcare concerns)

OUTCOME

Following the assessment, the HCP has several options, fit to interview, fit to interview with safeguard, currently unfit to interview and unfit at any stage (within the timeframe of their detention). As always, the outcome of the assessment should be explained to the individual. As discussed earlier, HCPs advise and the custody officer decides. Police can still interview someone who the HCP believes is unfit. In such cases, HCPs should discuss their concerns with the custody officer, investigating officer and inspector, as well as clearly document these in the custody and healthcare record.

Fit to Interview

There are no discernible reliability, vulnerability, intoxication or withdrawal concerns. This includes those with an earlier condition that has responded to treatment.

Fit to Interview with Safeguard

There are some reliability or vulnerability risks. Safeguards will depend on the risk but as a minimum include an appropriate adult. Other safeguards may include shorter interviews, specially trained officers or time limits when fitness to interview will require reassessment.

Currently Unfit to Interview

Where an individual may be temporarily unfit by illness, intoxication or withdrawal but likely to improve within a few hours, HCPs can suggest a medical rest period before re-evaluating. This approach may be applicable when it is uncertain whether a person's behaviour stems from substance use or mental illness.

Unfit at Any State to Interview

Individuals with severe learning disabilities or dementia-like illnesses, which are permanent and unlikely to improve with time, may be unfit to interview. This could also include those with mania or psychosis, which may respond to treatment but not within custody time limits. However, it should be noted the presence of psychosis or mania alone does not render someone unfit for interview and HCPs should consider their functional ability. It is also worth noting an interview is not a prerequisite to being charged and police may charge an individual who is unfit for interview.

CONCERNS RAISED DURING AN INTERVIEW

It may not always be possible to identify concerns before an interview, either because their condition has deteriorated, or the officer's questions elicited additional information. For example, someone suspected of possessing an offensive weapon may appear well initially but during the interview, advises officers they are on a mission from God to rid the world of evil demons. Therefore, it is important to re-assess where concerns have been raised and consider this new information.

| **SCENARIO 3.2** | Fitness to interview |

You are asked to assess fitness to interview for a 19-year-old arrested for the first time on suspicion of rape. He suffers with type 1 diabetes, generalised anxiety disorder and smokes cannabis most nights. When arrested he was intoxicated with alcohol but now appears sober. His blood glucose level is 6.1 mmol/l and he is up to date with his medication (insulin and citalopram).

1. *Describe your approach to the fitness to interview assessment.*

2. *Using the PHIT approach, what are the reliability vulnerabilities?*
   a. *Personal factors*
   b. *Health*
   c. *Interview*
   d. *Totality of circumstances*

3. *Are they fit to be interviewed?*
   a. *What is the most likely foreseeable risk(s)?*
   b. *Would you recommend an appropriate adult?*

FITNESS TO CHARGE

Where there is sufficient evidence for a realistic prospect of conviction, an individual may be charged with an offence. Depending on the offence charging decisions are made by the police or Crown Prosecution Service.[3] Once charged, individuals may be released or remanded for court.

Those fit to interview will be fit to charge, assuming no major changes. However, where officers have enough evidence to charge someone unfit for an interview, they may request a fitness-to-charge assessment.

DETERMINING FITNESS TO CHARGE

The assessment follows the standard process with the focus being on their ability to understand the statutory warning[4] and the offence they are charged with, see Box 3.15. Both may need to be explained in simple, layperson language.

| **BOX 3.15** | **STATUTORY CHARGE WORDING (ENGLAND AND WALES)** |

'You do not have to say anything. But it may harm your defence if you do not mention now something which you later rely on in court. Anything you do say may be given in evidence'

Source: Crown, 2019 / Public Domain.

---

[3] Crown Office & Procurator Fiscal Service – Scotland; Public Prosecution Service – Northern Ireland.
[4] The exact wording differs between the devolved nations, but remains substantially the same.

Fitness to charge

You are asked to assess fitness to charge for a 33-year-old male who is being charged with theft. They have a history of borderline personality disorder. They have been uncooperative during detention and refused to leave the cell for interview. When charged they denied understanding the wording. They agree to a brief assessment in the cell. They are hostile but appear sober, their speech is normal and they do not appear distracted.

1. *Describe your approach to the fitness-to-charge assessment.*

2. *Are they fit to be charged?*

FITNESS TO RELEASE (PRE-RELEASE RISK ASSESSMENT)

Suicide following release is a concern. Custody officers may request an assessment of fitness to release where someone has indicated they will harm themselves on release, self-harmed in custody, collateral information or the offence gives rise to concern. While often termed 'Fitness to release' the assessment is actually a pre-release risk assessment. Those arrested for sexually motivated offences, particularly those involving children, account for most documented suicides following custody and must always be considered to be a high index of suspicion of potential suicide prior to assessment.

When assessing fitness for release, it is essential to understand the limits of detention. Custody officers must release individuals once there are no grounds to charge. There are no powers in PACE or PACENI to continue to detain someone for their safety beyond this point. Although, in Scotland, where there is a clear and imminent danger, custody officers can deny release (Police Scotland 2019). Additionally, officers cannot rely on mental capacity legislation to continue to detain someone in custody. However, if charged with an offence, individuals can be remanded to court if the custody officer is concerned about their safety. However, this alone does nothing to mitigate the risk when released from court.

DETERMINING FITNESS TO RELEASE

The assessment follows the standard scheme focusing on their mental and emotional state, thoughts of self-harm, suicide and social circumstances. Identifying any protective factors, along with short and long-term plans following release. Consideration should be given to the offence and the impact this may have, especially if it is considered socially reprehensible, like child sexual offences or is possibly career ending, such as a road traffic offence for a lorry driver. Finally, consideration should be given to any post-release restrictions, like no access to a partner or child. For this reason and because assessments are dynamic, the individual should be informed about any charging decisions and post-release restrictions before the assessment.

Depending on the outcome of the assessment and the level of risk, there may be several options that vary across the force areas. In England and Wales, for those at immediate risk of significant self-harm or suicide, the police may detain them under section 136 of the Mental Health Act and transfer them to a health-based place of safety for assessment.[5] In Scotland, best practice would support a mental health referral if the person is considered to be at high, imminent risk of suicide and be assessed by a Mental Health Professional who can come to Custody, or transfer to Secondary Care premises by Police Scotland. For those considered to not be an immediate risk, a referral for a crisis mental health assessment either in custody, immediately following or later the same day. For those presenting as low risk with no immediate concerns, it may be suitable to signpost them towards their general practitioner and advise them of services available in crisis needed (i.e. ambulance service, Samaritans, crisis services or local third sector organisations). For further information on assessing self-harm and suicide risk, see Chapter 6 – Mental Health.

Concerns regarding a child's release should be discussed with an adult with parental responsibility and an urgent safeguarding referral made. As a minimum arrangement should be made to release children into a parent's or responsible adult's care. Children's crisis mental health services vary across the United Kingdom, so it is important to be familiar with the local in-hours and out-of-hours arrangements.

Fitness to release

You are asked to assess fitness to release for a 21-year-old male with a history of emotionally unstable personality disorder and self-harm. He has been charged with a domestic assault. He is being released now with conditions not to contact the victim (his partner). While in custody, he was observed at Level 4 due to repeatedly tying clothing around his neck. During interview, he said he would kill himself if he could not go back to his partner. On examination, he is upset and tearful, voicing 'I don't want to carry on without my partner' but denies any current suicidal plans or intent.

1. *Describe your approach to the fitness-to-release assessment.*

2. *Is he fit to be released?*
   a. *What are the foreseeable risks?*
   b. *What is your advice to the police?*

3. *What onward referral or sign-posting options are available?*

4. *What, if any, grounds are there to impose further assessment if he is not agreeable to seeing the mental health crisis services?*

---

[5] The devolved nations equivalent legislation Section 297 of the Mental Health (Care and Treatment) (Scotland) Act 2003 and Section 130 of The Mental Health (Northern Ireland) Order 1986 cannot be applied in police custody, because it is not considered a 'public place'.

FITNESS TO TRAVEL

Individuals may need to be transported, this may be a short distance (i.e. to the local court) or across the country (i.e. transferred from custody in Cornwall to a court in Scotland). Additionally, individuals may be transferred from one force to another, for example someone may be arrested in Liverpool for an offence being investigated in London.

DETERMINING FITNESS TO TRAVEL

The assessment follows the same principles of assessing fitness to detain. Is travel safe? Are there any reasonably foreseeable risks? Consideration should be given to who and how someone is being transported. Force-to-force transfers will likely involve a police vehicle, such as a car or a van, both with different levels of comfort. A prisoner transport agency will likely move those

SCENARIO 3.5	Fitness to travel

You are asked to assess fitness to travel for a 69-year-old male with a history of ischaemic heart disease and angina. He is prescribed isosorbide mononitrate, bisoprolol, atorvastatin, aspirin, clopidogrel and glyceryl trinitrate spray as needed. Medication is in custody. He is required to travel by prisoner transport agency from Leeds to London for court.

1. *Describe your approach to the fitness to travel assessment.*

2. *Are they fit to travel?*
   a. *What are the foreseeable risks?*
   b. *What advice would you provide to both the police and the prisoner transport agency?*

going to court. Consideration should be given to mobility, comfort and any medication needs, with instructions for the transporting agency to provide any necessary medication and advice on when they may need to see further medical assistance.

FITNESS TO PLEAD

Custody HCPs do not assess fitness to plead. Assessments typically occur in prisons or secure hospitals by a forensic psychiatrist, who evaluates an individual's capacity to participate effectively in their trial, often due to mental health issues or learning disabilities.

CONCLUSION

In conclusion, fitness assessments serve as a critical component in custody work, helping to guarantee those held in custody are appropriately fit for detention and interview. HCPs are instrumental in carrying out these assessments and must possess a thorough understanding of pertinent legislation, such as PACE, PACENI and CJA. By executing comprehensive and well-documented assessments, HCPs can contribute to the fair and ethical treatment of individuals while minimising the likelihood of adverse outcomes, such as miscarriages of justice, deaths in or following custody which would result in a coroner's inquest or a Fatal Accident Inquiry (Scotland).

Throughout this chapter, we delved into the intricacies and complexities of fitness assessments, emphasising the importance of taking factors such as drug or alcohol withdrawal, intoxication and thoughts of self-harm into account. By adhering to a stringent process, HCPs can ensure their assessments are precise and informative. The knowledge and practical guidance offered in this chapter will enable HCPs to confidently carry out their responsibilities.

LEARNING ACTIVITIES

1. Write a reflection where you assessed fitness to detain, but their condition deteriorated, or they became unwell and were transferred to the hospital. Consider if the deterioration was foreseeable and how your attitude, values and beliefs may have impacted your decision-making.

2. Prepare a statement on a difficult fitness-to-interview assessment. Now consider the strengths and weaknesses of your statement and potential cross-examination questions and responses.

3. Develop a mental health contacts list specific to your suite with local services (including suitable third-sector services), referral criteria, working hours and out-of-hours alternatives.

RESOURCES

Online

- College of Policing | Authorised Professional practice | Detention and custody – https://www.college.police.uk/app/detention-and-custody

- Royal College of Physicians | National Early Warning Score 2 – https://www.rcplondon.ac.uk/projects/outputs/national-early-warning-score-news-2

- Police and Criminal Evidence Act 1984 (PACE) Code C | Code of practice for the detention, treatment and questioning of persons by police officers – https://www.gov.uk/government/publications/pace-code-c-2019

- Police and Criminal Evidence (Northern Ireland) Order 1989 (PACENI) Code C | Code of practice for the detention, treatment and questioning of persons by police officers – https://niopa.qub.ac.uk/bitstream/NIOPA/483/1/16-06-pace-code-c-2015%20%281%29.pdf

- Police Scotland | Criminal Justice (Scotland) Act 2016 (Arrest Process) – https://www.scotland.police.uk/spa-media/dvlnu5og/criminal-justice-scotland-act-2016-arrest-process-sop.pdf

- Police Scotland | Care and Welfare of Persons in Police Custody – https://www.scotland.police.uk/spa-media/0mfjn3pa/care-and-welfare-of-persons-in-police-custody-sop.pdf

- Queen's Nursing Institute Scotland | Think COULD | https://www.qnis.org.uk/new-animation-think-could/

Organisations

- UK Association of Forensic Nurses and Paramedics – www.ukafnp.org

- Faculty of Forensic and Legal Medicine – www.fflm.ac.uk

- Royal College of Nursing | Nursing in Justice and Forensic Health Care Forum – https://www.rcn.org.uk/Get-Involved/Forums/Nursing-in-Justice-and-Forensic-Health-Care-Forum

REFERENCES

Cambridge Dictionary (2023). Cambridge dictionary. https://dictionary.cambridge.org (accessed 16 February 2023).

College of Policing (2020). Authorised professional practice; detention and custody; detainee care. https://www.app.college.police.uk/app-content/detention-and-custody-2/detainee-care/ (accessed 14 July 2022).

College of Policing (2022). Investigative interviewing. https://www.college.police.uk/app/investigation/investigative-interviewing/investigative-interviewing (accessed 16 February 2023).

Dorn, T., Janssen, A., de Keijzer, J.C. et al. (2018). Hospital referral of detainees during police custody in Amsterdam, The Netherlands. *Journal of Forensic and Legal Medicine* 57: 82–85.

Home Office (2019). *CODE C Revised Codes of Practice for the Detention, Treatment and Questioning of Persons by Police Officers*. London: Home Office. https://assets.publishing.service.gov.uk/government/uploads/system/uploads/attachment_data/file/903473/pace-code-c-2019.pdf (accessed 16 November 2021).

Miles, T., Webb, V., Kevern, P. et al. (2020). Custody early warning scores; Do they predict patient deterioration in police custody? *Journal of Forensic and Legal Medicine* 76: 102069.

Norfolk, G. (2001). Fit to be interviewed by the police – an aid to assessment. *Medicine, Science and the Law* 41 (1): 5–12.

Police Scotland (2016). *Pre Interview Review of Rights Aide Memoire*. Scotland: Police Scotland https://www.whatdotheyknow.com/request/645846/response/1544629/attach/5/Pre%20Interview%20Review%20of%20Rights%20Aide%20Memoire.pdf?cookie_passthrough=1 (accessed 13 February 2023).

Police Scotland (2019). Care and welfare of persons in police custody. https://www.scotland.police.uk/spa-media/0mfjn3pa/care-and-welfare-of-persons-in-police-custody-sop.pdf (accessed 21 November 2022).

Police Scotland and NHS Scotland (2013). *National Guidance on the Delivery of Police Care Healthcare and Forensic Medical Services*. Scotland: NHS Scotland https://www.nss.nhs.scot/media/1999/shpn-11-10-v10-jan-2014.pdf (accessed 10 December 2022).

FURTHER READING

Peel, M. (2015). Assessing fitness to detain in police custody. *Nursing Standard* 30 (11): 43–49.

Peel, M. (2017). Assessing an individual's fitness to be interviewed in police custody. *Nursing Standard* 31 (40): 42–50.

Vulnerability and Appropriate Adults

Chris Bath[1] and Roxanna Dehaghani[2]

[1] National Appropriate Adult Network, Ashford, UK
[2] Cardiff University, Cardiff, Wales

CHAPTER 4

AIM

This chapter explores the role and purpose of the appropriate adult (AA) safeguard, the concept of vulnerability related to the AA and the risks of not securing an AA. It will introduce readers to the AA and vulnerability across the United Kingdom (UK).

LEARNING OUTCOMES

After reading this chapter, you will be able to:

- Understand the role and purpose of the AA

- Understand the concept of vulnerability as it relates to the requirement for an AA

- Understand the risks of not identifying vulnerability or not securing an AA

SELF-ASSESSMENT

1. Define vulnerability in the context of police interviews.

2. Outline how the AA safeguard protects the individual, the police, the evidence and the justice system.

3. What are the obstacles to implementing the AA safeguard?

INTRODUCTION

The AA safeguard is a fundamentally important protection for vulnerable suspects. If not implemented when it should be, there can be significant risks to the individual and the investigation. Although the responsibility for identifying vulnerability and securing an AA in custody rests with the custody officer, healthcare professionals (HCPs) are often called upon for their advice. As such, HCPs must have a strong understanding of the AA's role and purpose, the definition of vulnerability and the risks of not identifying vulnerability or securing an AA. HCPs must also be aware of the requirements under the relevant legislation:

- Police and Criminal Evidence Act 1984 (PACE)

- Police and Criminal Evidence (Northern Ireland) Order 1989 (PACENI)

- Criminal Justice (Scotland) Act 2016 (CJA)

APPROPRIATE ADULTS

HISTORY AND LEGISLATIVE BASIS

Appropriate adults are used across the United Kingdom but with significant variations in definition and application. In all UK jurisdictions, the absence of an AA, when required,

---

can impact the reliability and therefore admissibility, of evidence.

England and Wales

The AA was formally introduced in 1986 with PACE 1984 and its Codes of Practice. PACE was introduced in response to a loss of public confidence in policing following high-profile miscarriages of justice, often linked to vulnerability. In a key case, two children and an 18-year-old with a learning disability were wrongfully convicted of various offences related to the death of Maxwell (also known as Michelle) Confait in 1972, following allegedly coerced confessions. This led to the Fisher Report in 1977, the Royal Commission on Criminal Procedure in 1981 and ultimately the PACE Act 1984.

Northern Ireland

In Northern Ireland, the AA exists in a similar guise as in England and Wales, but by virtue of the Police and Criminal Evidence (NI) Order 1980 and its accompanying Codes of Practice (Department of Justice 2015).

Scotland

In Scotland, a significantly different AA role has existed since 1991. Since 2019, AAs have been provided on a statutory basis under the Criminal Justice (Scotland) Act 2016 (Support for Vulnerable Persons) Regulations 2019.

APPLICABILITY

England, Wales and Northern Ireland

The AA safeguard applies to children and vulnerable[1] people of any age who are detained in police custody, attending a voluntary interview under caution or subjected to a search exposing intimate parts of the body (Department of Justice 2015; Home Office 2019).

Scotland

The AA safeguard applies to vulnerable people aged 16 or over[2] who are victims, witnesses, suspects or accused (Scottish Government 2020).

THE ROLE OF AN AA

ENGLAND AND WALES

The AA's role is to safeguard a person's interests, including their rights, entitlements and welfare (Crime and Disorder Act 1998, s. 38(4); Home Office 2019, 1.7A). Among other things, the AA is expected to:

---

[1] Definitions of vulnerability vary significantly between jurisdictions.
[2] For children under 16, a parent must be asked to come to the station and given access to their child subject to limited exceptions (Criminal Justice (Scotland) Act 2016, s38–s40). However, this is distinct from the role of an AA.

- support, advise and assist the person when they are given or asked to provide information, or participate in any procedure under the PACE Codes.

- help them to communicate whilst respecting their right to say nothing unless they want to.

- help them to understand their rights and make sure those rights are protected and respected.

- observe whether the police are acting properly and fairly and tell a more senior police officer if not (Home Office 2019, 1.7A).

The precise requirements around AA involvement are complex and detailed throughout the PACE Codes. However, a custody officer must secure an AA's attendance as soon as practicable after authorising detention. The AA has a role throughout detention, from rights and entitlements, identification (e.g. photographs, fingerprints and DNA), taking samples, charging decisions and related actions such as cautions, bail and child accommodation transfers. Subject to authorisation by a Superintendent, in cases of urgency where the delay could lead to significant harm, some procedures (such as interviews) can occur without the AA present (Home Office 2019).

Northern Ireland

In Northern Ireland, the AA's role is similar to England and Wales: advise the suspect, observe a proper and fairly conducted interview and facilitate communication. However, the communication element does not apply where a Registered Intermediary facilitates communication during the interview (Department of Justice 2015, 11.17, 13.1). The Registered Intermediary's role is distinct from that of an AA, focusing on communication strategy rather than general understanding. Therefore, it is important to remember a Registered Intermediary does not replace AA.

Scotland

In Scotland, the AA's role is focused purely on communication. It does not include rights and welfare. It is limited to helping the person understand what is happening and facilitating communication (Criminal Justice (Scotland) Act 2016 (Support for Vulnerable Persons) Regulations 2019, Regulation 3).

WHO CAN ACT AS AN AA

ENGLAND, WALES AND NORTHERN IRELAND

A child's AA can be a parent or guardian, a person from a local authority or voluntary organisation responsible for that child's care, or a social worker. Failing these, the AA may be some other 'responsible adult' (Department of Justice 2015, 1.7; Home Office 2019, 1.7).

For vulnerable people, an AA can be a relative, guardian or another person responsible for their care or custody;

someone experienced in dealing with vulnerable people; or failing these a 'responsible adult' (Department of Justice 2015, 1.7; Home Office 2019, 1.7). It is considered 'someone experienced or trained' may be 'more satisfactory' but if the person 'prefers a relative to a better-qualified stranger, or objects to a particular person their wishes should, if practicable, be respected' (Department of Justice 2015, Note for Guidance 1D; Home Office 2019, Note for Guidance 10D).

Exceptions to the above are set out in the PACE Codes (Department of Justice 2015; Home Office 2019) and have been reinforced in case law (Dehaghani 2020). The person must not be:

- anyone who has received an admission of guilt prior to attending

- involved in the offence in any way (i.e. co-accused, victim or witness)

- at the station acting in another capacity, such as the solicitor (or legal representative) or independent custody visitor

- a police officer, employed by the police, under the direction or control of the chief of police or a person who is providing services, under a contractual arrangement to the police, to assist with the chief of police's functions (including HCPs)

- a parent who is estranged from a child (if the child does not want them)

- the principal of a child's educational establishment (unless waiting would cause unreasonable delay and the offence is not against that establishment)

In practice, there are broadly three categories of persons acting as AAs:

1. **Relatives and friends (including but not limited to parents)**: They often have no prior experience or training in the AA role, which, without support, can make it a challenging role to fulfil effectively. The pre-existing personal relationship can bring significant benefits, such as trust and knowledge of the person's needs. However, the deeper emotional connections can also bring challenges that negatively impact the AA and the person (Quinn and Jackson 2007).

2. **Ad-hoc professionals**: For example, social workers, care home staff and youth and community workers, with whom the person has a pre-existing wider professional relationship. The benefits and challenges vary according to the nature and quality of the existing relationship. They are likely to rarely act in the AA role and often will not have received specific AA training and development.

3. **Dedicated AAs**: Volunteers, sessional staff or employees of an organised AA scheme. In England and Wales, local authorities have a statutory duty to provide AAs for children (Crime and Disorder Act 1998, s.38). Schemes are either delivered or commissioned by youth justice services. Publicly funded schemes for vulnerable people also exist in most areas, although no statutory duty exists. In Northern Ireland, a single AA scheme (NIASS) supports children and vulnerable people, funded by the Department of Justice and delivered by a charity using contracted and casual staff. In England, Wales and Northern Ireland, dedicated AAs do not have a pre-existing relationship with the person. However, they will have undertaken training and, increasingly, formal qualifications in the AA role (Dehaghani 2020). They will benefit from organisational support, coordination, supervision and professional development. Almost all AA schemes are National Appropriate Adult Network (NAAN) members. NAAN is a charity and membership organisation which acts as a centre of expertise for the AA role. This includes publishing national standards approved by the Youth Justice Board, Association of Directors of Social Services and Association of Police and Crime Commissioners (Scottish Government 2020).

SCOTLAND

By law, AAs are trained and provided by local authority schemes. They are coordinated by the Convention of Scottish Local Authorities (COSLA). Quality assessment is undertaken by the Care Inspectorate.

CHILDREN AND VULNERABLE PEOPLE
DEFINITION

The word 'vulnerable' is commonly used in policing, health and wider public discourse but with variable meaning. Healthcare practitioners working in police custody may experience multiple legal and theoretical frameworks, including:

- Fitness for detention or interview assessments

- Mental capacity assessments

- Mental health assessment

- Criminal justice liaison and diversion assessments

- Vulnerability Assessment Framework (the ABCDE system[3])

- Equality legislation (reasonable adjustments for disability)

Each jurisdiction has a specific definition and threshold to determine the need for an AA.

---

[3] Appearance, Behaviour, Communication capacity, Danger and Environment circumstances.

England and Wales

Definition The person:

- may have difficulty understanding or communicating effectively about the full implications for them of any procedures and processes connected with:
  - their arrest and detention; or
  - their voluntary attendance at a police station or presence elsewhere for a voluntary interview and
  - the exercise of their rights and entitlements; or

- does not appear to understand the significance of what they are told, of questions they are asked or of their replies; or

- appears to be particularly prone to:
  - becoming confused and unclear about their position;
  - providing unreliable, misleading or incriminating information without knowing or wishing to do so;
  - accepting or acting on suggestions from others without consciously knowing or wishing to do so or
  - readily agreeing to suggestions or proposals without any protest or question.

A person to whom one or more of the factors apply solely because they are under the influence of drink or drugs is not considered 'vulnerable' but should be re-assessed once they have recovered from the effects (Home Office 2019, Note 1G).

The PACE definition of vulnerability is not limited to a lack of basic understanding (e.g. of the current time, their location and/or what rights they have). A person is vulnerable if they may not understand the *full implications* (consequences) of processes and procedures, or decisions about whether and when to exercise their rights. Or if they do not appear to understand the *significance* (meaning and importance) of information given to them, what they are asked and what they say in response. PACE vulnerability should not be confused with mental capacity.[4]

Code C references 'mental health condition or mental disorder' as causal factors and links to the non-exhaustive list of 'clinically recognised conditions' in the Mental Health Act 1983 Code of Practice (Department of Health 2015).[5]

However, there is no requirement for a clinical diagnosis. Code C states; 'A person may be vulnerable as a result of having a mental health condition or mental disorder. Similarly, simply because an individual does not have, or is not known to have, any such condition or disorder, does not mean they are not vulnerable for the purposes of this Code' (Home Office 2019, Note 1G).

Threshold This complex definition is balanced with a low threshold. If there is '*any reason to suspect* a person of any age *may* be vulnerable', they must be treated as vulnerable unless there is 'clear evidence to dispel that suspicion' (Home Office 2019, 1.4). This is reinforced by the words 'may' and 'appears to', within the factors themselves (Home Office 2019, 1.13d). It need not be certain, or even likely, that one or more of the factors apply. If there is any *reason* to suspect the person may be vulnerable, an AA is mandatory.

Unlike legal advice, there is no provision for the AA to be waived by the individual. Mental capacity is irrelevant, as they are not being asked to make a decision. While a person can refuse to engage with an AA, the AA must be present when required under PACE.

Children An AA is always required if a person appears to be aged under 18 years, unless there is 'clear evidence they are older' (Home Office 2019, 1.5, 1G). It is advisable to exercise caution when determining the need for an AA when someone who looks over 18 but may in fact be under 18. It can be difficult to ascertain age; although unusual, children sometimes claim to be adults (Dehaghani 2019).

SCENARIO 4.1 AA refusal

You are asked to review an adult who was seen earlier by another colleague and is refusing to be interviewed with an AA. They have a history of schizophrenia, but there is no evidence of an acute deterioration. The custody officer would like you to assess his capacity to refuse an AA.

1. *Describe your approach to this request.*

2. *Can individuals with capacity refuse an AA?*

Reasonable enquiries Police must first make 'reasonable enquiries' to ascertain what information is available that is relevant to whether any of the vulnerability factors in PACE Code C apply. They must then record whether or not any factors apply and make that record available to anyone required, or entitled to communicate with the person (including HCPs, legal representatives and AAs) (Home Office 2019, Note 1.4).

The requirement for police to make reasonable enquiries about potential vulnerability applies equally to children.

---

[4] There is evidence the AA safeguard has erroneously not been applied because a person is judged to 'have capacity'. Most people who are 'PACE vulnerable' would have capacity in most contexts. However, a person deemed not to have capacity would likely meet the definition of vulnerability. A person may be considered to have capacity subject to having the support of an AA.

[5] Affective disorders, such as depression and bipolar disorder; schizophrenia and delusional disorders; neurotic, stress-related and somatoform disorders, such as anxiety, phobic disorders, obsessive compulsive disorders, post-traumatic stress disorder and hypochondriacal disorders; organic mental disorders such as dementia and delirium (however caused); personality and behavioural changes caused by brain injury or damage (however acquired); personality disorders; mental and behavioural disorders caused by psychoactive substance use; eating disorders, non-organic sleep disorders and non-organic sexual disorders; learning disabilities; autistic spectrum disorders (including Asperger's syndrome); behavioural and emotional disorders of children and young people.

Children in conflict with the law are likely to have specific additional vulnerabilities beyond age, for example related to mental health, learning disability, neurodiversity and speech language and communication needs (Hughes et al. 2012).

Code C provides police with a non-exhaustive list of sources of relevant information that may be available to them (Home Office 2019, Note 1GA), any of which could provide a reason to suspect vulnerability:

- what the child or adult says about themselves

- their behaviour, mental health and capacity

- information from relatives and friends

- information from police officers and staff, police records

- information from health and social care (in or outside custody) and other professionals who have had previous contact

Northern Ireland

The threshold for children is the same as in as England and Wales (Department of Justice 2015, 1.5).

In relation to vulnerable people, if an officer has any suspicion, or is told in good faith, that a person may be 'mentally disordered' or otherwise 'mentally vulnerable', or have 'significant communication difficulties',[6] in the absence of clear evidence to dispel that suspicion, they must be treated as vulnerable and an AA is required (Department of Justice 2015, 1.4). 'Mentally vulnerable' applies to any suspect who, because of their mental state or capacity, may not understand the significance of what is said, of questions or of their replies. 'Mental disorder' means 'mental illness, mental handicap and any other disorder or disability of the mind' (Department of Justice 2015, Note 1G).[7]

Scotland

An AA is required if, in the context of a criminal investigation or criminal proceedings (Criminal Justice (Scotland) Act 2016, s.42), a police constable believes the person is 16 or over and owing to 'mental disorder', they appear to be unable to:

- understand sufficiently what is happening, or

- communicate effectively

'Mental disorder' means 'any mental illness, personality disorder, learning disability however caused or manifested' (Mental Health (Care and Treatment) (Scotland) Act 2003 s.328). In practice, this includes people with acquired brain injury, autistic spectrum disorder and dementia (Scottish Government 2012).

---

[6] A person with significant communication difficulties must also be provided with a Registered Intermediary – a person with specialist communication skills who has been accredited by the Department of Justice.
[7] This definition was used in England and Wales prior to 2018, when replaced by the expanded functional test.

HEALTHCARE RESPONSIBILITIES

Police custody HCPs play an important role in identifying vulnerable people for whom an AA is required.

The custody officer is legally responsible for identifying people who may be vulnerable and implementing appropriate safeguards. This cannot be delegated to HCPs, either officially or in practice. Police can determine the need for an AA without an assessment from an HCP. However, both HCPs and the Liaison & Diversion (L&D) service (or equivalent) can provide the custody officer with information about a person's possible vulnerability and recommend an appropriate adult (NHS England 2019). Similarly, L&D services cannot assess fitness for interview but can provide information to support decision-making (NHS England 2019).

Neither the Code C of PACE nor the courts have defined what constitutes 'clear evidence' to dispel suspicion. A reasonable interpretation may be reliable information that removes the reason to suspect vulnerability. Police may seek to rely on information from HCPs as 'clear evidence to dispel' a suspicion. For example the fact a person has said they are vulnerable may be contrasted with an HCP selecting 'no AA recommended' on a 'Detained Persons Medical Form'. In cases where vulnerable people were not provided with an AA, HCPs have been called to court to explain their advice on why one was not recommended. It is, therefore, important HCPs:

- Understand the definition and threshold for treating a person as vulnerable.

- Understand where a person may be vulnerable, an AA is mandatory.

- Provide police information and advice rather than a decision.

- Do not advise police no vulnerability factors apply unless they have the appropriate professional competencies, have conducted appropriate assessments covering all vulnerability factors, or have consulted with a suitably qualified professional.

- Never advise police no AA is required if there is a reason to suspect the person may be vulnerable. HCPs should not be influenced against recommending an AA because the individual does not want one, they did not have one last time, there is no AA available, it is only a minor offence, or they intend to respond, 'no comment'.

SCENARIO 4.2   Query AA

You are asked to see a 34-year-old male with ADHD. He has been arrested for a domestic assault. The custody officer would like advice on the need for an AA, as the male had one last time. The custody officer does not think he needs one and the individual does not want one, stating it delayed their interview and release last time.

1. *Describe your approach to this assessment.*
2. *Should you recommend an AA?*
   a. *What are the risks to the individual, police and justice if an AA is not given?*
   b. *What are the risks of recommending an AA?*

RISKS TO JUSTICE

Failure to identify possible vulnerability, or to apply the AA procedural safeguard, having identified it, poses serious risks to the individual, the investigation and therefore to justice.

INDIVIDUALS

For individuals, the potential risks include:

- Breach of human rights (in particular, the right to a fair trial)
- Breach of rights under the Equality Act (reasonable adjustments for disability)
- Ineffective participation
- Providing false or misleading information (Home Office 2019, 11C)
- Anguish, time and stress
- Unfair application of a caution or conditional caution
- Wrongful conviction
- Potential deprivation of liberty through bail conditions or remand in custody

INVESTIGATIONS

For the investigation, the potential risks include:

- Inaccurate or misleading information complicating, misdirecting or delaying
- Wasted time and resources
- Exclusion of evidence at trial, for example confession deemed unreliable, exclusion of evidence that if admitted would result in unfairness
- Unsuccessful conviction where otherwise there may have been a finding of guilt (PACE 1984, s 76 and s 78; PACE(NI) 1989, s 74 and s 76)
- Conviction of an innocent party
- Guilty party not being held to account

Miscarriages of justice have occurred where a vulnerable suspect has been questioned without appropriate support, such as an AA (e.g. the *Confait* case). The AA safeguard aims to protect against unreliable or misleading confessions, avoiding miscarriages of justice and enabling vulnerable people to progress through the justice system where appropriate.

Case Study 1: *R v Aspinall* (1999)

A forensic physician had determined a man with schizophrenia to be fit for interview because he was on regular medication, anxious but lucid in thought, and orientated in time and space. No AA was secured and Mr Aspinall declined legal advice, saying 'the reason being I want to get home to my missus and kids'. A second doctor later said Mr Aspinall was likely to understand the nature of the procedure and questions, and would have been able to answer questions, but he would likely have been tired, under stress, worried and possibly depressed. He might have been less able to cope with questions and might have given answers that he thought would let him leave custody earlier. The Court of Appeal held the police had failed to consider the purpose, significance and extensive duties of the AA safeguard. They overturned the conviction because the lack of an AA made it unfair to admit the interview evidence.

Case Study 2: *Miller v DPP* (2018)

As noted earlier, the AA safeguard is not limited to interviews, and convictions have been quashed for a failure to apply the AA safeguard during other procedures and processes as required by PACE. For example, in the case of *Miller v Director of Public Prosecutions* (2018), the High Court considered a conviction for failing to provide a specimen of blood in custody. An HCP had said no AA was required; however, the custody record referred to mental health issues, learning difficulties and self-reported Asperger's Syndrome (an old diagnosis within Autism). The Court quashed the conviction as the AA would have had a calming influence on Mr Miller and would have been able to explain the purpose of obtaining a sample and the consequences of a failure to do so.

RESEARCH FINDINGS
CAUSES OF VULNERABILITY

Research has identified four groups of factors from which vulnerability can arise when combined with specific context and circumstances (Gudjonsson 2003: 61–75):

- mental disorder
- abnormal mental states (including anxiety, phobias, bereavement, intoxication, withdrawal and mood disturbance)
- intellectual functioning
- personality (such as suggestibility, compliance and acquiescence)

Some people may struggle with processes and procedures in police custody and may not give accurate or reliable

BOX 4.1	TYPES OF FALSE CONFESSIONS
Voluntary	Offered by individuals without any external pressure. These individuals might confess due to a desire for notoriety, or to offset guilt feelings. Some cannot differentiate between reality and fantasy, which is often linked to psychotic illnesses like schizophrenia. In some cases, these confessions might be given to protect the real culprit or to pre-empt the investigation of a more serious crime.
Accommodating-compliant	Arise from an individual's need for approval and to be liked. In these situations, the police use leading questions but are not coercive. People of all intellectual levels can be at risk, especially those who are excessively compliant.
Pressurised-compliant	Elicited during persuasive interrogation. In these cases, suspects see an immediate gain from confessing, such as ending the interrogation or being allowed to go home. These confessions are usually retracted once the immediate threat is over.
Coerced-reactive	Result from pressure by non-police individuals, like family or friends. The close emotional relationship between the confessor and the coercer adds additional pressure. In some relationships, non-compliance might lead to fear of emotional rejection or even violence.
Coerced-internalised	Occur where suspects are persuaded that they committed a crime they do not recall. This can happen when suspects have amnesia or when their memory and beliefs are manipulated by interrogators. Suspects might retract their confession when they realise or suspect their innocence. Susceptibility, whether due to naivety, low IQ, suggestibility, or other factors, plays a key role in facilitating internalisation.

Source: Adapted from Gudjonsson (2018).

evidence in interviews. As a result, they may be at a heightened risk of giving a false confession and therefore possibly a wrongful conviction (Gudjonsson 2018). There are five types of false confessions (see Box 4.1).

Context and Circumstance

Vulnerability exists along a continuum (Gudjonsson and Joyce 2011: 18). It varies significantly between individuals with the same condition. It varies over time, context and circumstance. For example being impacted by an individual's capacity to cope with police detention, interviews and other processes. A person who is not vulnerable in daily life, or even when first arrested, can become vulnerable after a period of detention or under questioning.

These in turn can be impacted by circumstances (the nature and seriousness of the crime, pressure on the police to solve the crime), interactions (between interviewer and suspect), personality and health (physical and mental) (Gudjonsson and MacKeith 1997).

Mental Disorders

A person diagnosed with a mental disorder may be more prone to experiencing difficulties with custody procedures and processes, more likely to be compliant, suggestible, or acquiescent and therefore may be more prone to false confession.

Physical Conditions

Physical conditions can make a suspect vulnerable. For example neurological conditions, such as, for example Parkinson's disease, stroke and dementia, can impact an individual's

cognitive abilities (JUSTICE 2017, 15). Physical illnesses such as epilepsy, diabetes and heart problems can result in heightened agitation and distress, thus affecting the accuracy and reliability of a confession (Gudjonsson et al. 1993, 16).

Trauma

Negative life events (e.g. trauma and adverse childhood experiences) can also make a person susceptible to misleading information. The more negative life events a person has experienced, the more easily they may accept the information put to them, even if this information is misleading and the more prone they may be to changing their answers because of interrogative pressure (Drake et al. 2008, 306).

Neurodivergence

Neurodivergence may also make a suspect vulnerable in the context of policy custody and interviews. For example autistic people, when compared to their neurotypical peers, may experience challenges in communicating and interacting with others (e.g. by providing too much or insufficient detail); may not understand how others think or feel or may not understand sarcasm or turns of phrase; may be easily overwhelmed, distressed or even physically pained due to the sensory environment in police custody; may experience significant and impairing anxiety when in unfamiliar situations and may take longer to process information (Cooper and Allely 2017). Anxiety may also result in silence or disengagement (shutdowns) and/or a loss of verbal and physical abilities (meltdowns). People with ADHD may be particularly prone to false confessions (O'Mahony et al. 2012, 302). Challenges include: impulsivity, boredom, memory, distractibility and difficulties with paying attention, appearing not to be listening, risk-taking, being chatty and difficulty following instructions and managing emotions.

CHALLENGES

Under-identification of Vulnerable Suspects

Clinical research conducted in the Metropolitan Police Service area indicated that 39% of detentions of adults involved a person with a mental disorder and 25.6% involved a person with psychosis, major depression, intellectual disabilities or whom researchers felt lacked capacity to consent to a questionnaire (McKinnon and Grubin 2013).

In comparison, only 8.7% of adult detentions in England and Wales and 12.4% in Northern Ireland were recorded by police as requiring an AA in 2022/23, with rates varying between forces from 0.3% to 21.7% (National Appropriate Adult Network 2023).

In 2018/19, police secured AAs for only 1 in 5 (19.4%) of adults identified as vulnerable by L&D services while in police custody (National Appropriate Adult Network 2020).

Application varies significantly according to diagnosis. In 2016/17, only 51–57% of people identified by L&D as having an acquired brain injury, dementia or schizophrenia had an AA. In comparison, only 15–19% of people with the higher prevalence diagnoses of anxiety, PTSD or depression had an AA (National Appropriate Adult Network 2019).

Barriers to the Identification of Vulnerability

Several barriers exist to implementing the AA safeguard for adults (Dehaghani 2019):

- The absence of – or deficiencies in – screening tools in custody, such as problems with the risk assessment
- Limitations in time and expertise of custody staff and HCPs
- An absence of information about the suspect
- Suspicion regarding self-reporting
- Drugs and alcohol complicating an assessment
- Reliance on previous assessments without considering individual changes over time – HCPs may overlook evolving circumstances, such as the impact of chronic alcohol misuse on memory. Alternatively, failing to take into consideration the individual circumstances surrounding the allegation and the individual's reaction to that allegation – for example someone arrested for child neglect may be very distressed

Problems with the Definition of Vulnerability

Custody staff and HCPs:

- Not understanding the definition of vulnerability
- Conflating assessments of fitness for interview and the need for an AA
- Not understanding what conditions fall under the definition of 'mental disorder'
- Developing their own definition of vulnerability which fails to align with the relevant definition

Problems with the Implementation of the AA Safeguard

- AA perceived or actual availability
- Limitations of police time and resources, particularly the perceived delays calling an AA would have to custody processes.
- Presuming that the lawyer can perform the role of the AA
- Letting the suspect decide whether to have an AA or not, or dissuading the suspect from having one
- Not implementing the AA for 'low-level' offences even when the suspect has been identified as vulnerable

---

SCENARIO 4.3 Query AA

You are asked to see a 30-year-old male who was argumentative at booking in, demanding an AA. He is demanding his sister be his AA. The custody officers advised he did have an AA last time, but he appears to understand everything said to him. The custody officer believes he is requesting an AA to reduce his culpability. He reports a history of memory issues following a traumatic brain injury.

1. *Describe your approach to this assessment.*

2. *How does the AA or identification of vulnerability affect an individual's culpability for the offence.*

3. *Should you recommend an AA?*
   a. *What are the risks to the individual, police and justice if an AA is not given?*
   b. *What are the risks of recommending an AA?*

CONCLUSION

The AA safeguard is pivotal in police custody for vulnerable individuals. Despite the low threshold for recommending an AA, many who need it are overlooked. While custody officers are primarily responsible for identifying vulnerability, HCPs play a crucial advisory role. Familiarity with the legislation (PACE, PACENI and CJA) is essential. The omission of an AA can endanger the individual and compromise the investigation. Thus, HCPs must actively champion the AA's role, ensuring those at risk are adequately protected. In the complex landscape of police custody, the AA serves as an essential safeguard and upholding it is a shared responsibility for all involved.

LEARNING ACTIVITIES

1. Write a reflection where you were asked to assess someone for an AA and you did not recommend one. Consider how your understanding, attitude, values and beliefs around the AA role may have impacted your decision-making.

2. Now, consider you have been asked to provide oral evidence in court regarding your decision. Outline the strengths and weak-nesses of your evidence and response to likely cross-examination questions.

3. Prepare a teaching session providing an update for your colleagues on the role of the AA, vulnerability and how HCPs can improve recognition and implementation of the AA.

RESOURCES

Online

- College of Policing | Authorised Professional practice | Children and young persons | https://www.college.police.uk/app/detention-and-custody/detainee-care/children-and-young-persons#appropriate-adults

- College of Policing | Authorised Professional practice | Response, arrest and detention | https://www.college.police.uk/app/detention-and-custody/response-arrest-and-detention#vulnerability

Organisations

- National Appropriate Adult Network | https://www.appropriateadult.org.uk

- JUSTICE | https://justice.org.uk

- University of Exeter Law School | Miscarriages of justice registry | https://evidencebasedjustice.exeter.ac.uk

REFERENCES

Cooper, P. and Allely, C. (2017). You can't judge a book by its cover: evolving professional responsibilities, liabilities and "judgecraft" when a party has Asperger's Syndrome. *Northern Ireland Legal Quarterly* 68 (1): 35–58.

Crime and Disorder Act (1998). Crime and Disorder Act 1998. https://www.legislation.gov.uk/ukpga/1998/37/contents (accessed 10 August 2023).

Criminal Justice (Scotland) Act (2016). Criminal Justice (Scotland) Act 2016. https://www.legislation.gov.uk/asp/2016/1/section/45/enacted (accessed 10 July 2023).

Dehaghani, R. (2019). *Vulnerability in Police Custody: Police Decision-making and the Appropriate Adult Safeguard*. Abingdon and New York: Routledge.

Dehaghani, R. (2020). Defining the "appropriate" in the appropriate adult': restrictions and opportunities for reform. *Criminal Law Review* 1137–1155. https://orca.cardiff.ac.uk/id/eprint/135417/.

Department of Health (2015). *Mental Health Act 1983: Code of Practice*. London: TSO https://assets.publishing.service.gov.uk/government/uploads/system/uploads/attachment_data/file/435512/MHA_Code_of_Practice.PDF (accessed 10 August 2024).

Department of Justice (2015). *Police and Criminal Evidence (Northern Ireland) Order 1989: Code C: Code of Practice for the Detention, Treatment and Questioning of Persons by Police Officers*. Belfast: Department of Justice https://www.justice-ni.gov.uk/sites/default/files/publications/doj/16-06-pace-code-c-2015.pdf (accessed 10 August 2023.

Drake, K.E., Bull, R., and Boon, J.C.W. (2008). Interrogative suggestibility, self-esteem, and the influence of negative life events. *Legal and Criminological Psychology* 13: 299–307.

Gudjonsson, G.H. (2003). *The Psychology of Interrogations and Confessions: A Handbook*. Hoboken, NJ: Wiley.

Gudjonsson, G.H. (2018). *The Psychology of False Confessions: Forty Years of Science and Practice*. Hoboken, NJ: Wiley.

Gudjonsson, G.H., Clare, I., Rutter, S., and Pearce, J. (1993). *Persons at Risk During Interviews in Police Custody: The Identification of Vulnerabilities. Royal Commission on Criminal Procedure Research Study No 12*. London: HMSO.

Gudjonsson, G.H. and Joyce, T. (2011). Interviewing adults with intellectual disabilities. *Advances in Mental Health and Intellectual Disabilities* 5 (2): 16–21.

Gudjonsson, G.H. and MacKeith, J. (1997). *Disputed Confessions and the Criminal Justice System*. London: The Maudsley https://mojoscotland.org/wp-content/uploads/2011/10/Disputed-Confessions-amd-miscarriages-of-justice.pdf (accessed 1 August 2023).

Home Office (2019). *CODE C Revised Codes of Practice for the Detention, Treatment and Questioning of Persons by Police Officers*. London: Home Office https://assets.publishing.service.gov.uk/government/uploads/system/uploads/attachment_data/file/903473/pace-code-c-2019.pdf (accessed 16 November 2021).

Hughes, N., Williams, H., and Chitsabesan, P. (2012). *Nobody Made the Connection: The Prevalence of Neurodisability in Young People Who Offend*. London: The Office of the Children's Commissioner https://assets.childrenscommissioner.gov.uk/wpuploads/2017/07/Nobody-made-the-connection.pdf (accessed 10 August 2023).

JUSTICE (2017). *Mental Health and Fair Trial*. London: JUSTICE https://files.justice.org.uk/wp-content/uploads/2017/11/06170615/JUSTICE-Mental-Health-and-Fair-Trial-Report-2.pdf (accessed 10 August 2023).

McKinnon, I.G. and Grubin, D. (2013). Health screening of people in police custody--evaluation of current police screening procedures in London, UK. *European Journal of Public Health* 23 (3): 399–405.

Mental Health (Care and Treatment) (Scotland) Act (2003). https://www.legislation.gov.uk/asp/2003/13/contents (accessed 10 August 2023).

Miller v Director of Public Prosecutions (2018). High Court of Justice Queen's Bench Division case CO/4533/2017 BAILII [Online] https://libguides.city.ac.uk/Harvardreferencinglawresources/cases (accessed 11 August 2023).

National Appropriate Adult Network (2019). There to help 2: ensuring provision of appropriate adults for vulnerable adults detained or interviewed by police – an update on progress 2013/14 to 2017/18. https://www.appropriateadult.org.uk/policy/research/there-to-help-2 (accessed 10 August 2023).

National Appropriate Adult Network (2020). *There to Help 3: The Identification of Vulnerable Adult Suspects and Application of the Appropriate Adult Safeguard in Police Investigations in 2018/19.* London: National Appropriate Adult Network https://www.appropriateadult.org.uk/policy/research/theretohelp3 (accessed 10 August 2024).

National Appropriate Adult Network (2023). Identifying vulnerability. https://www.appropriateadult.org.uk/policy/vulnerable-adults/identification (accessed 10 August 2023).

National Health Service England (2019). Liaison and diversion standards service specification 2019. https://www.england.nhs.uk/wp-content/uploads/2019/12/national-liaison-and-diversion-service-specification-2019.pdf (accessed 10 August 2024).

O'Mahony, B.M., Milne, B., and Grant, T. (2012). To challenge, or not to challenge? Best practice when interviewing vulnerable suspects. *Policing* 6: 301–313.

Police and Criminal Evidence (Northern Ireland) Order (1989). https://www.legislation.gov.uk/nisi/1989/1341/contents (accessed 10 August 2023).

Police and Criminal Evidence Act (1984). https://www.legislation.gov.uk/ukpga/1984/60/section/117 (accessed 10 March 2023).

Quinn, K. and Jackson, J. (2007). Of rights and roles: police interviews with young suspects in Northern Ireland. *British Journal of Criminology* 47 (2): 234–255.

Scottish Government (2012). Making justice work for victims and witnesses: victims and witnesses bill – a consultation paper. https://www.gov.scot/binaries/content/documents/govscot/publications/research-and-analysis/2013/01/making-justice-work-victims-witnesses/documents/social-research-report-making-justice-work-victims-witnesses/social-research-report-making-justice-work-victims-witnesses/govscot%3Adocument/00412912.pdf (accessed 15 January 2024).

Scottish Government (2020). Appropriate adults: guidance for local authorities. https://www.gov.scot/publications/appropriate-adults-guidance-local-authorities/ (accessed 14 January 2024).

FURTHER READING

Bath, C. (2022). *Police Searches of People: A Review of PACE Powers.* Ashford: National Appropriate Adult Network.

Dehaghani, R. and Bath, C. (2019). Vulnerability and the appropriate adult safeguard: examining the definitional and threshold changes within PACE Code C. *Criminal Law Review* 3: 213–232.

Gudjonsson, G.H. (2010). Psychological vulnerabilities during police interviews: why are they important? *Legal and Criminological Psychology* 15: 161–175.

Managing Long-Term Conditions

Vanessa Webb

Nurture Health and Care Ltd, Norwich, UK

CHAPTER 5

AIM

This chapter explores the management of long-term health conditions and associated risks, providing an aide memoir for healthcare professionals (HCP) caring for those detained in custody.

LEARNING OUTCOMES

After reading this chapter, you will be able to:

- To understand the management and risks associated with long-term conditions and to prioritise their care

- To consider management of medicines in relation to long-term conditions

- To look at specific conditions that are high risk in custody and their possible care plan, which may support their detention including their co-morbidity

---

SELF-ASSESSMENT

1. What are the key factors to consider when assessing fitness to detain in a person with a chronic health condition?

2. List three chronic health conditions and outline how they may impact an individual's fitness to be interviewed.

3. List the names of three medications that should not be stopped abruptly in custody and describe how you would access their medication.

INTRODUCTION

This chapter examines the crucial area of long-term health condition management in police custody. If the management of chronic health is not timely and effective, individuals will present with the sequelae of untreated conditions and are likely to require additional input and even hospital admission. It offers insights into frequent clinical situations, considering current legislation and best practices. Conditions such as hypertension, diabetes and epilepsy and their management will be reviewed and follow the principle their care should be equivalent to that in the community.

Confidentiality remains a healthcare professional's (HCPs) duty, except when relevant to custody case management.

Basic references to illnesses may suffice but online medication searches by police often reveal diagnoses.

Access to medications is essential; if refused, HCPs should be consulted. Although medication will be in police property, occasionally it can be stored elsewhere, but it is important this should be returned to the patient. Therefore, prompts can be vital.

Prescription verifications, including identity checks and medication protocols, are covered in Chapter 7 – Medicine Management.

Wider advice for the activities of daily living is also critical. Dietary information for conditions like diabetes is important, as are guidelines on managing conditions such

Police Custody Healthcare for Nurses and Paramedics, First Edition. Edited by Matthew Peel, Jennie Smith, Vanessa Webb, and Margaret Bannerman.
© 2025 John Wiley & Sons Ltd. Published 2025 by John Wiley & Sons Ltd.
Companion website: www.wiley.com/go/policecustodyhealthcare

as epilepsy, and consideration of factors such as stress and sleep deprivation. Care planning should consider those wider needs such as mobility and communication aids in custody.

Continuity of care continues to be part of the duty of care as HCPs, which creates complications as we do not wish to automatically disclose an individual has been in police custody. However, legal exceptions for sharing exist, especially in safeguarding situations and establishing care plans for reoccurring attendees is recommended.

Transfers between custodial settings require continuity of care and the use of the person escort record (PER), ensuring essential information is shared is an important part of the care plan.

Governance insights include:

- Complex cases are challenging to manage, especially when people have multiple diagnosis.

- Critical conditions are often missed and misdiagnosis due to intoxication common.

- Proper medication management is crucial, as missed doses can result in acute illness or legal implications, with insulin forming part of the NHS Never Events within Patient Safety (NHS Improvement 2018).

- Transferring patients from hospital to custody requires health team consultation.

Red Flags are dealt with in Chapter 19 – Emergencies. Opportunistic health promotion in custody should be encouraged and we know that often, our population does not access mainstream services, so making every contact count is important. Consider advice regarding:

- Diet, physical activity and reducing smoking/vaping

- Limiting alcohol and recreational drug use

- Participating in screening services such as blood-borne viruses and others

- Engaging in addiction services if appropriate remembering addiction can encompass gambling, drugs and alcohol but food, cosmetic procedures and image enhancers including steroid use, all form part of problematic practices

- Regular GP and dental visits

- Medication compliance

- Well-being strategies, particularly mental well-being and understanding our arousal response, emotions along with our behaviours

- Provision of informative resources

Each system has been considered separately for ease of reference.

CARDIOLOGY AND VASCULAR DISEASE

COMMON CONDITIONS

Common conditions include hypertension, ischemic heart disease encompassing conditions like angina, transient ischemic attacks (TIA) and strokes, heart failure, valve diseases, arrhythmias, particularly atrial fibrillation, emboli and pacemaker or implantable cardioverter defibrillator recipients.

RISK FACTORS

Risk factors for cardiology and vascular disease include hypertension, hyperlipidaemia, diabetes, obesity, smoking (tar staining can be noted), substance misuse especially stimulants, steroids and injecting substances (track marks can be noted), poor dental hygiene, rheumatic fever and family history of cardiac disease. Remember to consider Long QT syndrome, which can be associated with some medications (National Institute for Health and Care Excellence 2016).

BASELINE PHYSICAL ASSESSMENT

A baseline physical assessment should be undertaken in all assessments, which will include blood pressure (BP), pulse, oxygen saturation (SpO_2) and respiratory rate. Additional considerations include:

- Blood glucose

- Temperature

Signs and Symptoms

Remembering signs and symptoms can be part of a silent condition, so it may not have been diagnosed yet. Signs and symptoms which need to be considered as part of history taking and physical examination include:

- Fatigue

- Fever

- Dyspnoea (shortness of breath): note if on exertion, lying down or causes waking

- Palpitations: can ask the person to tap the rhythm

- Oedema

- Weight changes

- Muscle weakness

- Calf pain

Physical assessment can reveal that people are pale with poor peripheral circulation or cyanosis through hypoxia or indicators of acute presentations such as feeling cold and clammy, chest pain or severe breathlessness (see Chapter 19 – Emergencies) (see Box 5.1).

| BOX 5.1 | FEATURES AND THEIR RELATIONSHIP TO DIFFERENT CONDITIONS |

- Fatigue and weight gain can be associated with many cardiovascular presentations, particularly congestive heart failure

- Palpitations can indicate arrythmia

- Fever and weight loss may indicate pericarditis or endocarditis

- Muscle weakness can indicate a stroke (or TIA if temporary)

- Calf pain can be associated with deep vein thrombosis and with exercise can indicate peripheral vascular disease

- Xanthomata can indicate hyperlipidaemia

- Finger clubbing, splinter haemorrhages and other hand findings can be indicators of underlying conditions – consider GP review

Pulse rhythm is an important part of cardiovascular assessment:

- **Bradycardia**: Pulse <60 bpm is often seen due to varied causes such as opiate use, patients in heart block, certain medications and athletic individuals.

- **Tachycardia**: Pulse >100 bpm is often seen due to anxiety, but can be associated with stimulants in custody. Acute illness, hyperthyroidism and atrial fibrillation are also common, so if a new presentation is persistent, review in the Emergency Department (ED).

Remember to consider how parameters change over time as these are critical to effective management in custody and often missed in handovers in custody and not easily followed on e-notes systems.

MEDICATION

ACE inhibitors, Beta Blockers, Calcium Channel Blockers and Diuretics, are the mainstay of hypertension management. Beta-blockers can also be used in atrial fibrillation, anxiety and other conditions. Diuretics form part of the management of congestive heart failure. Statins and antiplatelets treat coronary artery disease. Anticoagulants are used in atrial fibrillation, heart valve disease and emboli. Glyceryl trinitrate (GTN) spray forms angina management and must be made available on request, so follow local policy.

Non-Steroidal Anti-inflammatory Drugs (NSAIDs) such as aspirin or ibuprofen can exacerbate heart failure.

FITNESS TO DETAIN, INTERVIEW, TRAVEL OR RELEASE

Individuals with cardiovascular disease, when well, typically are fit to detain and interview, providing they have their medications. Level 1 observations usually suffice in the absence of complications. If individuals decline medication, police must seek advice from HCPs.

Consideration can be given to breaks in interviews or reviews if presenting with severe cardiovascular symptoms, as stress can often worsen. An appropriate adult is usually not indicated unless other vulnerabilities are present.

It is unusual for those with cardiovascular disease to have concerns with fitness to release or travel.

Ensure medication for cardiovascular disease is continued in a timely manner and especially manage access to GTN spray, so it is immediately available.

Stimulants (e.g. cocaine, ecstasy and amphetamines) activate the sympathetic nervous system leading to:

- Tachycardia

- Blood pressure issues (dizziness and headache)

- Coronary artery vasospasm (chest pain)

Opiates (e.g. morphine and heroin) activate the parasympathetic nervous system causing:

- Bradyarrhythmias

- Hypotension (syncope)

Alcohol and cannabis have mixed effects on cardiovascular disease, but alcohol is specifically linked with atrial fibrillation.

Anabolic steroids are associated with myocardial hypertrophy, dyslipidaemia and arrhythmias.

MANAGEMENT OF UNCONTROLLED BLOOD PRESSURE

While isolated, high blood pressure does not typically necessitate an ED visit and often arises from missed medications. Therefore, this can be managed in custody with an individualised approach, but consider continuity of care plans. Remember, eclampsia should be ruled out in any woman of childbearing age (see Chapter 16 – Special Circumstances).

Hypertensive Emergency

A hypertensive emergency must be referred to the ED. Symptoms can include:

- Headaches

- Nausea and vomiting

- Visual changes

- Chest discomfort

- Non-specific neurological signs

- Seizures

A BP consistently over 180/110 mmHg, coupled with confusion, left ventricular failure, intravascular coagulation, renal dysfunction, haematuria or weight gain, signifies a hypertensive emergency. Additionally, neurological symptoms like seizures, visual disturbances and altered consciousness could indicate hypertensive encephalopathy.

SCENARIO 5.1 | Multiple medications

It is 02:00 and you have been asked to see a 62-year-old male who is intoxicated. They are accompanied with a bag of medication (boxed and labelled) and include:

- *Aspirin 75 mg, daily*

- *Atorvastatin 20 mg, daily*

- *Ramipril 10 mg, daily*

- *Bisoprolol 10 mg, daily*

- *GTN Spray, as needed*

1. *How do you approach this assessment?*
    a. *What factors will impact your decision?*

2. *How would you manage this patient?*

3. *Outline your advice to the police.*

RESPIRATORY DISEASE

COMMON CONDITIONS

Common conditions include asthma, chronic obstructive pulmonary disease (COPD) and pulmonary fibrosis (associated with smoking substances), sleep apnoea and infective diseases such as tuberculosis and lung cancer. On occasion, rarer conditions such as cystic fibrosis and bronchiectasis may be seen. Acute presentations are discussed in Chapter 19 – Emergencies and Chapter 8 – Minor Illness.

RISK FACTORS

Risk factors for respiratory diseases include family history and genetic conditions, environmental factors including travel, occupational exposure or related to hobbies and smoking, including inhaling recreational substances.

BASELINE PHYSICAL ASSESSMENT

A baseline physical assessment should be undertaken in all assessments, which will include BP, pulse, SpO_2 and respiratory rate (although note that co-morbidity can alter normal parameters). Observe breathing visually through the hatch if direct assessment is not feasible and include respiratory rate. Additional considerations can include:

- Peak flow

- Blood glucose

- Temperature

Check vaccination status, including influenza, pneumococcus, COVID-19 or tuberculosis

Signs and Symptoms

Signs and symptoms which need to be considered as part of history taking and physical examination:

- Inability to speak whole sentences is a red flag (see Chapter 19 – Emergencies)

- Wheeze

- Chest pain is typically an acute presentation of a respiratory problem rather than an indicator of a chronic problem

- Fatigue

- Dyspnoea (shortness of breath)

- Cough: can ask if this is a dry cough or a productive cough

- Haemoptysis (coughing blood)

- Weight change

Physical assessment can reveal people with cyanosis through hypoxia or indicators of acute presentations such as feeling cold and clammy, chest pain or severe breathlessness (see Chapter 19 – Emergencies) (see Box 5.2).

BOX 5.2 | FEATURES AND THEIR RELATIONSHIP TO DIFFERENT CONDITIONS

- **Dyspnoea**: Shortness of breath is associated with all respiratory conditions

- **Systemic symptoms**: Fatigue, weight loss and persistent cough can indicate lung cancer, albeit be seen in other conditions. But please remember this population may miss such signs on a background of smoking tobacco and cannabis.

- **Cough**: Productive cough can indicate pneumonia, COPD or dry, pulmonary fibrosis. It can also be a side effect of ACE inhibitors.

- **Haemoptysis**: Coughing blood is often linked to lung cancer or pulmonary embolism, so do not ignore. However, check for injuries to the mouth as often trauma is a source of blood.

- **Wheeze**: Sound on expiration, typical in asthma and COPD, but remember anaphylaxis.

- **Bruising and thin skin**: May indicate long-term steroid use.

MEDICATION

Short-acting beta-2-agonist inhalers such as salbutamol and terbutaline should be easily accessible, so follow local policies to ensure it is made available on request for those with asthma.

Long-acting beta-2-agonist inhalers such as salmeterol and formoterol and inhaled corticosteroid inhalers, such as fluticasone, budesonide and beclomethasone, and antimuscarinic inhalers, such as ipratropium and tiotropium, are all used for respiratory conditions.

Oral steroids (e.g. prednisolone) are often used in chronic exacerbations of respiratory conditions and occasionally drugs like theophylline.

Antibiotics including co-amoxiclav, doxycycline and azithromycin can treat respiratory infections and on occasion, even prescribed prophylactically.

Do not forget the link between oestrogen-containing medication and increased risk of pulmonary embolism.

FITNESS TO DETAIN, INTERVIEW, TRAVEL OR RELEASE

Generally, Level 1 observations suffice for individuals with respiratory conditions. Access to medications, especially short-acting inhalers, should be ensured in custody. If individuals decline medicines, it is essential for the police to consult with the HCP.

Individuals with respiratory disease, when well, typically do not face concerns regarding their fitness to interview. An appropriate adult is usually not indicated unless other vulnerabilities are present. It is unusual for those with respiratory disease to have concerns with fitness to release or travel.

Respiratory conditions frequently require the use of inhalers for management, especially in chronic cases. However, it is important to note inhalers not only open up the airways to increase substance absorption but can also be misused as storage for other substances.

Ensure medication for respiratory disease is continued in a timely manner and especially manage access to salbutamol or equivalent so that it is immediately available.

OBSTRUCTIVE SLEEP APNOEA

Obstructive sleep apnoea (OSA) causes intermittent cessations of breathing during sleep, prompting the brain to awaken the individual and restore breathing. This can occur numerous times overnight, leading to daytime drowsiness. Within a police custody setting, the resulting oxygen deprivation may affect the interview's quality, possibly rendering it inadmissible.

Risk Factors

- Obesity
- Male gender
- Aging
- Menopause
- Fluid retention
- Adenotonsillar hypertrophy
- Smoking

Treatment

OSA is commonly treated with continuous positive airway pressure (CPAP), using a device to deliver pressurised air via a face mask. This keeps the airway open, preventing obstruction.

Myths and facts

While there is a misconception that those with OSA can die in their sleep without their machine, this is inaccurate. While CPAP does prevent certain vulnerabilities and complications, lack of treatment mainly results in fatigue and confusion, not an immediate fatality.

Management

For diagnosed individuals:

- If they do not use a CPAP machine, no extra measures are necessary. There is no need for routine Level 2 (rousal) observations

- If they do use a device, assess if overnight detention is appropriate

For diagnosed *intoxicated* individuals: an individual care plan will need to be identified. Theoretically, CPAP will impact positively as when an individual is intoxicated; the airway is further compromised; however, agitation and behaviour increase the risk of harm, so currently, this requires a personalised approach.

In cases of serious crimes where detention is imperative:

- Obtain the CPAP device

- Ensure access to a plug socket, monitor for self-harm and consider a reclining chair for optimal sleep. Standard concrete beds may not be suitable.

- Place on constant close proximity observations (Level 4) as device and electrical cords can be a ligature or other hazard.

> **SCENARIO 5.2** Management of asthma
>
> *It is 05:00 and you are asked to see a 21-year-old male at the booking in desk who states he has asthma. He currently has no active respiratory symptoms. He refuses to allow officers to collect his inhaler or allow you to access his medical records. He is refusing to allow you to complete any assessment but wants an inhaler.*
>
> 1. *How do you approach this assessment?*
>
> 2. *Identify the risk factors you need to consider.*
>
> 3. *How would you manage this request?*

ENDOCRINE DISEASE

Endocrine disease, particularly diabetes, is a challenge within a custody setting and an area of high risk if poorly managed.

COMMON CONDITIONS

Common conditions seen include diabetes, Addison's disease and Cushing's syndrome, hyperthyroidism and hypothyroidism.

BASELINE PHYSICAL ASSESSMENT

A Baseline Physical Assessment should be undertaken in all assessments, which will include BP, pulse, SpO_2 and respiratory rate. Additional considerations can include:

- Blood glucose
- Temperature
- Ketones
- Skin condition

Signs and Symptoms

Key elements of history taking should include the patient's diagnosis, any signs or symptoms that reflect the severity of their condition, their current medication regimen, and any recent acute changes in their health. Endocrine conditions, when severe, lead to confusion and altered behaviour and can present with acute presentations that can be life threatening (see Chapter 19 – Emergencies). They are also associated with eye conditions, peripheral neuropathy and cardiovascular disease.

Often symptoms can be attributed to other causes, so always consider referral back to the GP for further assessment, where symptoms are persistent or where an abnormally high blood sugar has been identified (see Box 5.3).

MEDICATION

Diabetes is treated with insulin, metformin, sulfonylureas, DPP-4 inhibitors, GLP-1 receptor agonists, SGLT2 inhibitors and thiazolidinediones.

Thyroid disorders are treated with levothyroxine, carbimazole and beta blockers, which are medicines that may be prescribed in custody.

Addison's disease is treated with hydrocortisone, prednisone or fludrocortisone. **Not ensuring the continuity of steroids can lead to life-threatening adrenal crisis.**

Osteoporosis is managed with bisphosphonates, denosumab, raloxifene and hormone replacement therapy, and other endocrine conditions will have their own treatment regimes.

| BOX 5.3 | FEATURES AND THEIR RELATIONSHIP TO DIFFERENT CONDITIONS |

- Adrenocorticotrophic hormone regulates glucocorticoid production. Excess levels manifest as Cushing's syndrome and can present with cognitive changes, fatigue, muscle weakness, easy bruising, infections, stretch marks and acne due to steroid overload. Conversely, deficient levels in Addison's disease can lead to symptoms ranging from fatigue, dizziness and joint pain to fever and abdominal discomfort.

- Thyroid malfunctions can be subtle. Hyperactivity may cause nervousness, intolerance to temperature extremes, concentration issues and sleep disturbances. In contrast, hypothyroidism can lead to mood swings, fatigue, skin changes constipation and weight gain.

- Diabetes often presents with symptoms of increased thirst, frequent urination, weight changes and increased hunger. Other key symptoms include blurred vision, frequent infections, limb discomfort and persistent wounds.

Individuals can present with behavioural changes before diagnosis has been undertaken and present in custody; therefore, a holistic assessment of every person should exclude physical causes and not assume intoxication or other reasons.

In all cases, life-threatening presentations can present (see Chapter 19 – Emergencies).

FITNESS TO DETAIN, INTERVIEW, TRAVEL OR RELEASE

Most endocrine disorders, including well-managed diabetes, typically require Level 1 observations. Individuals with insulin pumps necessitate Level 4, close proximity observations. In instances of unstable blood sugars after insulin administration, Level 2 observations with rousals can be beneficial for a duration. An appropriate adult is usually not indicated.

A detailed management plan should be collaboratively established with the individual, healthcare professionals and custody staff, ensuring consistent care, especially during shift changes. Regular blood glucose testing and reviews are vital for those with insulin-dependent diabetes.

Individuals with endocrine disorders typically do not face issues regarding fitness to release or travel. However, effective insulin management is crucial. Therefore, it is imperative to complete the PER form and ensure continuity of care.

DIABETES

Type 1 diabetes (formerly known as insulin-dependent diabetes mellitus (IDDM)) or Type 2 diabetes (formerly known as noninsulin-dependent diabetes mellitus (NIDDM)) are commonly encountered in custody and provide some unique management challenges. In recent years, there has been a significant increase in the number of type 2 diabetics who require insulin. In addition to insulin, new medications and regimes, as well as methods of administration and continuous monitoring, add to the complexity of clinical decision-making.

Confirmation of diabetes through validation is critical, as merely possessing insulin does not guarantee an authentic diagnosis. Verification through electronic patient summaries or elevated blood sugar levels is imperative. Since insulin pens often lack pharmacy labels, detailed inquiries into the individual's diabetes history should be integral to the assessment.

During the assessment, ensure documentation of:

- Diabetes type
- Treatment approach: diet, medication or insulin regime
- Previous hypoglycaemic/hyperglycaemic incidents
- History of hospitalisation due to diabetes-related issues
- Medication details and next scheduled dose
- Blood sugar reading: average range and frequency

For type 2 diabetes, manage as with other chronic health conditions, administering medication based on the labelled prescription.

For insulin-reliant patients, deeper assessment is needed, covering:

- Medication location, if outside custody
- Timing of the last dose and meal
- Medication adherence
- Additional diabetic complications
- Signs indicating hypoglycaemia
- Concurrent or past medical issues

Upon detention, any patient identifying as having diabetes should be referred to the HCP. Detention management should factor in insulin delivery, dietary needs and blood sugar regulation, to prevent an acute episode, which can require hospitalisation if poorly managed in custody. Complaints and incidents are common from those with diabetes and include serious incidents and litigation where substandard care is given.

If detention extends over mealtimes and overnight, insulin must be retrieved from the patient's residence or an alternative source accessed.

Blood Sugar Targets

Aim for blood glucose levels between 4 and 12 mmol/l. If between 12 and 20 mmol/l and asymptomatic, conduct a thorough assessment. With suitable management, individuals can typically remain in custody. Check for ketones to rule out diabetic ketoacidosis (DKA). If above 20 mmol/l. See Chapter 19 – Emergencies.

There is currently no consistent approach to continuous glucose monitoring, although the National Institute for Health and Care Excellence (NICE) (2022) has issued guidelines recommending the wider use of flash and continuous glucose monitoring devices for individuals with diabetes. The Free-Style Libre system, a type of flash glucose monitoring, is specifically mentioned in the context of type 1 diabetes. The guidelines suggest all children with type 1 diabetes should be offered flash glucose monitoring and all adults with type 1 diabetes should have access to either flash or continuous glucose monitoring. This represents a significant shift in the approach as these devices can provide continuous or on-demand glucose data, potentially reducing the need for frequent finger-prick testing and improving awareness of hypoglycaemia. The use of such devices is aimed at empowering individuals to better manage their diabetes and potentially reduce the risk of complications. Flash glucose monitoring measures the glucose levels in the interstitial fluid, which lags behind blood sugar levels by up to 15 minutes and may not always match the blood glucose readings. Therefore, it is important to understand the readings from these two methods, which can be different and follow local policies to manage using smartphones to scan sensors or replace them with traditional blood sugar monitoring.

Individuals with well-regulated diabetes and stable blood glucose levels, as well as most other endocrine conditions, are typically fit for detention and interview. However, conducting interviews with patients with abnormal blood glucose readings, even in the absence of other symptoms, can risk impairing cognitive function, reasoning and memory, potentially rendering the interview inadmissible.

In cases where a person appears well but has abnormal blood sugar levels, especially after a hypoglycaemic event, the potential impact on the interview should be discussed with the custody team.

For serious offences where the integrity of the interview is crucial, consider management of their diabetes prior to interview.

According to the Care Quality Commission (2023), anyone on insulin should have a Care Plan encompassing:

- An evaluation of the individual's need for assistance in diabetes management
- Identification of who will provide additional support, if required
- Plan for blood glucose monitoring, specifying both frequency and acceptable ranges
- Actions to take if glucose levels deviate from the recommended range
- Recognising symptoms of both high and low blood glucose levels and their appropriate treatment
- Specific dietary needs and cultural needs tailored to the individual
- Document any measures or interventions required to help an individual effectively manage their diabetes

This comprehensive approach ensures the complex needs of those with diabetes are met responsibly, minimising risks and maintaining the highest standards of care and safety and should be mirrored in custody.

Should a patient who drives, present with hypoglycaemia or other worrisome symptoms, it is crucial to advise them against driving and recommend consultation with their GP.

Insulin

Inspect insulin, reviewing the insulin type, expiry date and maintain pens at room temperature to prevent altering absorption rates (insulin not already opened should be refrigerated). It is really important to understand the different types of insulin and their absorption rates to ensure appropriate management and reviews are considered, see Figure 5.1.

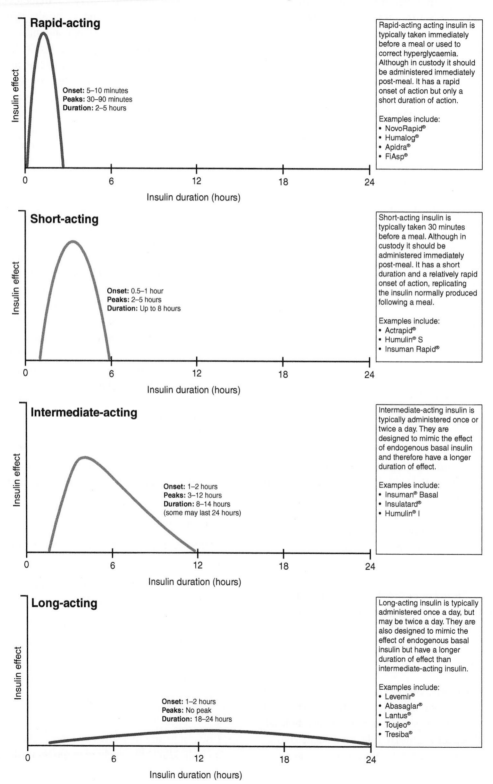

FIGURE 5.1 Types of insulin.

Administration Insulin can be life threatening, as an overdose might lead to hypoglycaemia; therefore, caution must be exercised in the self-administration. Custody staff should be aware of hypoglycaemia symptoms and be prepared to act, erring on the side of hypoglycaemia and administering glucose or food when in doubt.

Any alterations in behaviour or refusal to take meals or medication must be reported to the HCP for a potential adjustment in the management strategy.

As an HCP, ensure you understand the insulin type and the corresponding follow-up management and this can be reviewed in the British National Formulary (BNF). An agreement must be made regarding the doses through shared decision-making, considering their compliance, custody environment risks, potential changes in diet, stress and exercise levels. This mutual understanding of the insulin regimen ensures the necessary adjustments are made.

Insulin pumps Insulin pumps are often called continuous subcutaneous insulin infusions. Insulin pumps require robust management. Observe the pump's siting, confirm insulin type and settings and maintain Level 4 observations, which are close proximity cell watch. Staff must understand the pump features and related risks.

Dosing To prevent hypoglycaemia, titrate insulin against current blood glucose levels and carbohydrate intake, which is likely to differ from home arrangements.

It might be safer to keep blood glucose levels slightly higher than optimal to minimise the risk of hypoglycaemia during detention but ensure local policies are followed, as this is an area with no consistency in practice. Comply with local procedures for authorisation and administration. Provide sharps boxes for safe needle disposal. Insulin administration must only occur under the direct supervision of HCPs, considering whether detention officers should be present.

Custody-specific considerations In custody, consider a 'food first' approach, possibly reducing insulin units, as consideration of the possible low carbohydrate content of custody food should be accounted for. Management of requests for externally bought-in food varies across police forces.

Despite being in custody, the standards remain the same, always using insulin-specific syringes or commercial devices and avoiding extracting insulin with non-specific syringes, as this can lead to grave errors. Always write 'unit' in full when handling insulin to avoid confusion. Dispose of sharps in proper containers.

Device maintenance Blood sugar and ketone devices must be regularly calibrated, maintained and audited. Compliance with manufacturers' instructions and frequent quality assurance checks are vital including access to strips, which are in date and suitable for the device in the custody.

All HCPs should complete a self-assessment competency tool for blood glucose and ketone monitoring. Familiarity with blood sugar reading equipment and ketone assessment is essential for best practice.

| SCENARIO 5.3 | Management of insulin in a person with diabetes |

It is 18:00 and the custody sergeant asks you to see someone stating they are diabetic and on insulin; they have not had an evening meal. They are refusing to eat and will not tell you when they last ate. Their blood glucose if 5.0 mmol/l; all other observations are normal.

1. *How do you approach this assessment?*

2. *Identify the risk factors you need to consider.*

3. *How do you manage this scenario?*

   You are advised he is staying in custody overnight.

4. *How would you manage this scenario now?*

5. *Outline your care plan for this individual.*

GASTROINTESTINAL, RENAL, UROLOGY AND GYNAECOLOGY DISEASE

COMMON CONDITIONS

Common diagnosis seen in custody include gastro-oesophageal reflux disease (GORD), liver cirrhosis, gallstones, constipation, gastric/duodenal ulcers, irritable bowel disease, diverticulitis, hernias, pancreatitis, haemorrhoids, coeliac disease, ulcerative colitis, Crohn's disease, endometriosis, menorrhagia, polycystic ovary disease and prostatic disease, to name but a few. A variety of cancers are also seen.

RISK FACTORS

Risk factors for the conditions above are wide and varied. However, alcohol dependency and excess alcohol intake increase the risk of gastrointestinal malignancy (e.g. oesophageal and stomach cancer) and the development of alcoholic hepatitis/cirrhosis, along with other sequalae, particularly ulcers and pancreatitis. Intravenous drug use is also a risk factor for hepatitis.

Opiate use is associated with bowel conditions and their side effects of constipation and diarrhoea can sometimes mask serious pathology.

Ask individuals about their surgical and travel history, as they can give insight into the nature of their symptoms. Sexual history can be considered, although remember the medical records kept may be disclosed in court, so ask relevant focused history.

BASELINE PHYSICAL ASSESSMENT

A baseline physical assessment should be undertaken in all individuals, which will include BP, pulse, SpO_2 and respiratory rate. Additional considerations can include:

- Blood glucose
- Temperature

- Ketones
- Abdominal auscultation: Gurgling sounds are normal. If absent, it may be due to opiate use, but consider a wider differential diagnosis.

Note the location of the stoma bag(s), as this can provide clues as to the type of stoma (e.g. colostomies are typically located in the left iliac fossa, whereas ileostomies are usually located in the right iliac fossa. These then need the appropriate equipment to be managed in custody.

SIGNS AND SYMPTOMS

Signs and symptoms that need to be considered:

- Weight changes with rapid weight loss being particularly concerning
- Nausea and vomiting (and the possibility of dehydration)
- Haematemesis
- Confusion
- Fatigue
- Fever
- Jaundice
- Aphthous ulceration
- Haemoptysis (coughing blood)
- Pain (see Chapter 8 – Minor Illness for Abdominal Pain)
- Dysphagia
- Constipation
- Diarrhoea
- Malaena

Physical assessment can reveal abdominal distension, which may be due to constipation, pregnancy, ascites, obstruction or malignancy. Wider oedema can be seen in limbs. Anaemia might be seen by observing the skin colour and eyes for pallor. Jaundice presents as a yellowish skin and eye tint. Bruising can sometimes indicate clotting disorder associated with liver dysfunction (see Box 5.4).

MEDICATION MANAGEMENT

Loperamide forms part of the symptom management for opiate withdrawal, however, can be used for non-infective causes of diarrhoea.

Sodium alginate/calcium carbonate such as Gaviscon, proton pump inhibitors such as lansoprazole and H_2 receptor antagonists such as ranitidine are commonly taken both as a prescription but also over the counter for 'indigestion'.

Laxatives such as senna, lactulose or others are often prescribed or taken for constipation.

| BOX 5.4 | FEATURES AND THEIR RELATIONSHIP TO DIFFERENT CONDITIONS |

- Jaundice is linked to hepatitis, liver cirrhosis and biliary obstruction (e.g. gallstone and pancreatic cancer)
- Aphthous ulceration are ulcers inside the mouth, which are often benign (e.g. stress) but may indicate nutritional deficiencies or Crohn's disease.
- Vomiting is associated with various conditions, from intoxication, infections to GORD and bowel obstruction. Haematemesis, where blood is present either fresh or coffee ground needs further investigation. However, remember to examine the mouth for trauma or recent nose bleeds as this can often lead to blood in vomit.
- Gastro-oesophageal reflux, where the stomach content backflows due to lower oesophageal sphincter issues, causes epigastric discomfort.
- Dysphagia presents as difficulty in swallowing, potentially due to conditions line oesophageal cancer.
- Maleana can present as dark stools from upper gastrointestinal bleeding. Fresh red blood can be due to haemorrhoids.
- Scars may be visible, which can indicate prior abdominal surgeries or hernias.

It is important immunosuppressants are continued for serious conditions such as Crohn's disease and should be made available but also given as prescribed. These include corticosteroids, ciclosporin, methotrexate and other biologics.

Some over-the-counter drugs which may impact the gastrointestinal system, include aspirin and NSAIDs, which may worsen gastrointestinal bleeding and symptoms and contribute to gastric or duodenal ulceration.

FITNESS TO DETAIN, INTERVIEW, TRAVEL OR RELEASE

Level 1 observations usually suffice for individuals with the exceptions discussed below. Individuals with chronic disease, when well, typically do not face concerns regarding their fitness to interview. An appropriate adult is usually not indicated unless other vulnerabilities are present. Fitness to transfer and release are typically not impacted by the gastrointestinal conditions. However, where complexity such as stoma management or catheters exist, these may require a specific plan and ensuring continuity of care, so ensure the PER enables ongoing management to be understood.

Gender-appropriate practices are important in custody and therefore each police force will have female staff, feminine hygiene products but might benefit from the HCP's advice if they need more information. Cultural considerations may also arise.

Patients with coeliac disease may report abdominal pain, nausea and diarrhoea when eating gluten-containing foods and gluten-free alternatives should be sought.

Patients with gallstones or other pathology may report fatty foods trigger right upper quadrant pain and again alternatives should be sought.

Stoma bags and catheters can be managed in custody; however, this might require an increase in the level of observations if this is associated with a risk of self-harm or antisocial behaviours. Equipment needs collecting from peoples' homes, which may not be easy for the police to find, so it is important to liaise to ensure they understand the need for creams, stoma bags, de-odourisers, catheter bags, catheters, the gloves and other items that enable an individual to manage this independently.

On occasions, individuals may be transferred from hospital and may have drains, feeding tubes or other needs. This should be discussed prior to transfer from hospital to custody and a care plan put in place, including access to all the correct equipment, appropriate observation levels and as the care in custody should be equivalent to that in the community, district nurses or other staff can deliver care in custody, although this will need to be agreed and they must always be accompanied by a member of staff, preferably an HCP, so information sharing can be managed effectively.

SCENARIO 5.4 Management of a stoma

You are asked to assess fitness to detain an individual with a stoma.

1. *How do you approach this assessment?*
   a. *What questions you will ask as part of your assessment?*
   b. *What physical examination should be made?*

2. *List any key recommendations that ensure an individual will be fit to be detained overnight.*

NEUROLOGY

COMMON CONDITIONS

Common diagnosis seen in custody include epilepsy, the sequelae of head trauma, myalgic encephalomyelitis/chronic fatigue syndrome, neuralgia such as trigeminal neuralgia, multiple sclerosis, nerve palsy such as Bell's palsy, carpal tunnel syndrome, Parkinson's disease and stroke all present in custody, but Chapter 8 – Minor Illness and Chapter 19 – Emergencies give more information.

BASELINE PHYSICAL ASSESSMENT

Baseline physical assessment should be undertaken in all individuals, which will include assessment of consciousness, pupil size and reaction, BP, pulse, SpO_2 and respiratory rate. Additional considerations can include:

- Blood glucose
- Temperature
- Cranial nerve examination
- Assessment of muscle strength, sensation and movement

Signs and Symptoms

Neurological disorders manifest in a myriad of ways, each with its unique set of symptoms. Recognising an individual's specific presentation, understanding the effects of stress on their condition and knowing their symptom management techniques are crucial during history-taking. Often these involve taking recreational drugs such as cannabis for symptom control.

If someone has had a seizure without a prior epilepsy diagnosis, it should be documented as an 'unexplained seizure'. See Chapter 19 – Emergencies for the emergency management of seizures or Chapter 8 – Minor Illness for transient loss of consciousness.

A comprehensive neurological assessment typically involves:

- **Mental status examination**: This begins with an assessment of the patient's level of consciousness, orientation to time, place, person and attention span. The Mini-Mental State Examination or equivalent is frequently used to evaluate cognitive functions like memory and language comprehension.

- **Cranial nerve examination**: This evaluates the function of the 12 cranial nerves. The examination encompasses testing for visual acuity, pupil response, facial muscle strength, sense of smell, hearing and tongue movement.

- **Motor system examination**: This assesses muscle bulk, tone, strength and involuntary movements. Noting the symmetry of muscle bulk and looking for any atrophy or fasciculations. Power in various muscle groups is graded on a scale from 0 (paralysis) to 5 (normal strength).

- **Reflexes and sensory examination**: This can be considered (see Box 5.5).

- **Coordination and gait:** This can be included as part of assessment.

BOX 5.5	FEATURES AND THEIR RELATIONSHIP TO DIFFERENT CONDITIONS

Specific patterns of sensory or pain: Conditions like carpal tunnel syndrome present with tingling and numbness in the median nerve distribution of the hand. While cervical or lumbar radiculopathy might manifest as short, shooting pains radiating along the nerve pathway. Sciatica, a type of lumbar radiculopathy, typically presents as pain radiating down the back of the leg. Understanding the pattern of distribution can help identify possible causes.

MEDICATION MANAGEMENT

Epilepsy is treated with a spectrum of medications such as carbamazepine, valproic acid, lamotrigine, topiramate, levetiracetam, phenytoin, gabapentin and phenobarbital.

Parkinson's disease is treated with carbidopa-levodopa, dopamine agonists, monoamine oxidase-B inhibitors and catechol O-methyltransferase (COMT) inhibitors.

Multiple sclerosis may be treated with beta interferons, glatiramer acetate and dimethyl fumarate.

Alzheimer's disease treated donepezil, memantine and rivastigmine.

Botulinum toxin may also be given in neurological conditions.

The medication regime for neurological conditions is critical and medications should be accessed, and, but more importantly, are often time critical and medications should be from the same manufacturer.

FITNESS TO DETAIN, INTERVIEW, TRAVEL OR RELEASE

Most neurological conditions with the right advice regarding the management of their condition are fit to detain, fit for interview without an appropriate adult and fit to release and transfer. Level 1 observations are usually adequate where there is a neurological condition with no seizure history.

Timely access to medication is critical and any deviation to the prescribed medication management should be discussed with the HCP, including if a person has declined medication. Medication in relation to neurological conditions if delayed could lead to challenges in relation to fitness to interview.

When a seizure history exists, Level 3 observations with CCTV can be used to oversee individuals who have epilepsy, rather than Level 4 close proximity observations. Stress and lack of sleep may exacerbate seizures, so rousals should only be used where there are concerns due to the consumption of drugs and alcohol, or other considerations such as head injury.

Those who experienced a seizure and are in a post-ictal fatigue state are unlikely to be fit for interview for the minimum of 12 hours and may be unfit for detention.

On occasions where memory issues, cognitive challenges, difficulties concentrating and other cognitive changes are present in neurological conditions, an appropriate adult may be required.

Where communication is a barrier such as aphasia in a stroke, the use of family members may provide a communication aid and act as an appropriate adult; other forms of communication, such as the written statement, might be appropriate.

It is unusual for those with neurological disorders to have concerns with fitness to release or travel. However, information sharing is critical in medicines management and at times, the type of police transport vehicle may need to be considered, so complete the custody record and PER to ensure continuity of care.

A holistic, person-centred assessment is essential for those with neurological issues, helping create an effective care plan. Rather than making assumptions, it is crucial to approach each neurological case with a fresh perspective, ensuring no acute symptoms are overlooked.

Engage individuals in conversations about how their disorder impacts their daily life, covering aspects like daily routines, emotional health, substance use history, social relationships and challenges with employment or housing. Always consider an individual's cultural, socioeconomic and religious background, as these factors can influence symptom perception and treatment preferences.

Take the time to understand both the challenges and strengths of those with neurological conditions, including their perspectives on well-being, strategies for symptom management and any home aids they might require. Ensure discussions about care and support plans for those in custody are aligned with risk assessments, custody duration and interview schedules.

DRIVING

There are clear guidelines regarding seizures and driving, which are accessible online (see Resources). It is the legal responsibility of the person with epilepsy to inform the DVLA about their condition. People with epilepsy, who are seizure free for a year (though this may vary depending on individual circumstances and licence type held, e.g. HGV), are usually issued with short-term licences, for periods of up to three years. However, if at any point during that time, they have a seizure, they must cease driving and inform the DVLA, who will revoke their licence until certain criteria are met.

EPILEPSY

Epilepsy is a neurological condition marked by recurring seizures stemming from abnormal brain activity. These seizures can arise without a discernible cause (idiopathic) or from specific underlying issues (secondary). Secondary epilepsy can be associated with past head injuries, infections of the central nervous system, strokes, brain tumours, congenital or genetic brain malformations and traumatic births. Epilepsy is also associated with learning disabilities.

Classification of Seizures

- Simple partial seizure → Focal, aware seizure

- Complex partial seizure → Focal, unaware seizure

- Absence → Generalised, non-motor seizure

- Tonic–clonic seizure → Generalised, motor seizure

During focal, unaware seizures, an individual might display peculiar behaviours or fail to respond predictably. It is essential to distinguish between diagnosed epilepsy and other causes like acute head injuries, alcohol misuse, drug reactions, infections or non-epileptic attack disorders, when an individual experiences 'fits' in custody.

Key history includes:

- Seizure type and onset date

- Frequency and duration

- Last occurrence

- Potential triggers

- Warning or aura signs

- Post-seizure characteristics

- Prescribed medications and adherence

- Specialist consultations

- Driving status

Awareness of medication compliance, substance use, other health conditions and current health status can guide management, while the individual is in custody.

Management of a seizure is covered in Chapter 19 – Emergencies and temporary loss of consciousness within Chapter 8 – Minor Illness.

Individuals with epilepsy should have a clear care plan for custody staff.

Medication

It is paramount to ensure continuity of medication for those with neurological conditions. Missing antiepileptic drugs can risk seizure occurrence, affect interview robustness and have legal implications. However, where individuals inconsistently take their medicine, it is crucial to exercise caution when administering it in custody.

The Epilepsy Society (2022) recommends

- For once-daily doses, take the missed one immediately

- For twice-daily doses, if it is less than six hours late, take it immediately. If over six hours late, miss dose and continue as scheduled

Although NICE has sanctioned cannabis for epilepsy treatment, its application is narrowly defined, making it a rarity in custody. Yet, many people self-medicate with cannabis or other drugs and withdrawal can lead to agitation.

Risk Management

Ideally, individuals diagnosed with epilepsy should be placed in CCTV-equipped cells with low benches. Showering should be supervised for safety reasons. Provide clear indicators for recognising seizures, especially non-typical ones, to aid custody staff. Well-regulated epilepsy patients should be routinely checked every half hour, but avoid waking them, as disrupted sleep can prompt seizures. Those showing signs of intoxication or head injuries should be observed continuously and roused at half-hour intervals.

To ensure safety, provide custody staff with comprehensive guidelines to manage neurological conditions. This might involve acquiring specific equipment, offering fall prevention tips, addressing facial paralysis, limb positioning and dietary considerations for swallowing issues, among other essential recommendations.

SCENARIO 5.5	Management of medication for epilepsy

It is 03:00 and you are asked to see a 29-year-old male who has a history of epilepsy. He is visiting your area and lives 200 miles away. He has no medication with him and the police are unable to collect. He is cooperative with an assessment and reports he has seizures when his medication is omitted. He is not under the influence of substances and has normal physical observations. The seizures are usually focal, so he becomes unaware of his environment and describes lip smacking and an unusual smell, which can progress to a 'tonic clonic seizure'. You are able to verify his medication as lamotrigine 200 mg twice a day.

He reports taking his dose at normal at 17:00 the previous day. He had a strip of lamotrigine with him, but it is not in his property and he does not know where he lost it. He would normally take his next dose when he wakes up. He is likely to remain in custody till early afternoon.

1. *Identify the risk factors you need to consider.*

2. *How do you manage this scenario?*

MUSCULO-SKELETAL CONDITIONS

Musculo-skeletal conditions present in custody range from chronic pain conditions to sequelae of old injuries, fibromyalgia, rheumatoid disease and are often part of co-morbidity of wider diseases. Acute musculoskeletal conditions are covered in Chapter 9 – Minor Injuries.

PAIN MANAGEMENT

Chronic or Persistent Pain

Chronic or persistent pain endures for a more extended period, generally exceeding three months. This form of pain includes conditions like back pain, arthritis or pain linked to nerve damage. Unlike acute pain, the intensity of chronic pain does not always reflect the extent of tissue damage, making it a complex and challenging issue to address.

Persistent pain might initiate with an injury but continue long after healing, or it may arise without a clear origin. Moreover, it is not usually indicative of ongoing tissue damage and conventional pain medications might only offer partial relief.

Individuals may seek alternative pain management strategies such as recreational cannabinoids and other non-prescribed pharmaceutical medicines.

In managing chronic pain, especially within the custodial environment, a comprehensive and person-centred approach becomes crucial (Royal College of General Practitioners 2019). This approach should include the following.

Referral and continuity of care Signposting patients for further evaluation by their GP and maintaining continuity of care for those with validated prescriptions.

Consideration of specific conditions Conditions like gout, rheumatoid arthritis or migraine necessitate tailored management plans, whereas non-specific pain might lead to more generalised requests for analgesics.

Comprehensive assessment A personalised assessment of those presenting with chronic pain to identify contributing factors and the pain's effects on the individual's life enables a well-designed management plan.

Recognise factors such as anxiety, fear and uncomfortable custody conditions might amplify pain perceptions and drug-seeking behaviours whilst understanding the impact of pain on daily activities, well-being and social relationships, while considering the influence of cultural, economic and ethnic backgrounds on the patient's symptoms and treatment choices is important.

Creation of a custody-specific care plan Developing a comprehensive care and support plan tailored to the custodial environment, considering risk assessment, duration of custody and interview timing will be required for those with pain management requests.

For those with mobility difficulties, toileting needs, sleep aids and wider disability, each individual should be discussed with the custody team and a management plan should be put in place. Constant observations, whether in close proximity or through CCTV, may be required where risks are increased by the presence of equipment.

Most individuals with chronic pain and musculo-skeletal conditions can be managed on Level 1 observations, with advice. However, consideration should be given to rousals, if there is any possibility of overdose.

Interviews can be compromised by the presence of pain, equally sedation from medication could undermine interviews. The risk assessment should include fitness to interview, with a management plan that ensures medication regimes consider this impact.

It is unusual for those with musculo-skeletal disorders to have concerns with fitness to release or travel. However, information sharing is critical in medicines management and at times, the type of police transport vehicle may need to be considered.

Continuity of care in pain management is of paramount importance, especially in safeguarding vulnerable individuals. It is crucial to maintain consistency across healthcare teams, ensuring there is a unified approach to patient care (see Box 5.6). Effective information sharing is essential, particularly when risks of overdose or other concerns arise.

INFECTIOUS DISEASES INCLUDING SEXUAL HEALTH

Infection Prevention and Control (IPC) procedures form part of the governance processes within police and other organisations, and as occurred in the COVID pandemic, subject to alteration by national strategy (see Box 5.7).

Stigma and discrimination are often experienced with infections, particularly blood-borne viruses and it is important to ensure confidentiality is maintained, where it is not relevant to the case.

For each infection, it is important to be able to identify:

- The name of the infection
- The mode of transmission
- Understanding of isolation needs and special precautions

Medications play a pivotal role in treating infections:

- Antibiotics treat bacterial infections and should be administered in full courses
- Antivirals treat viral infections
- Antifungals treat fungal infections
- Antiparasitic medications address parasitic infections

To mitigate infection risks, vaccines are employed. Prophylactic treatments and post-exposure prophylaxis are becoming increasingly common in preventing infections. Sexual health medications, while unnamed, bear an ID number and should be timely administered, adhering to local protocols, as they are crucial and have a low diversion risk.

BOX 5.6	MUSCULO-SKELETAL MEDICATION

Medication

As part of the history taking, a detailed medication history is critical, including which medication is prescribed, taken over the counter, or accessed via internet or other sources. What formulation is the medication taken? When was the medication last taken? Where is their medication now?

Many pain medications are sedative in nature and present a risk in the intoxicated person, so a risk assessment often leads to medications being omitted when intoxication is present. Alternatively, late ingestion can occur on arrest or concealment, so this should be considered in the management plan.

Even where prescribed, diversion means that, on occasion, medications are not taken as prescribed, so ensure a thorough risk assessment is undertaken.

Medication that are associated with musculo-skeletal conditions:

- Paracetamol
- Non-steroidal anti-inflammatory drugs
- Topical NSAIDs, capsaicin and OTC 'Deep Heat'
- Opioid based medication, tablet, liquid and patches
- Benzodiazepines
- Antiepileptic and antipsychotic drugs including gabapentinoids and amitriptyline have been prescribed in relation to pain
- Corticosteroid trigger point injections, prednisolone and steroid-based local anaesthetics
- Disease Modifying medication for rheumatoid conditions

Opiate-based medication, tend to be Class B controlled drugs, pregabalin and gabapentin (gabapentinoids) are Class C controlled substances (under the Misuse of Drugs Act 1971) and scheduled under the Misuse of Drugs Regulations 2001 as Schedule 3.

First-line formulary choice

Lowest risk of harm and minimal diversion potential, so full dose paracetamol should be prescribed and supplemented with non-steroidal drugs (NSAIDs), if available on the formulary.

Second-line formulary choice

Should only be used when first-line treatment is inappropriate or unsuccessful.

Where paracetamol is provided, ensure robust documentation to minimise the risk of duplication of administration, as accidental overdose is one of the possible consequences seen in custody.

Relevant safety information, NICE guidance, BNF and other resources are available for all medications, but always review to ensure that you have the most up-to-date information.

Patches should be examined and continued in custody and observation of any removal and reapplication supported, but recognise the high potential for diversion.

BOX 5.7	COMMON INFECTIONS

Name of infection (chronic)	Mode of transmission	Isolation needs and special precautions
Athletes foot	Close contact	No isolation of special precautions
Body, head or pubic lice	Contact	No isolation is required, but recommendation of chemical insecticide may be appropriate and materials washed at high temperature
Shingles	Contact (less infectious than chickenpox and not airborne) 90% of adults in the UK are considered immune, however, review guidance in relation to chickenpox	For shingles (where the rash is on an exposed site), the infectious period is from the onset of the rash until crusting of lesions. Minimise movement of an individual is preferable.
Cold sores (herpes simplex)	Contact	Isolation not required
Hepatitis B and C	Blood borne so sexual contact and contact with body fluids including saliva Vertical transmission	Isolation not required, but to ensure health promotion includes advice on needle exchange programmes, vaccination and screening.
HIV	Blood borne so sexual contact and contact with body fluids, although saliva is very low risk Vertical transmission	Isolation not required, but to ensure health promotion includes advice on needle exchange programmes
Scabies	Contact	Isolation not required. Material washed at high temperature
TB (Mycobacterium tuberculosis)	Active pulmonary disease is infective until fourteen days of treatment is given. Seek advice from Respiratory Consultant or ED	No isolation is required
Sexually acquired infections	Each infection has a different transmission profile	No isolation is required

Source: Adapted from Health Protection Agency.

SEXUALLY ACQUIRED INFECTIONS AND EVIDENCE PROCEDURES

In the context of custody, diagnosing infections can be pertinent to serious offences like rape. A robust chain of evidence must manage these diagnoses, which may involve virus sequencing, viral load assessment, initial tests, confirmatory tests and tests of cure. Consulting sexual health experts, or those within sexual offence services, is vital for diagnostic screening and usually does not occur in a custody environment.

HANDLING SHARPS AND BODILY FLUIDS SAFELY

Staff could face exposure risks from prisoners using bodily fluids as weapons, self-harm activities and unsanctioned use of sharps. Healthcare professionals often address potential exposures to blood-borne viruses like Hepatitis B, Hepatitis C and HIV. Managing such exposures effectively and following local policies are vital. Some regions, take blood samples for risk assessments, while others refer to local services.

The crucial factor post-potential exposure is the infection route, categorised as:

- Parenteral (e.g. needle-sticks and bites)

- Mucous membranes (e.g. mouth and eyes)

- Contaminated, non-intact skin

Risk assessment and management should be determined based on the fluid's risk level. High-risk fluids comprise blood, semen and vaginal secretions, whereas saliva, urine and vomit are low risk, unless tainted with blood. Hand hygiene and skin care and using personal protective equipment, all form part of the management of infection prevention strategies. Although chronic infections typically do not influence interview fitness, infection control precautions are essential.

In instances of 'dirty protests' where a person soils their cell, police protocols typically handle the situation. However, health assessments might be necessary, in which case, if there is a perceived risk, an observation-only assessment is recommended.

OTHER CONSIDERATIONS

MULTIPLE CO-MORBIDITY, FRAILTY, CANCER AND PALLIATIVE CARE

Increasingly, individuals detained may be arrested for historic offences, which brings complications from multiple co-morbidities and frailty. Equally, younger individuals may be arrested with life-limiting illnesses. These individuals require access to their medication and their care needs to be met whilst in detention. HCPs must also recognise where these needs are identified on a backdrop of drugs and alcohol misuse, or behavioural challenges, care is taken to ensure

individuals are not over-medicated, their prescribed medications and wider needs are prioritised.

It would be unusual for a detained individual known to be at imminent risk of cardiac arrest to remain detained in police custody, even if presenting with a terminal diagnosis. An acute deterioration of their condition would still require management in a hospital or appropriate setting.

For each police force, a policy should consider how to manage a cardiac arrest in a custodial setting for an individual who has stated they state they do not wish to be resuscitated. To apply cardiopulmonary resuscitation (CPR), would deprive the person of a dignified death. These are known as 'Do Not Resuscitate' (DNR) orders (otherwise known as Do Not Attempt Resuscitation – DNAR or Do Not Attempt Cardio-Pulmonary Resuscitation – DNACPR). Concerns about not responding to a cardiac arrest should be considered preferably prior to detention and this should include conversations about advance care planning and end-of-life care that protects people's human rights while managing the legal obligations of the police and their duty of care (see Box 5.8). These may be known as a ReSPECT (Resuscitation Council) form which details the individuals wishes.

It will be essential that in assessing fitness for detention in custody, the care plan includes a full awareness of the police process and timelines, and communicates the status of the patient, the findings and the intended management and the presence of a DNACPR decision as part of the management of care.

When undertaking the assessment for those with social care needs and multiple long-term conditions, the HCP should always consider the person's perspective on the impact and preferences in relation to their condition while ensuring access to continuity of medications.

Older people and those with co-morbidity, especially if frail, require special care and consideration from prescribers and for those involved in the administration, or supervision of medicines along with their wider needs.

BOX 5.8	JOINT GUIDANCE FROM THE BRITISH MEDICAL ASSOCIATION, THE RESUSCITATION COUNCIL (UK) AND THE ROYAL COLLEGE OF NURSING

Where no explicit decision about CPR has been considered and recorded in advance, there should be an initial presumption in favour of CPR. However, in some circumstances where there is no recorded explicit decision (e.g. for a person in the advanced stages of a terminal illness where death is imminent and unavoidable and CPR would not be successful), a carefully considered decision not to start inappropriate CPR should be supported.

Source: With permission of Resuscitation Council UK.

When individuals receive multiple drugs for their co-morbidity, this greatly increases the risk of drug interactions, as well as adverse reactions and may affect compliance. The balance of benefit and harm of some medicines may be altered in the elderly. Therefore, elderly or frail patients' medicines should be given as prescribed and be aware of caution when utilising PGDs, or as prescribers of new medicines.

Frail individuals may have difficulty swallowing tablets, so they should always be encouraged to take their tablets or capsules with enough fluid whilst in an upright position, or may be given liquid alternatives. Liquid medications will require management as local processes identify.

Pharmacokinetic changes can markedly increase the tissue concentration of a drug in the elderly or those who have multiple co-morbidities, especially in those who are frail or have co-morbidity. The most important effect is reduced renal clearance. Many excrete drugs slowly and are highly susceptible to nephrotoxic drugs. Acute illness can lead to rapid reduction in renal clearance, especially if accompanied by dehydration. Hence, a patient stabilised on a drug with a narrow margin between the therapeutic and the toxic dose (e.g. digoxin) can rapidly develop adverse effects when other illnesses occur. The hepatic metabolism of lipid-soluble drugs is reduced because there is a reduction in liver volume. This is important for drugs with a narrow therapeutic window.

Drug-induced effects can include confusion as the presenting symptom, which is caused by almost any of the commonly used drugs; other manifestations are constipation (with antimuscarinics and opiate-based medication) and postural hypotension and falls (with diuretics and psychotropics). Many hypnotics with long half-lives have serious hangover effects, including drowsiness, unsteady gait, slurred speech and confusion. All of these can be problematic if given in custody therefore be cautious in the use of medicines.

Bleeding associated with aspirin and other NSAIDs is more common and more likely to have a fatal or serious outcome in the frail. NSAIDs are also a special hazard in patients with cardiac disease or renal impairment, which may again place this population at particular risk.

In addition, many individuals are also carers of the frail or those with additional needs, but may not see themselves as such so ensure the police are aware of any caring responsibilities which they are unaware of.

OPHTHALMOLOGY, EAR, NOSE AND THROAT AND DERMATOLOGY

Glasses and contact lenses should be part of the police risk assessment. Contact lens cases are part of the police role to provide. However, certain conditions such as glaucoma may require an explanation of the nature of sight loss and this can include support to administer eye drops.

Once again, ensure you understand the disability and the impact from the perspective of the individual with the condition. Many disabilities, providing access to aids and devices, prevent little barriers to managing their detention. Do not assume all people with a particular diagnosis need the same support.

Find out what communication formats and media the person prefers and consider British Sign Language interpreters for those who are deaf. Communicate with them using their preferred format. Ensure the format allows them to use any inclusive terminology relevant to them.

Eczema, dry skin and acne are all common skin conditions and accessing creams, emollients and other treatments is important. However, this should be undertaken in the context of the police risk assessment, noting recreational substances can be hidden in creams and therefore sealed containers are important, even if over the counter.

CONCLUSION

This chapter has provided a comprehensive guide to managing long-term health conditions in police custody, highlighting the unique challenges and responsibilities faced by HCPs in this setting. This included outlining the necessary knowledge and skills needed to effectively care for those in custody with chronic health conditions, ensuring their safety and well-being.

The detailed exploration of various conditions, such as cardiovascular, respiratory, endocrine, neurological and aspects such as frailty, among others, reminds us of the complexity and diversity of healthcare needs in the custodial environment. The chapter's focus on medication management, risk assessment and continuity of care underscores the critical importance of maintaining high standards of healthcare comparable to those in the community.

Confidentiality, legal considerations and the integration of health promotion strategies all enhance the reader's ability to make informed decisions in complex custodial settings, equipping them with the tools and understanding necessary to manage long-term health conditions effectively. It encourages a holistic, empathetic approach to healthcare, acknowledging the importance of considering the physical, mental and emotional needs of those detained.

> ## LEARNING ACTIVITIES

1. Write a care plan for a repeat attender with at least one significant co-morbidity.

2. Write down three risks associated with insulin management in custody and write how you can reduce these.

3. Write down three risks associated with those with epilepsy and write how you can reduce these.

RESOURCES

Online

- British National Formulary | https://bnf.nice.org.uk/

- Geeky Medics | https://geekymedics.com/

- Gov | Epilepsy and driving | https://www.gov.uk/epilepsy-and-driving

- Resuscitation Council UK | ReSPECT | https://www.resus.org.uk/respect

Organisations

- Faculty of Forensic & Legal Medicine | www.fflm.ac.uk

- National Institute for Health and Care Excellence (NICE) | https://www.nice.org.uk/

- Royal College of General Practitioners: Secure environments group (rcgp.org.uk)

REFERENCES

British Medical Association, the Resuscitation Council (UK) and the Royal College of Nursing (2016). Decisions relating to cardiopulmonary resuscitation. https://www.bma.org.uk/media/1816/bma-decisions-relating-to-cpr-2016.pdf (accessed 22 February 2024).

Care Quality Commission (2023). Diabetes mellitus and insulin use in adult social care. https://www.cqc.org.uk/guidance-providers/adult-social-care/diabetes-insulin-use (accessed 22 February 2024).

Department of Health (2011). Prevention of infection and communicable disease control in prisons and places of detention. https://assets.publishing.service.gov.uk/media/5a7d6d8840f0b6262bad4f2b/Prevention_of_infection_communicable_disease_control_in_prisons_and_places_of_detention.pdf (accessed 22 February 2024).

Epilepsy Society (2022). If you are taking medication. https://epilepsysociety.org.uk/about-epilepsy/epilepsy-treatment/medication/anti-seizure-medication-asm/if-you-are-taking-medication#:~:text=For%20anti%2Dseizure%20medication%20(ASM,or%20accidentally%20miss%20a%20dose (accessed 22 February 2024).

National Institute for Health and Care Excellence (2016). Physical health of people in prison. https://www.nice.org.uk/guidance/ng57/evidence/full-guideline-pdf-2672652637 (accessed 22 February 2024).

National Institute for Health and Care Excellence (2022). Type 1 diabetes in adults: diagnosis and management. https://www.nice.org.uk/guidance/ng17/resources/type-1-diabetes-in-adults-diagnosis-and-management-pdf-1837276469701 (accessed 22 February 2024).

NHS Improvement (2018). Never events list 2018. https://webarchive.nationalarchives.gov.uk/ukgwa/20200707050656/https://improvement.nhs.uk/resources/never-events-policy-and-framework/#h2-revised-never-events-policy-and-framework-and-never-events-list-2018 (accessed 22 April 2024).

Royal College of General Practitioners (2019). Safe prescribing in prisons. https://elearning.rcgp.org.uk/pluginfile.php/176185/mod_book/chapter/620/RCGP-safer-prescribing-in-prisons-guidance-jan-2019.pdf (accessed 22 February 2024).

FURTHER READING

British Thoracic Society | Guidelines | https://www.brit-thoracic.org.uk/quality-improvement/guidelines/

Faculty of Forensic & Legal Medicine | Managing blood-borne virus exposure in Custody | https://fflm.ac.uk/wp-content/uploads/2022/05/Managing-blood-borne-virus-exposures-in-custody-FFLM-May-2022.pdf

Faculty of Forensic & Legal Medicine | Recommendations – Management of epilepsy in Custody | https://fflm.ac.uk/resources/publications/recommendations-management-of-epilepsy-in-police-custody/

Faculty of Forensic & Legal Medicine | Recommendations – Management of Diabetes Mellitus in Custody | https://fflm.ac.uk/resources/publications/recommendations-management-of-diabetes-mellitus-in-custody/

NHS England | Never events | https://www.england.nhs.uk/publication/never-events/

Specialist Pharmacy Service | Identifying risk factors for developing a long QT interval | https://www.sps.nhs.uk/articles/identifying-risk-factors-for-developing-a-long-qt-interval/

Mental Health

Vanessa Webb[1] and Abdulla Kraam[2]

[1] Nurture Health and Care Ltd, Norwich, UK
[2] North Lincolnshire CAMHS, Scunthorpe, UK

CHAPTER 6

AIM

This chapter explores mental health and how to manage, assess and refer in police custody, including fitness to detain, interview, charge, release and travel. It will introduce the approach to holistic assessments to help readers effectively perform assessments, ensuring safety and adherence to legal and ethical standards.

LEARNING OUTCOMES

Upon completion of this chapter, readers should be able to:

- Identify the key components of a holistic assessment, considering the mental and emotional well-being of individuals in custody

- Understand the legislative frameworks that apply in police custody in relation to mental health

- Understand how to manage fitness to release, risk formulation and safety planning in relation to self-harm and suicide

---

SELF-ASSESSMENT

1. List the three common mental health conditions and outline how they may impact an individual's fitness to be interviewed.

2. Outline the legal guidelines and frameworks healthcare professionals must be familiar with when assessing fitness to release.

3. Describe a mental status examination and describe the presentation of a person that you have seen in custody.

INTRODUCTION

Mental health is central to every assessment in police custody. It is essential to distinguish between good mental well-being, encompassing self-worth, trust, emotional depth, ability to adapt and other characteristics, and the diagnosis of mental health conditions, which focus on recognising emotional, cognitive and behavioural signs and symptoms. Within the custody environment, prevalent conditions include anxiety, depression, substance abuse and psychosis. Often the arrest process can exacerbate these conditions due to the inherent stress and potential for re-traumatisation.

This chapter has used the Diagnostic and Statistical Manual of Mental Disorders, fifth edition (DSM-5) (American Psychiatric Association 2013).

Personality and psychotic disorders are notably more prevalent among those in custody than in the general populace (National Institute for Health and Care Excellence (NICE) 2017). While the links between crime and mental illness remain unclear, factors like homelessness or substance misuse might lead to criminal activities such as theft. Hence, healthcare professionals (HCPs) must efficiently assess and devise appropriate management and referral plans.

Understanding the mental health landscape entails recognising signs and risk factors, ensuring continuity of care, developing risk formulations and safety plans and being familiar with local care pathways. It is crucial to be informed about the Mental Capacity Act (2005) and the Mental Health Act (1983) for England and Wales and their counterparts across the United Kingdom.

Partners such as Liaison and Diversion (L&D) are not available in all countries or every custody but have a primary function to include identifying vulnerabilities, screening for risks, assessing using a trauma-informed approach and referring individuals to suitable health and wider services.

ASSESSMENT

Approach those with a mental health diagnosis or emotional distress with compassion, respect and dignity.

Healthcare professionals should conduct a mental health assessment, evaluating the person's mental state and related functional and interpersonal challenges (see Box 6.1). If under the effects of drugs and alcohol, a full assessment should wait until an individual is optimally responsive. With dependencies, withdrawal management is paramount, but mental health evaluations can be done once an individual is interview-ready.

The HCP's role is to identify, not diagnose, the nature and severity of the disorder, assessing symptom gravity and functional impairment in a custody context. For critical disorders like psychosis or suicide risk, immediate assessment is vital. Chronic conditions require medication continuity and broader needs assessment.

The assessment should also consider the impact of custody on vulnerable individuals and children. If needed, follow local safeguarding measures. Additionally, consider antenatal and postnatal mental health and exclude risks in those groups. See Chapter 4 – Vulnerability and Appropriate Adults and Chapter 14 – Safeguarding

MENTAL STATUS EXAMINATION (MSE)

MSE offers a systematic assessment of a patient's mental health. It covers:

- Appearance and Behaviour
- Speech
- Mood and Affect
- Thoughts
- Perception
- Cognition
- Insight and Judgement
- Risk

Its goal is to capture a snapshot of a patient's mental functioning at a given point.

BOX 6.1	MENTAL HEALTH REVIEW

Initial questions include:

- Has the person consulted a healthcare professional for mental health (e.g. psychiatrist, GP, psychologist and counsellor)?
- Have they been admitted to a psychiatric hospital? If so, details about the recent discharge, hospital and consultant, and if so, is this a voluntary patient or under section?

Further questions could encompass:

- Past mental health disorders
- Chronic physical health issues, learning disability and educational experiences
- Treatment history and its effectiveness
- Interpersonal relationships quality
- Living conditions and potential social isolation
- Family history of mental illness
- History of abuse or adverse childhood experiences
- Employment and immigration status

For those on mental health medication, inquire about:

- The medicine name
- Current dosage and compliance levels
- The last dose taken

Common questions which may be helpful are:

- 'What's been on your mind recently?'
- 'Are you worried about anything?'
- 'Do you sometimes have thoughts that others tell you are false?'
- 'Do you have any beliefs not shared by others you know?'
- 'Do you ever feel people are out to harm you?'
- 'Do you ever feel specific events in the world relate to you somehow?'
- 'Are there any thoughts you have a hard time getting out of your head?'
- 'Do you sometimes feel the need to perform certain behaviours repetitively, despite understanding these are irrational?'
- 'Do you ever think about ending your life?'
- 'Have you ever felt your life was not worth living?'
- 'Have you ever harmed yourself to cope with difficult emotions'?
- 'Do you ever think about harming others?'
- Examine the custody record, considering if it current and the source of data.

Appearance and Behaviour

Evaluate self-neglect, clothing appropriateness for weather and setting, signs of self-harm or disease and evidence of being underweight or having a high Body Mass Index. Note how individuals engage, their eye contact, facial expression, body language and consider signs of paranoia and psychomotor activity (i.e. restless or fidgety).

Speech

Observe rate (pressured or slow), quantity (limited or excessive), tone (monotonous or tremulous), volume and fluency.

Mood and Affect

Affect is observed emotion, whereas mood is the patient's described emotional state. Ask about feelings, current mood or recent emotional changes. In mania, for example the person's mood is high (elated), they speak fast and have grandiose ideas (e.g. that they have special status or powers); the person might present as very active, unable to sit still or pause. Conversation can be difficult because they jump from one topic to another (flight of ideas). A depressed person will express the loss of pleasure in activities they used to enjoy (anhedonia). People give up hobbies. They complain about low energy levels. They might struggle to fall asleep (initial insomnia) or have interrupted sleep or both. Or they might sleep a lot more than usual for them. Their mood might be worse in the morning and improving gradually towards afternoon and in the evening (sometimes dramatically so). This is called diurnal mood variation. Feelings of guilt and worthlessness are not unusual for depression. Enquire about crying. They might struggle to change their emotional response depending on the topic of the conversation or the situation. This is called reduced affective modulation. For example they could be just sad and depressed throughout and any attempts by the health care professional to change that (e.g. by smiling, saying something positive or funny if appropriate) are to no avail. If the affect stays the same, it is referred to as flat affect.

Thoughts

Assess the speed, coherence and content of thoughts by listening to what our patients say to us.

This helps us notice signs like disjointed ideas that are not linked (loose associations), thoughts that veer off topic and are unconnected to our conversation and if rapid (flights of ideas), overly grand self-beliefs (grandiosity) and unusual experiences like feeling that thoughts are being removed, placed into their mind by others or broadcasted publicly (thought deletion, insertion and broadcasting), which are indicators of acute psychosis.

We also ask about any fixed false beliefs (delusions), repetitive thoughts (obsessions), the need to perform specific actions repeatedly (compulsions) and any thoughts of harming themselves or others.

Perceptions

We also check for experiences like seeing or hearing things that are not there (hallucinations), similar experiences the patient knows are not real (pseudo-hallucinations), misinterpretations of real sensory events (illusions), feelings of being detached from one's self (depersonalisation) and feelings of the world not being real (derealisation). Hearing voices discussing the person from outside their head are called third-person hallucinations. Record where a person is responding to unseen stimuli, such as taking to someone who is not there.

Hallucinations can involve other sensory modalities like smell or touch.

Cognition

We are familiar with identifying if an individual is orientated to date, time and place. Still, we should consider if people can pay attention, have any memory impairment or lack understanding. Consider tests like the mini-mental state exam or abbreviated test for in-depth assessment, a set of questions designed to give the HCP a screening tool for cognition, see Box 6.2. An extended version is utilised in psychiatric services.

One point is scored for each correct answer in the mental test score as long as the criteria are fulfilled, for example the time is given correct to the nearest hour.

A score of 8–10 is normal. A score of 7 is probably abnormal although it is recognised the stressful environment and anxiety could explain deviation. Less than 7 should be

---

BOX 6.2 **ABBREVIATED MENTAL TEST SCORE (AMTS)**

Score one point for each correct answer: (maximum score 10)

- Age in years

- Time of day (to the nearest hour)

- Name of building

- Address for recall at the end of the test (this should be repeated by the patient to ensure it has been heard correctly) – 42 West Street

- Year

- Recognition of two persons (doctor, nurse and police officer)

- Date of birth

- Year of the First World War – 1914

- Name of present Monarch

- Count backwards from 20 to 1

- *Test recollection of earlier address*

Source: Adapted from Hodkinson (1972).

considered as evidence of cognitive challenges and if new onset, referral is required to their GP or further assessment is required. In custody, this can help identify those people who might have dementia and could present with their first offence in custody as an older person, recognising early onset dementia. Those with alcohol dependency may experience Korsakoff's syndrome, a chronic memory disorder caused by severe deficiency of thiamine (vitamin B-1). One of the key symptoms of Korsakoff's syndrome is confabulation, where individuals make up stories to fill gaps in their memory. This condition is most commonly caused by alcohol misuse, but it can also arise from conditions that affect the absorption of vitamin B. The assessment of cognition as part of your assessment to identify individuals who need an appropriate adult is valuable.

Insight and Judgement

Evaluating insight involves understanding a patient's self-awareness, especially regarding their mental health condition. Assessing judgment focuses on their ability to make decisions effectively. By asking questions about what they believe caused their problems, their awareness of these issues, whether they think they need help or how they would react to imaginary situations, we can gauge how they handle risks and challenges. This approach helps us determine the necessity for more detailed assessments.

By focusing on the essentials, the MSE remains a comprehensive yet succinct method of describing the presentation of mental health symptoms.

OTHER VALIDATED TOOLS

NICE (2011) does not 'approve' diagnostic tools but recommends methods based on evidence. For mental health, this includes structured interviews and symptom checklists. When assessing mental health disorders, consider measures like PHQ-9,[1] HADS[2] or GAD-7[3]. Always refer to a current Diagnostic Classification System, usually DSM-5 or International Classification of Diseases, Tenth Revision (ICD-10), currently being updated and NICE guidelines for updated information.

In custody, these questions can be useful:

- During the last month, have you often been bothered by feeling down, depressed or hopeless?

- During the last month, have you been bothered by feeling nervous, anxious or on edge, which stops you from doing the things you need to do?

---

[1] Patient Health Questionnaire-9.
[2] Hospital Anxiety and Depression Scale.
[3] Generalised Anxiety Disorder-7.

ASSESSING RISK OF HARM TO SELF AND OTHERS

Initial risk assessment for those in custody:

- Directly ask about suicidal ideation and intent

    If there is a risk of self-harm or suicide:

- Assess their awareness of help sources and social support.

- Provide a safety plan based on risk formulation and clinical judgement.

- Advise them to seek further assistance if conditions worsen.

    Note: NICE (2022) recommendations on risk assessment tools and scales state that these should not be used to predict suicide or repetition of self-harm.

A care and safety plan and a risk formulation (formerly risk assessment) should be developed collaboratively through shared decision-making to prevent escalation of self-harm, address each of the risks identified, improve any associated mental health conditions, including emotional distress and consider on release how we can improve social and occupational function and their quality of life. Ensure each person has a safety plan including self-management strategies and how to access services during a crisis when self-management fails.

Specific Assessments

Self-harm and suicide risk assessment

- Assess feelings of hopelessness, suicidal thoughts or plans, see Box 6.3.

- Note any severe concerns about self-harm based on responses, observations including extreme agitation and emotional distress.

BOX 6.3	SELF-HARM AND SUICIDE: QUESTIONS TO CONSIDER

- 'Have you thought about harming yourself?'

- 'Do you plan to act on those thoughts?'

- 'When you thought about this last time, what protected you?'

- 'What are you planning for the next couple of weeks?'

- 'Who is in your life that makes you feel better?'

- 'Sometimes, when people are going through difficult things, they might have thoughts of wanting to harm themselves. Is this something you have experienced?'

- 'People can sometimes hurt themselves to manage overwhelming emotions or feelings of numbness – is this something you have ever done? If so, how do you cope with these feelings?'

- Consider the influence of internet usage and social media.

- Document the impact of their arrest if this is their first detention and the nature of their offence.

- Review their self-harm history, most recent incident and the most severe incident and any formal care or safety plans which are in place.

- Assess substance misuse, self-neglect, physical health needs and the impact of chaotic behaviours.

Make referral to mental health professionals a priority when:

- the person's levels of concern or distress are rising, high or sustained.

- the frequency or degree of self-harm or suicidal intent is increasing.

- the HCP is concerned.

- the person is asking for further support from mental health services.

As part of our duty of care, consider informing the GP to ensure continuity of care, particularly where there are vulnerabilities and the threshold to access services has not been met and consider signposting to local services or resources such as The Samaritans, Papyrus (children and under 35 years) and more bespoke services.

Risk to Others

Consider the nature of the crime in relation to the risk to others, but the following questions may be useful:

- 'Have you ever felt like harming someone else?'

- 'Do you plan to act on those thoughts?'

When an individual declares that they may harm others, we must inform others.

CARE PLANNING AND PRE-RELEASE RISK ASSESSMENT

For every individual seen, an HCP recommends a care plan, considers appropriate adult requirements (Chapter 4 – Vulnerability and Appropriate Adults) and includes continuity of care and fitness to release, including a safety plan if required.

This should be in collaboration with the person and the police. Every HCP involved in creating the plan should ensure it aligns with care plans from other services.

LEVEL OF OBSERVATIONS

Most individuals with a mental health disorder will be managed on level 1 observations. However, each person is unique and therefore, level 3 observations with CCTV or level 4 close proximity observations may be required. See Chapter 3 – Fitness Assessments for more information on Levels of observation.

OUR APPROACH

We should use a trauma-informed approach, recognising violent outbursts and unhelpful behaviours are often associated with triggers, so part of the assessment process could consider what early warning signs and strategies individuals use to manage their emotions and implement de-escalation techniques. Share this information with the custody team.

Individuals may:

- Feel overwhelmed by sensory experiences such as noise and smell.

- Exhibit poor communication skills, answering questions bluntly or misunderstanding nuanced queries, which can be perceived as rudeness.

- Struggle with interpreting and regulating their emotions.

- Demonstrate poor impulse control and may react indifferently to the consequences of their actions.

- Perceive a lack of autonomy in their lives, view their actions as futile and find it challenging to set and achieve goals.

- Have a sense of self that is influenced by those around them.

- Experience difficulties in social functioning, so might not cooperate with others or result have manipulative behaviour.

- Be unable to articulate their thoughts clearly, leading to frustration.

HCPs should provide guidance on recognising, assessment and managing emotional distress, including those who self-harm and talk about suicidal tendencies. They should also be skilled in de-escalation techniques to reduce the need for restrictive practices and be attentive to behavioural changes that might signal the onset or alteration of mental health conditions. It is essential to have knowledge of effective mental health pathways and to understand strategies such as establishing safe boundaries and building rapport.

For individuals taken directly to a cell, recognise the accompanying risk as their behaviours may signal neurological or mental health issues. Consider toxicity of overdose, acute behavioural disturbance and escalating behaviours when assessing someone who has gone straight to the cell, often using observation only and documenting what can be seen accurately.

SCENARIO 6.1	Mental health presentation (adult)

You are asked to see a 25-year-old male, who has been arrested for a public order offence. It was believed they were under the influence of substances on arrest as they were aggressive, shouting at everyone and had threatened someone.

They have now been in custody overnight for seven hours and have not improved. They continue to be aggressive, appear to be talking and shouting at someone in the cell who is not there and the police have not been able to establish their identity.

1. *Describe the assessment approach you would undertake.*

2. *What possible options have you for managing this individual?*

3. *How would you manage his fitness to detain, observations and whether they are fit for interview?*

CHILDREN AND ADOLESCENTS IN POLICE CUSTODY

The terms Child, Young, Youth, Adolescent, Juvenile, Older Adolescent, Young Adult are commonly used interchangeably, but they can cover different age ranges within and outside the legal and criminal justice system. Review Chapters 4 and 16 in relation to children and vulnerable adults.

THE DEVELOPING BRAIN

One way to think of the brain is that it consists of different layers with each layer representing a different evolutionary age. The oldest part is our 'reptilian brain' and includes parts like the brain stem. This is followed by the limbic system responsible for emotions. The outermost layer is regarded as the youngest and most complex to develop and is called the neocortex. It has a whole range of important functions located in different parts (frontal, parietal, temporal and occipital lobes). For our purposes, the relevant part is the frontal lobe, specifically the structure called prefrontal cortex. Its responsibilities are vast and crucial for our ability to communicate (language), reason, make decisions, plan things, solve problems (executive functioning) and our cognitive functioning (attention, focus, working memory, ability to store information temporarily while performing a task). It also influences our emotional regulation and social behaviour.

Interestingly, research has also shown that the prefrontal cortex is the latest to mature during the development of the human brain and continues to develop until the mid-20s. However, most recent research shows that we might have to revise this view, Kolk and Rakic (2021) state that although neurons of the prefrontal cortex are generated before birth, their differentiation and development of synaptic connections (notably 'pruning') extend to the third decade of life.

It is not surprising that we often encounter young people or young adults in or outside the custody setting who do not behave or reason like 'responsible adults' without having an impairment like learning disability.

THE DEVELOPMENTAL AND SYSTEMIC PERSPECTIVE

The developmental perspective takes into account that the child and young person will, at any given time, be on a journey of maturation. Their chronological age might be totally deceptive and lead to exaggerated expectations. More often than not, we encounter children and young people in the criminal justice system where there is a discrepancy between their ability to communicate, interact, behave, control, regulate their emotions and impulses and deal with different challenges; in short, their overall presentation and their expected level of maturity is different to that based on chronological age as sole determinant.

We have to make the necessary personal, relational and environmental adjustments. In addition, external or internal causes and triggers need to be identified. A young person who is part of a violent criminal gang and presenting as highly agitated in custody might have very legitimate reasons for their presentation because of the threat posed by the members of their own or a rival gang. This acute reaction to an external stressor might resolve as soon as that young person feels safe.

It is not uncommon however for young people in custody to come from disadvantaged socioeconomic backgrounds, having experienced violence and abuse during their upbringing. In the above scenario, the young person might continue to display agitation despite being in a 'safe environment'. The reason might be that for the young person, the environment itself constitutes a trigger for fear and agitation because it has evoked traumatic memories of abuse.

When we encounter a (young) person behaving in a way that we do not understand immediately, it is advisable to take a broader perspective and remain curious and inquisitive. It is also helpful to understand the 'language' and cultural background because the 'rules of the game' might be different from what we assume. This is called a systemic perspective.

DEVELOPMENTAL TRAUMA

The traditional view of trauma is that a discrete/single adverse incident produces the classical debilitating symptoms/signs of hyperarousal, flashbacks and avoidance within a specific time period. It is based on the 'road traffic accident trauma model' and while useful for explaining the effect of these single and discrete events, it is inadequate for an understanding of the experiences of most children and young people who are in contact with the criminal justice system and present in custodial settings.

Van De Kolk proposed a model which has proven to be clinically useful and although not formally recognised by the different psychiatric classifications. An accepted definition of complex trauma involves traumatic stressors that are repetitive and prolonged, involve direct harm and neglect by caregivers, occur at developmentally vulnerable stages of life (early childhood) and have great potential to severely compromise a child's development. Children who experience rage, betrayal, fear, resignation, defeat or shame are at higher risk of developing complex trauma disorder. It has been found that children experiencing trauma repeatedly lose the ability to regulate their emotions when they encounter any traumatic cues and in turn feel bad about themselves, do not trust their caregivers and also external agencies like social care.

Complex post-traumatic stress disorder (PTSD) and their presentations include alterations in regulation of affect and impulses (e.g. excessive risk-taking); alterations in consciousness or attention (e.g. pathological dissociation); alterations in self-perception' (e.g. shame); 'alterations in relations with others' (e.g. distrust, victimising others); somatisation (e.g. unexplained physical complaints) and 'alterations in systems of meaning' (e.g. distorted beliefs). Often one of the most clinically pressing aspects of a complex PTSD presentation is 'self-destructive thoughts and behaviours', including anger, aggression and self-harm.

COMMON CONDITIONS SEEN IN CUSTODY

DEPRESSIVE DISORDERS

Characterised by persistent sadness, hopelessness, loss of interest in activities, significant weight or appetite changes, sleep disturbances, fatigue, feelings of worthlessness and may be associated with recurrent thoughts of death or suicide.

Formal diagnosis identifies that symptoms should be present for at least two weeks and each symptom should be present at sufficient severity for most of every day.

ANXIETY DISORDERS

Anxiety is a normal response to an unusual or stressful event; it is the psychological component of the 'flight or fight' response.

Anxiety is considered abnormal when:

- It is excessively severe or prolonged
- It occurs in the absence of a stressful event
- It impairs social, physical or occupational functioning

In custody, we often see panic attacks marked by palpitations, sweating, trembling, feelings of shortness of breath and fears of dying.

Generalised anxiety disorder (GAD) is a common disorder, of which the central feature is excessive worry about a number of different events associated with heightened tension. It should be present for at least six months and should cause clinically significant distress or impairment in social, occupational or other important areas of functioning.

Formal diagnosis requires symptoms to occur more days than not, for at least six months (excessive anxiety and worry about a number of events and activities, and difficulty controlling the worry) and are associated with restlessness or feeling keyed up or on edge, being easily fatigued, difficulty concentrating or mind going blank, irritability, muscle tension and sleep disturbance.

Other anxiety disorders can be diagnosed and more information identified.

SUBSTANCE-RELATED AND ADDICTION DISORDERS

Disorders related to the use of substances like alcohol, caffeine, cannabis, hallucinogens, inhalants, opioids, sedatives, stimulants, tobacco and gambling are all considered as part of the addiction disorders. These are covered in Chapter 10 – Substance Use and Misuse.

Non-substance-related disorders such as gambling may be seen in custody, associated with the need to gamble with increasing amounts of money, restlessness or irritability when attempting to stop, and loss of control over gambling behaviours and theft or other crimes being committed.

Dual Diagnosis

Although this is not a DSM-5 category, many of those detained in custody have the co-occurrence of substance use and another mental disorder. Dual diagnosis, also known as co-occurring disorders, refers to the coexistence of substance misuse disorders and mental health disorders within an individual. Substance misuse can exacerbate mental health symptoms, while mental health disorders can lead to substance misuse as a form of self-medication.

Traditionally, dual diagnosis presents challenges for the HCP as traditional treatment models were designed for either substance misuse or mental health disorders. Services that are integrated treatment approaches are difficult to access.

PERSONALITY DISORDERS

Personality disorders (PDs) represent a complex topic in the realm of psychology and psychiatry. PDs are not merely 'bad' behaviours; they are deeply ingrained patterns of thinking, feeling and behaving.

Definition

PDs are long-standing patterns of thoughts, feelings and behaviours that differ significantly from cultural expectations and can cause distress or impairment in social, occupational or other areas of functioning. Unlike acute mental disorders, such as major depressive disorder or schizophrenia, personality disorders are defined as resistant to changing easily as they form the core of who individuals are as people.

They are classified as:

- **Cluster A**: Paranoid, schizoid and schizotypal

- **Cluster B**: Which are often seen in custody such as antisocial PD (challenges with problem-solving, emotion regulation, impulse control and interpersonal relationships), borderline PD (emotional instability, disturbed thought patterns, impulsive behaviour and unstable relationship), histrionic and narcissistic PD

- **Cluster C**: Avoidant, dependant, obsessive compulsive

Illness vs. Traits

From a clinical standpoint, PDs are considered psychiatric illnesses because they cause significant distress or impairment. They are listed in diagnostic manuals and, therefore, form part of the illness spectrum.

However, PDs can also be viewed as extreme or maladaptive variations of common personality traits. For example, everyone may experience moments of narcissism, but not everyone meets the criteria for narcissistic personality disorder.

The development of a PD is believed to result from a combination of genetic, biological, environmental and social factors. Traumatic experiences, childhood adversity or inconsistent parenting may contribute.

Treatment and Management

PDs can be challenging to treat, partly because individuals often do not see their own behaviour as problematic and require insight to change their own thoughts, feelings and behaviours. Awareness of PDs can help staff create management strategies in a custody setting, such as setting clear boundaries, ensuring consistency in interactions and using a multidisciplinary approach for complex cases.

Individuals with PDs aren't necessarily 'choosing' to act in difficult ways, and therefore, empathy, patience and consistent boundaries are crucial.

Collaboration with mental health professionals is essential for effective management and potential treatment.

NEURODEVELOPMENTAL DISORDERS

Neurodevelopmental disorders, as classified by DSM-5, encompass a group of conditions that typically manifest early in a person's development. These disorders are characterised by developmental differences that produce impairments of personal, social, academic or occupational functioning. These vary from very specific limitations of learning or control of executive functions to global impairments of social skills or intelligence. In custody, we see young people and adults who often need to be considered in relation to

these diagnoses and to recognise how 'neuro-diversity' will create challenges in being within the custody environment but also the strengths that arise from our differences.

In custody, we see both young people and adults who will be undiagnosed but may be suspected by the HCP or self-identify with a diagnosis, along with those who have a diagnosis. Where any concerns arise, understanding their perception of their challenges or, where needed, discussing with their caregivers to ensure that our care plans align with their needs.

Intellectual disabilities are characterised by barriers in abilities, such as reasoning, problem-solving, planning, abstract thinking, judgment, academic learning and learning from experience. These result in challenges in adaptive functioning, requiring support for the individual to be independent and responsible. IQ scores are now outdated and assessment is of skills and functionality.

Autism spectrum disorder (ASD) identifies challenges with social communication and social interaction, alongside restricted, repetitive patterns of behaviour, interests or activities and are sensitive to many sensations: light, sound and busy environments, touch, spatial awareness, taste including the volume and textures of food and fluids, thus impact on routine and the need to seek self-soothing behaviours.

Attention-deficit/hyperactivity disorder (ADHD) is characterised by a persistent pattern of inattention and/or hyperactivity-impulsivity that interferes with functioning or development, although it is now also associated with other capabilities which can be seen as assets. Medication should be continued in custody if prescribed, but individuals often struggle with concentration and focus, being enclosed and not being able to follow instructions.

Specific learning disorder involves difficulties learning such as dyslexia, but can be associated with written expression or mathematics.

Stereotypic movement disorder, and tic disorders such as Tourette's syndrome, communication disorders and other neurodevelopmental disorders will all be seen in custody and each present in an individual manner.

SCHIZOPHRENIA AND OTHER PSYCHOTIC DISORDERS

Schizophrenia is characterised by delusions, hallucinations and disorganised thinking, which can be seen in the speech of individuals which is grossly disorganised and is often accompanied by negative symptoms where people feel depressed or are unable to feel their emotions, isolating themselves, without pleasure or motivation to undertake activities.

Psychosis: Encompasses various disorders where psychosis (hallucinations and delusions) is a feature, including drug-associated psychosis, which is a common presentation in custody.

BIPOLAR AND RELATED DISORDERS

Bipolar affective disorder is a condition where there are periodic swings of mood periods of months or years between manic episodes and depressed episodes. The DSM-5 identifies Bipolar I and Bipolar II where the latter do not experience mania, but have periods of hypomania, along with depression.

Bipolar disorder is characterised by episodes of mania (abnormally elevated mood or irritability and related symptoms with severe functional impairment or psychotic symptoms and lack of sleep along with depression (hence the designation, bipolar). Arrest may be related to the behaviour which presents alongside mania.

TRAUMA- AND STRESSOR-RELATED DISORDERS

It is important to be able to consider how trauma impacts on those detained with adverse childhood experiences and trauma in adulthood commonplace.

The DSM-5 categorises trauma- and stressor-related disorders as a group of mental health conditions that are directly related to the experience of trauma or significant stress. These disorders are characterised by the emotional and psychological responses individuals have to traumatic or stressful events.

Acute stress disorder may be seen in our population in response to their arrest or the circumstances linked to this and their symptoms occur immediately after the trauma and last from three days to one month, which is considered part of the healing process. If symptoms persist beyond one month, the diagnosis may evolve into PTSD. Adjustment Disorders are responses to a significant life change or stressor, such as divorce, job loss, a death in the family, but can also include being arrested and the sequelae. Symptoms can include depressive symptoms, anxiety and also include behavioural changes.

PTSD is characterised by the development of specific symptoms following exposure to one or more traumatic events. Symptoms include intrusive thoughts, flashbacks, nightmares, severe anxiety, as well as persistent avoidance of stimuli associated with the trauma, negative alterations in cognition and mood and marked changes in arousal and reactivity are seen. The diagnosis requires that symptoms last more than one month and cause significant distress or impairment in social, occupational or other important areas of functioning. Complex PTSD is seen where multiple traumas have occurred.

Reactive attachment disorder occurs in children who have not formed healthy emotional attachments with their primary caregivers, often due to severe early neglect or mistreatment and persist into adulthood and therefore reviewing attachment theory might give insight into the relationships and connections those in custody might experience.

ATTACHMENT THEORY

Attachment theory is vital for understanding human functioning. Early relationships with caregivers impact how we think, feel and act. Babies rely on caregivers to teach them about the world. Through numerous interactions, we make sense of things for proper brain growth and understanding of thoughts, feelings and behaviours. Interference can cause 'attachment disruption', leading to 'Insecure Attachment', while good care results in 'Secure Attachment' (Bowlby 1969). Understanding the 'Attachment Style', often helps us make sense of an individual's behaviours.

The DSM-5 emphasises the importance of the individual's subjective experience of the event in the diagnosis of these disorders. The impact of the trauma or stressor includes the duration and severity of symptoms and is considered in relation to the individual's cultural, historical and personal background.

OTHER CLASSIFICATION

The remaining categories related to Mental Health in DSM are:

- Obsessive–Compulsive Disorders
- Disassociated Disorders
- Somatic Symptom and Related Disorders
- Feeding and Eating Disorders
- Elimination Disorders
- Sleep–Wake Disorders
- Sexual Dysfunction
- Gender Dysmorphia
- Disruptive Impulse Control and Conduct Disorder
- Neuro-Cognition Disorders and includes Traumatic Brain Injury (Chapter 5 – Managing Long-Term Health Conditions)
- Paraphilic Disorders
- Medication-Induced Disorders

In addition, there is identification of diagnosis in respect of relational, abuse and neglect, education and occupational, housing and economic, related to social environment, related to crime or interaction with criminal justice system, environmental, personal history, lack of access and non-adherence.

For more information, when an individual presents with a disorder, these can be reviewed in the DSM-5 or alternative guidance, but the Royal College of Psychiatrists has information for patients that is easily understandable.

Mental health presentation (child)

A 15-year-old girl, who is in foster care, has been arrested for throwing a brick at the foster parent's window and stealing. She refuses to speak to the custody team, so she has not answered the booking in questions and has been moved to the area, so they have no previous history on their system.

The detention officer asks if she has a mental health condition that they should be aware of. The foster parents are not in custody, but they have a social worker attending soon.

1. *Describe the assessment approach you would undertake.*

2. *What possible options have you for managing this individual.*

3. *How would you manage her fitness to detain, observations and whether they are fit for interview.*

UNDERSTANDING WHY PEOPLE MAY NOT BEHAVE AS EXPECTED?

BEHAVIOURAL THEORY

Behavioural theory posits that all behaviours are learned through interaction with the environment, primarily through the processes of classical conditioning (learning by association) and operant conditioning (learning through consequences, such as rewards and punishments) (Skinner 1953). As we learn behaviour by modelling and copying others, responding to positive or negative reinforcement and risk and reward, varied upbringing often seen in looked-after children or inconsistent adult behaviours where parenting has been difficult, leads to individuals who struggle to identify the appropriate behaviour to a situation.

COGNITIVE DEVELOPMENT

Cognitive development as above concerns thinking, problem-solving, planning and sense-making. In custody, it is important to consider whether factors have impacted the cognitive growth of the individual and it is possible, that due to multiple factors, individuals are immature in certain aspects of development. This can aid development of strategies for managing behavior and distress.

THE ROLE OF ADRENALINE

Adrenaline-driven behaviours in response to stress or trauma are a well-documented phenomenon grounded in the body's physiological reaction to perceived threats. This response is facilitated through the limbic system. The surge of adrenaline and other stress hormones like cortisol increases heart rate, blood pressure and energy supplies while diverting resources away from non-essential functions to prioritise immediate survival. When we are in custody and might be frightened or challenged, the body's stress response creates a 'fight, flight, freeze or friend' response, which can often be seen in the heightened emotional state of those in custody.

In trauma-informed practices, strategies for understanding and dealing with trauma-related behaviours include being non-judgemental, calm, compassionate and consideration of techniques such as grounding, giving time as well as distraction can all be useful.

CO-OCCURRING CONDITIONS

This client group often has multiple diagnoses, and management plans, therefore, need to be individualised to each person and the impact of their diagnosis discussed with them to ensure we address their requirements.

COMMON TREATMENTS FOR MENTAL HEALTH

NICE (2011) references psychological therapies, often including cognitive behavioural therapy (CBT), computerised CBT, other cognitive and therapeutic models, counselling, psychotherapy, structured group programmes, peer support programmes, psychoeducational groups, relaxation, mindfulness and social activities and exercise.

MEDICATION

Medication is often the second line and includes the following.

Antidepressants

These are used to treat conditions like depression, generalised anxiety disorder and certain obsessive–compulsive disorders. Common types include selective serotonin reuptake inhibitors (SSRIs), such as fluoxetine and citalopram, serotonin and norepinephrine reuptake inhibitors (SNRIs), like venlafaxine.

Antipsychotics

These are often used to manage conditions like schizophrenia, bipolar disorder and severe depression. Examples include quetiapine, olanzapine and risperidone.

Mood Stabilisers

These are used for bipolar disorder to prevent episodes of mania, hypomania and depression. Lithium and certain anti-convulsants like lamotrigine are examples.

Anxiolytics

These are primarily used to treat anxiety disorders. Benzodiazepines, such as diazepam and lorazepam, fall in this category, but they are usually used for short-term relief of acute symptoms.

Stimulants

These are mainly used for ADHD and Methylphenidate is commonly prescribed.

Hypnotics

Used to manage insomnia and other sleep disorders and Zopiclone is commonly prescribed short term.

MENTAL HEALTH LEGISLATION

Key Mental Health Acts and Amendments to be considered in custody include:

- **England & Wales**: Mental Capacity Act (2005), Mental Capacity (Amendment) Act (2019), Mental Health Act (1983)
- **Scotland**: Adults with Incapacity (Scotland) Act (2000), The Mental Health (Care and Treatment) (Scotland) Act (2003) amended in 2017 by the Mental Health (Scotland) Act (2015)
- **Northern Ireland**: Mental Health Order (1986), Mental Capacity Act (2016)

DETENTION UNDER MHA 1983 (ENGLAND AND WALES)

Section 2

Allows for admission of someone suspected of having a mental disorder to a hospital for up to 28 days for assessment. It requires the agreement of an Approved Mental Health Professional (AMPH) and two doctors of which one must be 'Section 12 approved'.

Section 3

Permits admission for treatment up to six months in the first instance. It must be agreed necessary by an AMPH and two doctors, of which one must be 'Section 12 approved'.

Section 4

Emergency hospital admission lasting 72 hours when only one 'section 12-approved' doctor is available, for urgent cases.

Section 5

Provides holding powers for doctors or nurses with mental health/learning disability registration, to briefly detain inpatients for MHA 1983 assessment, excluding emergency departments.

Roles and Responsibilities

Detaining 'mentally disordered' individuals under the MHA 1983 is termed 'sectioning'. An AMHP and medical practitioners decide on detaining someone. The AMHP considers other alternatives before sectioning. Voluntary hospital admission does not result in sectioning, but if consent is absent or impossible, the AMHP, with medical backing, can 'section' the individual.

Doctors' Qualifications

'Section 12-approved' doctors possess specific training and experience in mental health.

Police Involvement (Which Varies Across the Four Countries)

Police powers include:

- **Section 17 of the Police and Criminal Evidence Act 1984**: Enter premises to save life or limb; otherwise, an MHA 1983 s 135(2) warrant is needed
- **Section 135**: Remove a mentally disordered individual from their residence (with a warrant)
- **Section 136**: If someone seems mentally disordered and is at risk to themselves or others, they can be moved to a Place of Safety. Section 136(1A) details where this power applies and excludes private dwellings

Place of safety and transfer Individuals, if they are taken to a place of safety, will require further assessment to identify if they are safe to be discharged or fit for release.

Police cells are not suitable places to detain people thought to have mental health problems. A person's condition may be exacerbated by being held in this environment and increasingly, police custody has been excluded as an appropriate place, unless there are exceptional circumstances.

As part of section 136, a healthcare presence must be maintained, with healthcare checks conducted every 30 minutes. If the custody sergeant is unable to comply with this requirement, they must arrange for the individual to be transferred to another safe location. Management of this process varies by police force, so local protocols should be adhered to.

An individual may be transferred to different places of safety for assessment, ideally by ambulance, and can be detained for up to 24 hours from the time of arrival at the first location. During this period, a police officer's presence is not required under the MHA 1983 S 136.

Detention under MHA 1983 S 136 ends in one of the two ways after a clinical assessment: either the doctor confirms the individual does not have a mental disorder or the AMHP arranges the necessary treatment or care.

If a doctor determines that the individual is not mentally disordered, they must be immediately discharged from detention.

An individual might be considered mentally disordered under Police and Criminal Evidence Act (PACE) Code C but not require further detention or care under the MHA 1983. For instance, a suicidal person with an effective community-based care plan may not need further detention. This can lead to a difference of opinion.

Section 34(2) of PACE mandates the release of a person from police detention if a decision is made not to charge them.

If releasing someone under PACE poses a risk to their health and safety due to mental health issues, detention under S 136 may be used. This decision should be made as if the person had just been encountered. Under PACE, individuals should not be held in police custody solely pending a mental health assessment or the identification of a hospital bed.

If an MHA assessment is completed in police custody and no hospital bed is available, the custody sergeant must decide whether to release the individual. This decision may require consultation with the investigating officer, their supervisor and potentially the Crown Prosecution Service for a statutory charging decision.

In some cases, a pre-release risk assessment reveals that an individual is extremely vulnerable, posing a credible risk, such as suicide, upon release. If the AMHP cannot or will not make an application, the custody officer is legally required to release the individual from police detention. The custody officer should inform the investigating officer and AMHP of their legal obligations so they can take necessary actions.

Forces may decide, based on the risk assessment and to preserve the dignity and safety of the individual, to allow them to remain at the police station (without legal detention) while escalating the issue to managers for resolution.

SCENARIO 6.3   Mental health scenario

A 34-year-old female has been arrested for theft and entering properties. On arrest, the police have felt her behaviour was really odd as she is stating that she has to gather plants together for an experiment as she is researching climate control and she is leading the world as a global leader in ecology and the impact on plants. She is jovial but aggressive when questioned. You overhear the booking assessment and she is speaking rapidly, cannot concentrate on any questions and is changing topics from one thing to the other.

You ask if you can see her after booking in.

1. *Describe the assessment approach you would undertake.*

2. *What possible options have you for managing this individual?*

3. *How would you manage her fitness to detain, observations and whether they are fit for interview?*

CONSIDERATIONS FOR CHILDREN AND INTOXICATED INDIVIDUALS (WHICH VARIES ACROSS THE FOUR NATIONS)

Children should not be taken to police stations as a place of safety. The child's welfare is the priority, and consideration of the Children Act's police protection order (PPO) or its equivalent across the four counties should be considered. This approach helps prevent unnecessary institutionalisation or stigmatisation and a PPO offers flexibility and is used if a police officer has reasonable cause to believe the child would otherwise likely suffer significant harm.

Individuals Who Are Under the Influence of Substances

There is no legal reason that the MHA S 136 cannot be used for someone intoxicated by drugs or alcohol. However, officers should be cautious in attributing behaviour to a mental health issue when the person has consumed significant amounts of alcohol or drugs, as this alters behaviour and typically, a formal mental health assessment is delayed to exclude this.

The Mental Health Crisis Care Concordat states that the presence of alcohol and/or drugs should not typically be a reason for a health-based place of safety to refuse admission to a person experiencing a potential mental health crisis (HM Government 2014). Additionally, the Concordat specifies that it is inappropriate and unacceptable for healthcare staff to use breathalysers to inform their decisions.

SCOTLAND AND NORTHERN IRELAND

Both have different, yet parallel legislation for detaining individuals with mental disorders.

LOCAL PATHWAYS FOR MENTAL HEALTH

Forces should collaboratively create local care pathways, often led by L&D or equivalent if available.

The pathways should facilitate:

- Access to Mental Health Act assessments through AMHP

- Effective sharing and communication about care with other professionals, including GPs

- Established pathways for referral across the diagnosis and level of need for mental health

We recognise those with mental health disorders who do not meet thresholds for service delivery, benefit from social, educational or vocational support and signposting may be beneficial.

- Educating about self-help groups, support circles and local and national resources

- Befriending or rehabilitation programmes for individuals including drugs and alcohol

- Access to Citizens Advice, Housing, educational and job-related support services

- Local resources like Improving Access to Psychological Therapy (IAPT), crisis services and local third-sector organisations such as MIND

Street triage may be available, allowing mental health professionals to offer immediate support to police officers handling situations involving individuals with potential mental health issues.

ADDITIONAL CONSIDERATIONS

It is important that we recognise the unique challenges faced by healthcare professionals and the police working in high-stress environments like police custody. As an HCP, promote the importance of self-care practices, such as stress management techniques, debriefing and supervision sessions and access to well-being support services and help professional colleagues to maintain their well-being.

CONCLUSION

Effective mental health assessment and management in police custody is paramount for the safeguarding and well-being of individuals in this environment. This chapter explores the complexity of mental health issues prevalent in custody, ranging from common disorders like anxiety and depression to more severe conditions such as psychosis and personality disorders. It underscores the importance of distinguishing between general well-being and specific mental health conditions, with an emphasis on the role of healthcare professionals in conducting comprehensive assessments and creating tailored care plans.

The discussion includes vital elements like the Mental Health Act, the role of Liaison and Diversion services if available, and the necessity of understanding various psychological theories and approaches. Additionally, the chapter emphasises the significance of continuity of care, risk assessments and safety planning and the Mental Status Examination, along with the consideration of the legal frameworks and ethical interfaces.

Overall, it calls for a compassionate and trauma-informed approach to mental health, recognising the unique challenges and responsibilities of healthcare professionals in this setting. This comprehensive approach aims not only to address immediate health concerns but also to contribute to the long-term well-being of individuals and reducing inequalities.

LEARNING ACTIVITIES

1. Can you describe a referral that you made for a Mental Health Act assessment and reflect on how this was facilitated in your local area?

2. Can you identify a plan that you made whilst in custody for an individual with a personality disorder and any suggestions that were included for the police?

3. Could you reflect on self-care that you have undertaken yourself in response to a case that you connected to in some way?

RESOURCES

Online

- Geeky Medics | Mental State Examination | https://geekymedics.com/mental-state-examination/

- NHS England | Health and Justice | https://www.england.nhs.uk/commissioning/health-just/

- Royal College of Psychiatrists | Mental illness and mental health problems|https://www.rcpsych.ac.uk/mental-health/mental-illnesses-and-mental-health-problems

Organisations

- Mind | https://www.mind.org.uk

- Mental Health Foundation | https://www.mentalhealth.org.uk

- Rethink Mental Health | https://www.rethink.org

REFERENCES

American Psychiatric Association (2013). *Diagnostic and Statistical Manual of Mental Disorders: DSM-5*, 5ee. Arlington, VA: American Psychiatric Publishing.

Bowlby, J. (1969). *Attachment and Loss. Vol. 1: Attachment.* New York: Basic Books.

HM Government (2014). Mental Health Crisis Care Concordant. https://s16652.pcdn.co/wp-content/uploads/sites/24/2014/04/36353_Mental_Health_Crisis_accessible.pdf (accessed 12 August 2024).

Hodkinson, H. (1972). Evaluation of a mental test score for assessment of mental impairment in the elderly. *Age and Ageing.* 41 (3): iii35–iii40.

Kolk, S.M. and Rakic, P. (2021). Development of prefrontal cortex. *Neuropsychopharmacology* 47 (1): 41–59. https://doi.org/10.1038/s41386-021-01076-5.

National Institute for Health and Care Excellence (2011). Common mental health problems: identification and pathways to care. https://www.nice.org.uk/guidance/cg123 (accessed 22 April 2024).

National Institute for Health and Care Excellence (2017). Mental health of adults in contact with the criminal justice system. https://www.nice.org.uk/guidance/ng66 (accessed 22 April 2024).

National Institute for Health and Care Excellence (2022). Self-harm: assessment, management and preventing recurrence. https://www.nice.org.uk/guidance/ng225 (accessed 22 April 2024).

Skinner, B.F. (1953). *Science and Human Behavior.* New York: Macmillan.

FURTHER READING

British Medical Journal | How to approach the mental state examination | https://www.bmj.com/content/357/sbmj.j1821

Health and Social Care Act |Section 20 Regulation, code of practice and guidance Regulation of regulated | https://www.legislation.gov.uk/ukpga/2008/14/part/2

Mind | Personality disorders | https://www.mind.org.uk/information-support/types-of-mental-health-problems/personality-disorders/about-personality-disorders/

National Institute for Health and Care Excellence | Violent and aggressive behaviours in people with mental health problems |https://www.nice.org.uk/guidance/qs154/resources/violent-and-aggressive-behaviours-in-people-with-mental-health-problems-pdf-75545539974853

Care Act | Assessment of an adult's needs for care and support | https://www.legislation.gov.uk/ukpga/2014/23/section/9

Medicine Management

Vanessa Webb[1] and Dipti Patel[2]

[1] Nurture Health and Care Ltd, Norwich, UK
[2] Mountain Healthcare Ltd, Stevenage, UK

CHAPTER 7

AIM

This chapter provides an in-depth understanding of medicine management within police custody. It focuses on the role of healthcare professionals (HCPs) in assessing the suitability of patients' medications for administration or self-administration. The chapter outlines the various categories of medication, such as General Sales List (GSL), Prescription Only Medicines (POM) and Controlled Drugs (CD), highlighting their differences and associated regulations. Additionally, it explores the processes involved in authorising, supplying and administering medication, including using Patient Group Directions (PGD) and prescriptions.

LEARNING OUTCOMES

On completion of this chapter, readers should be able to:

- Explain the processes and legal considerations involved in authorising, supplying and administering medications in police custody

- Identify which medications are time-critical and understand the importance of continuing essential medications

- Apply knowledge of medicines management to ensure safe, effective and legal healthcare practice within police custody

SELF-ASSESSMENT

1. Define the roles and responsibilities of HCPs, Custody Officers and Detention Officers managing medications in police custody.

2. How do PGDs differ from standard prescriptions, and in what situations are they typically used in police custody healthcare? What are the limitations of PGDS?

3. What factors should be considered when determining whether a medication is time-critical and essential to continue while in custody?

INTRODUCTION

Healthcare professionals (HCPs) are the primary individuals responsible for how medicines are administered in custody, including the self-administration of medication following a thorough risk assessment. It is therefore crucial that HCPs are familiar with the terms used within this chapter, as outlined in Box 7.1.

HCPs must adhere to the Human Medicines Regulations 2012, the Misuse of Drugs Regulations 2001, the Controlled Drugs (Supervision of Management and Use) Regulations 2006, and the Police and Criminal Evidence Act 1984 (PACE) Codes of Practice (applicable in England and Wales), or other relevant legislation in Scotland and Northern Ireland.

The custody officer has the ultimate responsibility for safeguarding any medication brought into custody and included in their property. They must ensure the individual has the opportunity to access any medication prescribed during or prior to detention, provided it is approved by an appropriate HCP. The manner in which this is carried out may vary between police forces.

Police Custody Healthcare for Nurses and Paramedics, First Edition. Edited by Matthew Peel, Jennie Smith, Vanessa Webb, and Margaret Bannerman.
© 2025 John Wiley & Sons Ltd. Published 2025 by John Wiley & Sons Ltd.
Companion website: www.wiley.com/go/policecustodyhealthcare

| BOX 7.1 | TERMS USED |

- **Patient Group Direction (PGDs)**: A written group direction that allows the supply or administration of a specific medicine by a named authorised HCP

- **Prescribe**: Authorise the legal supply of a medicine by appropriately qualified HCPs (non-medical prescribers)

- **Supply**: Supply a medication in line with a prescription, protocol or PGD

- **Dispense**: A legal activity carried out by pharmacists or dispensing doctors

- **Administer**: Select and give medication to a person for them to take themselves from a labelled container

- **Self-administration**: Refers to the practice where individuals are allowed to take their prescribed or supplied medication themselves under supervision. This may be under the supervision of an HCP or police staff. It is an important process to understand as it is how those detained in custody primarily receive their medication

The process for obtaining medications varies locally according to each Police Force and across the four countries. HCPs must understand these local arrangements.

- Purchased by the police or an outsourced provider, stored in a locked medicine cabinet within the medical room, and provided on a prescriber's instructions, or administered/supplied via a medicines protocol or Patient Group Direction (PGD).

- Previously prescribed medication which may be retrieved by the police or brought in by a friend or relative.

- Collected from a supervising pharmacy in relation to supervised doses of opioid substitute medication.

- Collected by the police using a prescription issued by a prescriber, which may be private, or through their GP or an alternative service.

Under medicines legislation, Prescription Only Medicines can be administered to a person by non-clinical staff if they act according to the instructions of an appropriate prescriber. PACE Code of Practice C (last updated November 2019) (applicable in England and Wales) does not allow custody staff to administer medication but does permit the supervision of self-administration (except for Schedule 1, 2 or 3 drugs). Similar regulations apply in Northern Ireland and Scotland.

The method of administration depends on several factors, including the type and authorisation of the medication, the clinical condition of the person, and the availability of qualified staff.

HCPs are required to make contemporaneous records of any medicines taken from the medicine stock, in line with local policy and regulatory requirements.

MEDICINES LEGISLATION

There are three classes of medicinal products for humans under the Human Medicines Regulations (2012).

1. **General Sale Medicines (GSL)**: available over the counter for self-selection

2. **Pharmacy Medicines (P)**: available to buy from a registered pharmacy premises

3. **Prescription Only Medicine (POM)**: medicines that are subject to a restriction of requiring a prescription by an appropriate practitioner

Controlled drugs (CDs) are POMs with further restrictions under the Misuse of Drugs Regulations (2001). The regulations classify CDs into five schedules according to the different controls attributed to each:

- **Schedule 1**: most have no therapeutic use

- **Schedule 2**: diamorphine, morphine, methadone etc.

- **Schedule 3**: buprenorphine, gabapentin, pregabalin and tramadol

- **Schedule 4**: diazepam, zopiclone etc.

- **Schedule 5**: codeine, dihydrocodeine etc.

HOW PATIENTS CAN ACCESS MEDICINES

Local medicines processes have **no consensus in practice** across the four countries and between providers.

We have highlighted key areas of practice, but local policies and procedures need to be followed to ensure the continuity of medicines is facilitated (see Box 7.2).

| SCENARIO 7.1 | Authorising medication |

You are asked to see a 24-year-old male who has been arrested for a serious assault. Officers have brought in a strip of Sodium valproate (Epilim®) 500 mg tablets. The batch number and expiry date are visible but it is not boxed and labelled. The patient states he is not from around here and is staying for the weekend, so he just brought a strip. You can confirm on the Summary Care Record (or equivalent) that he is prescribed one tablet, 500 mg, twice daily.

1. *How do you approach this assessment?*
   a. *What factors will impact your decision?*

2. *What are the risks and benefits of:*
   a. *Authorising?*
   b. *Not authorising?*

3. *Outline the options available and your rationale for choosing or declining that option.*

BOX 7.2	VERIFICATION, ADMINISTRATION AND STORAGE OF MEDICATION

Verification of the person and their prescription	Verification of the medicine	Administration or supply processes	Governance processes in relation to medicines	Storage and disposal of Medicines
Critical Medicines and those that are time sensitive must be provided.				
Medicines should always be administered in a timely manner and should not be delayed due to the unavailability of the HCP. Custody staff should be told to contact the HCP if there are any queries regarding the medication, or there are delays.				
Incidents have occurred where individuals have given false names – always triangulate identity	The medicine should be able to be identifiable preferably in a boxed and labelled format that is in dated and named.	Patient's own medications can be self-administered or administered from their own supply, the formulary or from a pharmacy through a prescription	Instructions should include: • name of patient; • name of the supplying organisation; • medication name, form, strength, dose, frequency and total quantity; • date (unless recorded in clinical system automatically) • any special instructions (e.g. before, with or after food; with plenty of water; swallowed whole) Other local processes may involve recording batch numbers, or other additional information such as patient information leaflets, but vary between providers.	Any medicine that is supplied to the patient using a PGD is subject to the requirements for labelling stipulated under the EU Labelling and Leaflet Directive 92/27. If the medicine is a POM, then it must be supplied in an appropriately labelled pack (i.e. with full directions and other legally required information), with a patient information leaflet made available to the patient and obtained from a licensed provider.
Verification of prescribed medicine should include patient summary care record, GP verification, prescription, clinic letter or locally agreed criteria, including clinical presentation	Local processes should be followed for: blister strips, which are identifiable, bottled medication, loose medication, multi-compartment compliance aids, injectables, creams and other formulations	Providers and police forces will vary in their approach to the supervision of oral medication, injectables and emergencies so understanding where, by whom and how medicines are managed should be understood.	The HCP should ensure the custody staff understand any risks or special circumstances associated with the medication.	Medications should be provided in suitable, appropriately labelled containers and ensure appropriate, storage facilities in place for medication they have authorised or supplied. The storage requirements of each medication must be adhered to (e.g. temperature requirements).
Evidence of concordance should be established if possible	Medications that are unfamiliar should be reviewed in the British National Formulary and advice sought if needed	Patient own medication must not be taken out of their prescribed box and put in bags with label. This is secondary dispensing and therefore NOT LEGAL, follow your local processes.	Instructions must be written, clear and unambiguous without abbreviations, using the computerised clinical record system where possible and understood by non-clinical staff.	Unused medicines must be disposed of appropriately. Arrangements should be in place for the disposal of pharmaceutical waste through a service contract for the supply, regular collection and replacement of a specialist bin from a registered provider.
The allergy status of the patient must be checked with the prescribed treatment (including dressings, antiseptic solutions/wipes and plasters) prior to administration or supply.				

(Continued)

BOX 7.2	(CONTINUED)

Sufficient medication should be supplied where appropriate, to last until such time as the patient requires further clinical HCP review or is due to leave police custody.

The HCP should be informed promptly if the patient refuses medication and this must be recorded in the custody record by the custody staff. The HCP cannot require someone with the capacity to take medication; however, understanding whether the medication is critical or if the consequence of omission is important and may impact the management plan of an individual.

Medication for the patient to take home, or transferred with them to court or prison, will have local processes to support continuity of care but consider the risk of misuse and diversion. There will be occasions when medication is not used (e.g. because the patient is released or transferred), before a dose is due or a patient may refuse to take medication offered.

For clarity and to avoid claims of unauthorised use, the HCP should advise in each case what action is to be taken, with recording and disposal of the 'spare' medication. The police must record compliance on the custody record (medication form).

Options are:

- to be given to patient on release. This should include instructions regarding dosage

- to be given to escort service (travel with patient). This should include instructions, including information on the Person Escort Record (PER), regarding dosage and the prescriber should ensure appropriate instructions are included for the supervised self-administration of medication to patients, while in both the escort service and any future custodial service (e.g. courts, immigration centres)

- to be disposed of in a specialist pharmaceutical waste bin

HOLISTIC ASSESSMENT

Ensuring that safety underpins practice, competent staff will need to conduct high-quality assessments, identifying and communicating the monitoring and re-assessment needs. This includes considering mental capacity, identifying any relevant medical history, presenting complaints, and signs of intoxication or withdrawal is crucial.

As part of the risk assessment, the timing of arrest in relation to recent consumption of psychoactive substances, including alcohol, is a key factor in risk and includes monitoring for delayed drug effects. This should be a dynamic process as the clinical condition of an individual can change rapidly and may necessitate urgent interventions.

Intoxication and withdrawal can pose significant risks, including medical, psychiatric, and legal complications, and deaths in custody are often linked to substance misuse and alcohol dependency.

In order to ensure an accurate assessment and determination of the need for medical intervention, the following will be included:

- undertaking a competent holistic assessment of needs and risks, which includes ensuring key background information from the custody officer and other sources is considered

- ensuring the rights of the individual are respected, with particular attention to the issue of consent and thorough recording of decision-making

- providing equivalency of care to that of a person in the community, including appropriate prescribing

- ensuring continuity of necessary treatments and care

- maintaining good communication with relevant services and the police

HOW TO MANAGE PATIENT'S OWN MEDICINES

Patient safety is the overriding consideration for the administration of medicines. However, patients can expect to receive the same standard of clinical treatment given to someone not detained (see Box 7.3).

The HCP has a professional responsibility to conduct a relevant clinical assessment before the administration of any medication, including the patient's own medications. However, if it is clinically inappropriate, medication may be withheld, delayed, or adjusted (with prescriber authority).

Before providing medication to an individual under the influence of substances, including prescribed or illicit drugs and alcohol, a clinical risk assessment must be conducted. The interactions between these substances can increase the risk of oversedation and other serious harm.

BOX 7.3	STANDARD OF TREATMENT

'The standard of clinical treatment is expected is expected to be equivalent to that given to any person in a non-custodial setting'

Source: With permission of Royal College of General Practitioners (2018).

PGD'S OR PRESCRIBING IN CUSTODY

Independent prescribers may prescribe from a locally agreed formulary and within their scope of competence. Nurse-independent prescribers can prescribe any medication (within their competence), including unlicenced drugs and CDs in Schedules 2–5, whereas paramedic-independent prescribers are more constrained and are able to prescribe from a limited number of CDs.[1]

Other HCPs can authorise the supply or administration of a prescription-only medicine via other mechanisms such as PGDs. Local medicines policies may include PGDs. They are named individuals, specifically authorised for each PGD drawn up by the organisation.

The administration of medication under PGD cannot be delegated to another individual. For example, an HCP at one suite cannot authorise medication under PGD for the HCP at another station to administer. However, where medication is supplied via PGD, this then becomes the patient's own medication, for which self-administration can be delegated.

The HCP must be aware of these imitations and seek a further opinion where required. Different providers manage medicines through remote assessment, verbal orders and use of technology to provide medicines, so it is important to understand your local processes.

MANAGEMENT OF CONTROLLED DRUGS

The Police and Criminal Evidence Act 1984 (PACE) and the PACENI Code of Practice C state that police officers are prohibited from administering or supervising the self-administration of Schedule 2 and 3 CDs (Misuse of Drugs Regulations 2001). Patients may only self-administer these drugs under the direct supervision of an HCP. However, in Scotland, police can supervise the self-administration of some Schedule 3 drugs, excluding opioids (Police Scotland 2019).

HCP stocks of Schedule 2 and 3 CDs must be stored in accordance with the standards for CDs. Records for Schedule 2 drugs must be maintained in a Controlled Drug (CD) register. Although not legally required for other Schedule CDs, it is considered good practice to keep such records.

The destruction of CDs must be recorded in an appropriate register and witnessed by one of the following: a police officer, the provider company's Home Office Licence authorised responsible person (where applicable), or the authorised deputy of the Controlled Drugs Accountable Officer from the relevant NHS Regional Team (England), Health Board (Scotland), Health Board (Wales) or Department of Health (Northern Ireland). Each force area will have specific processes for managing patient-owned medications, such as methadone.

Anyone collecting Schedule 2 or 3 CDs from a pharmacy on behalf of a patient must have a process that includes the named individual authorising the third party to collect the medication on each occasion. This requirement applies to police officers collecting methadone or buprenorphine for individuals.

COMMON MEDICATIONS GIVEN IN CUSTODY

HCPs must be familiar with their own drug formulary. See Box 7.4 for a list of common medication. However, this will differ nationally. Further information is available in the relevant chapters on the management of medical conditions. Some medications are considered time critical (see Box 7.5).

Salbutamol and GTN are single-use items and, therefore, must be either given to the patient on release or disposed of in the pharmaceutical waste.

Borderline substances, such as food for intolerances and carbohydrate-appropriate food for diabetics, may be considered prescriptions for police custody and requested.

Renal impairment, hepatic impairment, palliative care, care of the elderly, pregnancy, breastfeeding and children all require consideration in relation to medicine (see Chapter 5 – Long-Term Management of Conditions).

ACCURACY OF DOCUMENTATION AND HOW TO RECORD ON POLICE SYSTEMS

For each medication, the HCP creates a new medication form in the HCP field of the person's custody record. This should include clear instructions about the type and amount of medication, how many times it can be administered and disposal instructions. This should also include any other recommendations such as take with food.

Medicines are an area where mistakes are made, so there is required a clear handover of medication to the police

BOX 7.4	COMMON CUSTODY MEDICATIONS
Emergency medicines	Oxygen, naloxone, adrenaline (anaphylaxis) and glucagon
Analgesia	Paracetamol as a minimum
Respiratory medicine	Salbutamol inhaler
Cardiovascular medicine	Glyceryl trinitrate spray (GTN) and aspirin
Minor illness	Antibiotic, antihistamine and antacid
Substance misuse	See local formulary, but dihydrocodeine typically forms part of the management of opioid dependency but varies across the four nations and providers.
Alcohol dependency	Benzodiazepine (typically chlordiazepoxide or diazepam)

---

[1] Morphine, diazepam, midazolam, lorazepam and codeine phosphate.

BOX 7.5	CRITICAL MEDICINES WHERE TIMELINESS OF ADMINISTRATION IS CRUCIAL TO PREVENT HARM FROM MISSED OR DELAYED DOSES

Area	Medicine
Cardiovascular system	Anticoagulants
	Nitrates
Respiratory system	Adrenoceptor agonists
	Antimuscarinic bronchodilators
	Adrenaline for allergic emergencies
Central nervous system	Antiepileptic drugs
	Drugs used in psychoses and related disorders
	Drugs used in Parkinsonism and related disorders
	Drugs used to treat substance misuse
Infections	As clinically indicated but especially antivirals, TB medication and other anti-infectives
Endocrine system	Corticosteroids
	Drugs used in diabetes
Obstetrics, gynaecology and urinary tract disorders	Emergency contraceptives
Malignant disease and immunosuppression	Drugs affecting the immune response
	Sex hormones and hormone antagonists in malignant disease – depot preparations
Nutrition and blood	Parenteral vitamins B and C
Eye	Corticosteroids and other anti-inflammatory preparations
	Local anaesthetics
	Mydriatics and cycloplegics
	Glaucoma treatment

Source: With permission of National Institute for Health and Care Excellence (NICE) (2016).

staff and custody staff, will also be required to keep accurate custody records of the medicines that have been self-administered, including those who have been declined.

INSTRUCTIONS FOR CUSTODY STAFF ON SUPERVISING MEDICATION SELF-ADMINISTRATION

The patient must be observed taking the medication to minimise the risk of hoarding.

The HCP may advise that some medications (e.g. asthma inhalers, angina sprays and topical creams) are retained by the patient (after checking to exclude tampering, concealed substances or other items capable of causing harm) within their cells. The HCP should consider the possible risk of harm (to self or others) with some devices.

Other medication should be left with the patient only on the advice of an HCP following clinical assessment.

There are differences of practice in relation to medicines, across providers and models of delivery such as embedded and non-embedded suites. Some areas use single doses and review as part of administration, whereas others approach the dispensing of medication, as a course with appropriate labelling.

Secondary dispensing however is not legal, this is where a medication that has already been dispensed into a container with a prescribed label to the individual, is then removed and placed into a new container. This is why patients own medication needs to remain in the original packaging.

It is clear that medicines are managed differently across the force areas. It is important to follow the policies and procedures of your organisation which will have been overseen by a pharmaceutical adviser and have a formal arrangement in place for the governance and the development of the infrastructure to support safe medicines handling, including the storage, prescription, supply and administration of medicines within the law.

There will be a clear communication process about each medication, changes to medication and lines of accountability clearly laid down in policies and procedures, including the handling of medicines and where medicines are supplied for supervised administration, ensuring they are labelled in line with legislation and professional guidance.

PRIVATE PRESCRIPTION

Most custody healthcare services are not NHS-commissioned and, therefore, will not have access to the typical FP10 prescription pad. Any prescription for medication will be charged at cost and not a national dispensing fee. There should be an agreement between police and healthcare providers as to who is responsible for meeting this cost.

Prescribers can write a prescription (with the exception of Schedule 2 and 3 CDs) on headed paper which contains the following details:

- The form must contain the prescriber identification and follow the BNF prescription requirements.

- Non-medical prescribers must have assessed the patient, albeit remote assessment would be considered appropriate.
- If needing to prescribe Schedule 2 or 3 CDs, independent prescribers will need their own individual prescribing pad (FP10PCD in England).

SCENARIO 7.2 Prescribing query

You are asked to see a 32-year-old female who has been arrested and will be remanded over the weekend for court. She has a history of injecting drugs, heroin dependency and bilateral deep-vein thrombosis. She is taking 20 mg rivaroxaban daily. She has no medication with her and states it cannot be collected.

1. *How do you approach this assessment?*
   a. *What factors will impact your decision?*

2. *What are the risks and benefits of:*
   a. *Getting prescribed?*
   b. *Not getting prescribed?*

3. *Outline the different options available and your rationale for choosing or not choosing that option.*

PATIENT SAFETY

Medicine management requires a robust and auditable trail, so at all points, it is clear where the responsibility and accountability of medicines lie and this system needs to be consistent and the same process followed regardless of how busy the custody is, or if the HCP is on site.

Incidents in relation to medicines should be reported through local incident reporting structures and analysed for themes. Adverse drug reactions should be reported to the Yellow Card scheme, online https://yellowcard.mhra.gov.uk/.

BEING HELPFUL, prevents clear ownership of tasks. Clinical incidents frequently occur when there is a lack of clarity of roles and responsibilities, so when medicines are handed over, the custody staff are then accountable, so follow your local processes to avoid errors occurring.

Regular audits should be undertaken in relation to medicines, including checking expiry dates, fridge monitoring temperature and room temperature.

CONTINUITY OF CARE INCLUDING PERSON ESCORT RECORD

The HCP may deem it necessary to provide medication for the patient to use at court, during transfer to prison, or upon release. This is especially crucial for critical medications required within the next 24 hours (e.g., insulin, antiepileptics and medications for substance use disorders). An appropriate record of treatment (including the name of the drug, dose, administration time, and by whom it was administered) should be recorded to ensure continuity of care if ongoing treatment is necessary. Although a police process, contributing to the PER can ensure best practice. The Royal Pharmaceutical Society guidance, 'Keeping patients safe when they transfer between care providers – getting the medicines right' can provide guidance (see Resources).

SCENARIO 7.3 Continuation of medication

Police are transferring a 56-year-old man with type 2 diabetes from Ipswich to Carlisle. He has been prescribed an intermediate-acting insulin, Humulin I, 34 units in the morning and 42 units in the evening. He will be due his evening dose about halfway through his journey.

1. *How do you approach this assessment?*
   a. *What factors will impact your decision?*

2. *What are the risks and benefits of:*
   a. *Instructing the police to supervise his insulin administration?*
   b. *Not instructing the police to supervise his insulin administration?*

3. *Outline the different options available and your rationale for choosing or not choosing that option.*

CONCLUSION

Medicine management is an area of forensic clinical practice that has legislative frameworks that underpin our practice and from which we will have professional consequences if we do not follow them.

In addition, police have legislative frameworks, approved professional practice and policies and protocols that identify how medicines can be managed in a police custody setting.

In addition, patient safety underpins clinical decision-making and guides evidence-based practice, ensuring that those in custody do not suffer adverse detriment from their detention and there is an equivalency of care.

Clinical decision-making is therefore critical. This requires robust recording of the decisions made, the medications prescribed, supplied, administered, self-administered and how they are stored, disposed of and the quality governance around practice.

1. Write a reflection about where you felt pressured, either by a patient or police staff, to authorise or supply a medication that you did not feel suitable. Include your attitude, thoughts and beliefs and consider how you responded to such pressure.

2. Prepare a table of commonly encountered critical medication for you and your colleagues. Include the risks and benefits of omission or administering.

3. Facilitate a group discussion around the legal and ethical implications of medicines management. Following the discussion, present a practice scenario where the group must collaboratively develop a plan for managing a patient's medication regimen, considering all legal, ethical, and health-related aspects.

RESOURCES

Online

- General Medical Council | Patients' fitness to drive and reporting concerns to the DVLA or DVA | https://www.gmc-uk.org/professional-standards/professional-standards-for-doctors/confidentiality---patients-fitness-to-drive-and-reporting-concerns-to-the-dvla-or-dva/patients-fitness-to-drive-and-reporting-concerns-to-the-dvla-or-dva

- Medicines and Healthcare products Regulation Agency | Patient group directions (PGD) | https://www.gov.uk/government/publications/patient-group-directions-pgds

- Royal College of General Practitioners | For advice on Safer Prescribing – RCGP Secure Environments | Safer prescribing in prisons | https://www.rcgp.org.uk/getmedia/400e7a75-7b46-4a24-8151-d3ea4a2cf5a1/SPiP-Final-v10-20-Email-Friendly.pdf

- Royal College of Nursing | Medicines management | https://www.rcn.org.uk/library/Subject-Guides/medicines-management

- Royal Pharmaceutical Society | Keeping patients safe when they transfer between care providers – getting the medicines right | https://www.rpharms.com/Portals/0/RPS%20document%20library/Open%20access/Publications/Keeping%20patients%20safe%20transfer%20of%20care%20report.pdf

- Specialist Pharmacy Service | An introduction to PGDs: definition and examples of use | https://www.sps.nhs.uk/articles/what-is-a-patient-group-direction-pgd/

Organisations

- British National Formulary | https://bnf.nice.org.uk

- Electronic medicines compendium | https://www.medicines.org.uk/emc

REFERENCES

Controlled Drugs (Supervision of Management and Use) Regulations (2006). *SI 2006/3148*. London: The Stationery Office.

Human Medicines Regulations (2012). *SI 2012/1916*. London: The Stationery Office.

Misuse of Drugs Regulations (2001). *SI 2001/3998*. London: The Stationery Office.

National Institute for Health and Care Excellence (2016). NICE guideline [NG57] Physical health of people in prison. https://www.nice.org.uk/guidance/ng57/chapter/recommendations#managing-medicines (accessed 10 January 2024).

Police Scotland (2019). Care and welfare of persons in police custody. https://www.scotland.police.uk/spa-media/0mfjn3pa/care-and-welfare-of-persons-in-police-custody-sop.pdf (accessed 21 November 2022).

Royal College of General Practitioners (2018). Equivalence of care in secure environments. https://www.rcgp.org.uk/representing-you/policy-areas/care-in-secure-environments (accessed 10 January 2024).

FURTHER READING

Department of Health | Drug misuse and dependence; UK guidelines on clinical management | https://assets.publishing.service.gov.uk/government/uploads/system/uploads/attachment_data/file/673978/clinical_guidelines_2017.pdf

Faculty of Forensic & Legal Medicine | Safe and secure administration of medication in police custody | https://fflm.ac.uk/wp-content/uploads/2023/02/Safe-and-Secure-Administration-of-Medication-in-Police-Custody-C-Cooke-and-J-Payne-James-Feb-2023.pdf

National Institute for Health and Care Excellence | Patient group directions | https://www.nice.org.uk/guidance/mpg2/evidence/full-guideline-pdf-4420760941

Royal College of Nursing | Medicines management | https://www.google. com/url?sa=t&rct=j&q=&esrc=s&source=web&cd=&ved=2ahUKE wjI7ZDk9dKDAxXdUUEAHZBcD1MQFnoECBsQAQ&url=https% 3A%2F%2Fwww.rcn.org.uk%2F-%2Fmedia%2Froyal-college-of-nursing%2Fdocuments%2Fpublications%2F2020%2Fjanuary%2 F009-018.pdf&usg=AOvVaw31NYb1rJ23v4BUvb43mqKF& opi=89978449

Royal Pharmaceutical Society | Safe and secure handling of medicines | https://www.rpharms.com/recognition/setting-professional-standards/ safe-and-secure-handling-of-medicines

Royal College of Psychiatrists and Faculty of Forensic & Legal Medicine | Detainees with substance use disorders in police custody: Guidelines for clinical management (fifth edition) | https://fflm.ac.uk/ wp-content/uploads/2020/12/college-report-cr227.pdf

Minor Illness

CHAPTER 8

Matthew Peel[1], Samantha Holmes[2], and Nick Skinner[2]

[1] Leeds Community Healthcare NHS Trust, Leeds, UK & UK Association of Forensic Nurses and Paramedics
[2] Leeds Community Healthcare NHS Trust, Leeds, UK

AIM

This chapter aims to provide readers with the knowledge and skills necessary to effectively identify, assess and manage minor illnesses in police custody, emphasising the importance of recognising when an individual may not be fit for detention.

LEARNING OUTCOMES

Upon completion of this chapter, readers should be able to:

- Define and identify minor illnesses in the context of police custody and differentiate them from more serious conditions

- Apply effective assessment techniques to determine the health status of individuals and recognise red flags indicating they are not fit for detention

- Implement best practice guidelines in the management and communication concerning individuals with minor illnesses

SELF-ASSESSMENT

1. Define what is a minor illness.

2. List three common minor illness conditions you see and outline the assessment and management along with any national guidelines or recommendations.

3. Antibiotic stewardship is a coordinated program promoting the appropriate use of antibiotics to improve patient outcomes and reduce antibiotic resistance. What role do custody healthcare professionals (HCPs) have in promoting the appropriate use of antibiotics and reducing antibiotic resistance?

INTRODUCTION

Those with minor illnesses typically remain fit to detain. It is beyond the scope of this text to cover all conditions. Instead, we offer an overview of some common complaints. The focus of managing any minor illness is being aware of and recognising the red flags, which point away from the condition being minor to major and needing a hospital referral. Amber flags indicate where additional treatment, referral or signposting may be indicated.

ASSESSMENT

HISTORY TAKING

In addition to the standard assessment outlined in Chapter 3 – Fitness Assessments, use the SOCRATES acronym for a detailed history of the presenting complaint (see Box 8.1).

Police Custody Healthcare for Nurses and Paramedics, First Edition. Edited by Matthew Peel, Jennie Smith, Vanessa Webb, and Margaret Bannerman.
© 2025 John Wiley & Sons Ltd. Published 2025 by John Wiley & Sons Ltd.
Companion website: www.wiley.com/go/policecustodyhealthcare

BOX 8.1	SOCRATES

Site or symptom	• Where is the pain?
	• What are the symptoms?
Onset	• Sudden? Gradual?
	• When did it first start?
	• Have they experienced this before?
Character	• Describe the pain or symptoms
	• Is it continuous or intermittent?
Radiation	• Does the pain go anywhere else?
Associations	• Any other associated signs or symptoms?
Time course	• Has the problem changed over time?
Exacerbating or relieving factors	• Does anything make them feel worse or better?
Severity	• On a scale of 1–10?

EXAMINATION

Complete a full set of observations and measure against the National Early Warning Score 2 (NEWS2) (if completed locally). Further examination will depend on the presenting complaint.

SAFETY NETTING

Safety netting is a strategy to manage minor illnesses, where patients are advised to monitor their symptoms and seek further review if they do not improve or worsen. In custody, safety netting advice should also be shared with the custody officer. Ensuring patients and custody staff know the potential risks associated with their condition and the importance of seeking further care if necessary.

HEADACHE

Headaches are a common complaint associated with various conditions ranging from stress to meningitis. There are many types of headaches; the most common in custody is likely tension-type headaches. The priority is ruling out red flags needing hospital (see Box 8.2).

Tension-type headaches present as tight or band-like headaches, occurring towards the end of the day or following a stressful event. They are common and can last between 30 minutes to several days. Examination is usually unremarkable, except for cranial or posterior cervical muscle spasm or tenderness. They respond well to simple analgesics.

BOX 8.2	HEADACHE RED AND AMBER FLAGS

Red flags

Refer to the hospital

- Blood pressure over 200/115 mmHg (or 140/90 mmHg if pregnant)
- Sudden onset severe headache (thunderclap)
- Drowsiness or altered conscious level (including confusion)
- Meningism: neck stiffness or photophobia
- Neurological symptoms: double vision, uncoordinated or sensory disturbance
- Persistent headache following head injury
- Red and painful eye

Amber flags

Advise GP follow-up

- New onset of headaches:
  - Aged over 50 years old or
  - History of cancer or HIV
- Worsening or persistent headaches

HISTORY

Ask about any history of:

- Nausea and vomiting
- Visual disturbance
- Photophobia
- Neck stiffness
- Fever
- Rash
- Head injury

EXAMINATION

Inspect the pupils for size, symmetry and reaction to light. Note the presence or absence of any rash (meningitis) or head injury.

MANAGEMENT

Typically, headaches remain fit to detain unless a red flag or other concern is noted. There is no need for routine Level 2: intermittent observations. Non-pharmacological approaches include reassurance, fresh air and relaxation techniques in addition to regular food and fluids (avoid caffeine). Offer simple analgesia, such as paracetamol or ibuprofen. For migraines consider high-dose aspirin (900 mg) or ibuprofen (800 mg) and prochlorperazine (5–10 mg). Alternatively, if available, administer their own medication, such as sumatriptan, promptly following onset.

TOOTHACHE

Poor dentition is common among those in custody. Toothache can be excruciating and distracting but rarely affects fitness to detain. However, severe pain may negatively impact their fitness to interview. There are numerous reasons for toothache, including broken or missing teeth, infections or dislodged fillings and crowns.

HISTORY

Has the individual seen a dentist? Are they already taking antibiotics? Deterioration in an individual already taking antibiotics is concerning.

EXAMINATION

Inspect the mouth, noting general dentition and any abscesses, broken or missing teeth. Note their ability to speak, swallow and open their mouth normally.

MANAGEMENT

Toothache, including dental abscesses, are typically fit to detain in the absence of red flags (see Box 8.3). Offer regular

BOX 8.3	TOOTHACHE RED AND AMBER FLAGS

Red flags

Refer to the hospital

- Difficulty swallowing, speaking or breathing
- Drooling
- Sepsis
- Limited mouth opening (trismus)
- Significant facial/neck swelling

Amber flags

Consider antibiotics if abscess and delayed access to dentist

- Diabetic
- Heart valve disease
- Immunocompromised

simple analgesia (paracetamol and ibuprofen). Opioids are not effective at alleviating toothache.

Individuals should be signposted to a dentist. Out-of-hours, or those without a dentist should contact 111 in England, Wales and Scotland. In Northern Ireland, see the Health and Social Care website 'Emergency Dental Treatment'.

Routine antibiotics are not recommended for dental abscesses. However, those with an amber flag, who cannot access timely dental treatment (i.e. those remaining in custody for several days), may require antibiotics. The first-line treatment is amoxicillin or metronidazole if penicillin allergy. Arrangements should be made to review after 3 days.

CHEST PAIN

Chest pain covers several conditions with various treatment options (see Box 8.4). The priority is to determine whether a hospital referral is necessary (see Box 8.5).

ABDOMINAL PAIN

The differential list for abdominal pain is wide and ranges from immediately life-threatening to benign. While most presentations will not be serious, HCPs must take a detailed history and examination.

HISTORY

Enquire about any previous surgical operations or previous similar episodes. Correlate the location of pain with likely differential (Box 8.6).

EXAMINATION

Measure blood glucose. Examine the abdomen for swelling, masses and tenderness. If able, note bowel sounds. Perform urinalysis using urine analysis test strips, and always test for pregnancy test in women of childbearing age.

MANAGEMENT

Management will depend on the history, presentation and examination. Those with suspected serious pathology or red flags (see Box 8.7) should be referred to the hospital. Non-concerning abdominal pain may be treated with simple analgesics. Abdominal cramps may benefit from an antispasmodic such as mebeverine. Finally, reflux symptoms may benefit from an antacid such as Gaviscon.

SCENARIO 8.1 Abdominal pain

You are asked to see a 30-year-old female who reports generalised abdominal pain, nausea and some diarrhoea. She is normally fit and well. She is a little tachycardic and her temperature is 37.5°C. She appears anxious but comfortable at rest and walking to the medical room.

1. *Outline your clinical history and examination.*

2. *Outline any tests to be performed in custody.*

3. *What is the most likely cause?*

4. *Outline your advice to the female and the police.*

DIZZINESS

Feeling dizzy, while commonly reported, is rarely serious. However, there are some serious conditions which such be excluded: hypotension, hypoglycaemia and arrhythmias. Other causes may be neurological or vestibular (inner ear). Most likely, dizziness in custody is related to anxiety or panic attacks.

HISTORY

It is important to establish what exactly individuals mean when they report feeling dizzy, the term can mean different things to different people.

BOX 8.5	CHEST PAIN RED AND AMBER FLAGS

Red flags

Refer to the hospital

- Suspected ACS
- Angina not relieved with GTN
- Suspected PE
- Suspected pneumothorax
- Significant chest trauma
- New hypoxia (SpO$_2$ < 94%)

Amber flags

Advise GP follow-up

- Worsening stable angina
- Pleurisy

BOX 8.4	CHEST PAIN DIFFERENTIALS

Acute coronary syndrome (ACS)	Including myocardial infarction and unstable angina, this is an emergency condition requiring immediate treatment and ambulance transport to hospital (see Chapter 19 - Emergencies)
Stable angina	A history of angina, chest pain is precipitated by exertion or stress presenting as a central, dull chest pain, and quickly relieved by glyceryl trinitrate (GTN). Individuals may remain fit to detain depending on the presentation and effectiveness of treatment (see Figure 8.1).
Pulmonary embolism (PE)	A clot in the pulmonary circulation can be life threatening. It commonly presents as breathing difficulties with localised chest pain (can often point to it with a finger), exacerbated with inhalation. It is associated with a history of deep vein thrombosis (DVT). Any suspected PE should be treated as an emergency and referred to hospital.
Pleurisy	Inflammation of the lung lining usually caused by a virus. It can be very painful, but is rarely serious and is managed with analgesia, most commonly non-steroidal anti-inflammatory drugs (NSAIDs).
Spontaneous pneumothorax	A collapse of one of the lungs, presenting with a sharp, unilateral chest pain, commonly at the apex of the lung, there may also be breathing difficulties. Suspected pneumothorax will require transport to hospital.
Respiratory tract infection	Upper respiratory tract infection An infection affecting the nose, throat, and sinuses. Commonly caused by viruses, such as the cold or flu, and resulting in symptoms like a runny nose, sore throat, and coughing. Treatment includes simple analgesics. Lower respiratory tract infection An infection affecting the lungs and bronchial tubes. It is more serious than upper respiratory tract infections and can lead pneumonia or bronchitis. Infections can be viral or bacterial, and symptoms often include shortness of breath, cough, and fever. Treatment may include antibiotics.
Musculoskeletal chest pain	Pain originating from the structures of the chest, such as the muscles, ribs, or cartilage. It is not related to the heart or lungs and is often reproducible by palpation or movement. Treatment involves analgesia.

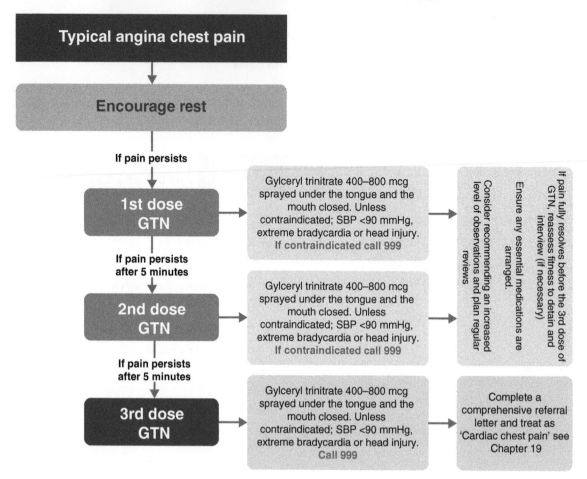

FIGURE 8.1   Angina chest pain management.

BOX 8.6	ABDOMINAL PAIN DIFFERENTIALS	

Right upper quadrant	**Epigastric**	**Left upper quadrant**
• Gallstones	• Gastro-oesophageal reflux disease	• Spleen rupture
• Cholangitis	• Perforated ulcer	
• Hepatitis	• Pancreatitis	
• Cardiac or pulmonary		
Right lumbar	**Umbilical**	**Left lumbar**
• Renal colic	• Appendicitis (early)	• Renal colic
• Pyelonephritis		• Pyelonephritis
• Ovarian pain		• Ovarian pain
Right lower quadrant	**Pelvic/lower abdomen**	**Left lower quadrant**
• Appendicitis	• Urinary retention	• Diverticulitis
• Crohn's disease	• Urine infection	• Ulcerative colitis
• Ectopic pregnancy	• Testicular torsion	• Constipation
• Renal colic		• Ectopic pregnancy
• Hernias		• Hernias
		• Renal colic
Generalised abdominal pain		
• Pancreatitis	• Bowel obstruction	
• Diabetic ketoacidosis	• Opioid withdrawal	
• Gastroenteritis	• Irritable bowel syndrome	

EXAMINATION

Measure a blood glucose level and note their current mental state. Note their gait on walking to and from the medical room.

BOX 8.7	ABDOMINAL PAIN RED AND AMBER FLAGS

Red flags

Refer to the hospital

- Severe pain
- Sudden onset testicular pain
- Upper abdominal or chest pain on exertion (angina)
- Fever or rigors
- Pregnant
- Urinary retention
- Appears unwell

Amber flags

Advice GP follow-up

- Losing weight (without dieting)
- Recurrent abdominal pain (over weeks)
- Rectal bleeding

MANAGEMENT

Individuals who walk to the medical room with a steady gait, looking well or appear anxious and whose dizziness settles with reassurance is reassuring. If dizziness is accompanied by any red flags (see Box 8.8) or symptoms appear cardiac or neurological (see Box 8.9), transfer to the hospital.

BOX 8.8	DIZZINESS RED AND AMBER FLAGS

Red flags

Refer to the hospital

- Neurological symptoms: double vision, uncoordinated or sensory disturbance
- Headache
- Recent head injury
- Chest pain or cardiac symptoms

Amber flags

Advise GP follow-up

- Family history of sudden adult cardiac death
- Low blood pressure (and taking antihypertensive medication)

BOX 8.9	CORRELATION OF SYMPTOMS AND LIKELY CAUSE

Symptom	Cardiac	Neurological	Anxiety	Presyncope
Nausea	+	+	±	+
Vomiting	+	+	±	±
Breathlessness	++	−	++	−
Palpitations	++	±	++	±
Chest pain/tightness	++	−	+	−
Tinnitus	±	+	+	+
Deafness/pressure in ears	−	+ (bilateral)	−	−
Difficulty speaking	−	+++	−	−
Greying or loss of vision	+	+	−	++
Double vision	−	++	−	−
Ataxia	−	+++	−	−
Pallor	++	−	−	++
Paraesthesia	−	++	+	±

Key: +++ Almost universal; ++ Very common; + Common; ± May be present; − Unlikely.

Source: Davison et al. (2009)/with permission of John Wiley & Sons.

TRANSIENT LOSS OF CONSCIOUSNESS (COLLAPSE)

It is not uncommon to see individuals who have suffered a transient loss of consciousness (TLOC). The most likely causes are syncope, psychogenic or factitious unresponsiveness (see Box 8.10) and are relatively benign. However, there are some serious conditions that can present with TLOC. Therefore, psychogenic or fictitious unresponsiveness can only be considered when all other conditions are excluded.

The leading cause of TLOC is syncope, a transient, self-limiting loss of consciousness, which resolves spontaneously. Syncope is typically associated with a vasovagal response, or postural hypotension and may be precipitated by some medications, dehydration, lack of diet, heat, pain or stress.

Psychogenic and factitious unresponsiveness both present identical; however, they are distinct. Psychogenic unresponsiveness is an unconscious manifestation of an individual's psychosocial distress and beyond their control (Posner et al. 2019). Factitious unresponsiveness refers to where an individual deliberately feigns being unconscious or unresponsive. In both, despite the appearance of unconsciousness, the individual is physiologically awake.

HISTORY

Eyewitness accounts are helpful. In addition, ask the individual:

- Do you remember falling?
- What happened during and after the event?

EXAMINATION

Record a blood glucose level. Inspect the pupils for size, symmetry and reaction to light. Check limb tone and response to pain. Consider lying and standing blood pressure. If able, review any CCTV footage of the collapse.

MANAGEMENT

Syncope, psychogenic and factitious unresponsiveness will typically remain fit to detain, assuming no red flags (see Box 8.11).

Syncope

Once recovered, identify triggers and attempt to mitigate them. This may include offering food, increasing fluids or encouraging rest. It may be appropriate to briefly increase the level of observations and additional CCTV monitoring.

BOX 8.10   SIGNS AND SYMPTOMS

Syncope	Psychogenic or factitious unresponsiveness
Symptoms	*Symptoms*
• Brief loss of consciousness	• Usually, a history of recent emotional upset
• Resolves spontaneously	• May have history of anxiety or personality disorder
• Occurs shortly after standing or having been stood up a long time	*Signs*
• Occurs during or following a painful or emotional event	• Eyes are usually closed
• Prodromal symptoms (feeling like they are going to pass out)	• Does not withdraw to painful stimuli
Signs	• May hold breath or hyperventilate
• Sweating	• Normal vital signs and good colour
• Pallor	• Resists eye-opening
• Hypotension	• Bell's phenomenon (eyes deviate upwards when opened against resistance)
	• No resistance to passive movements of limbs, normal tone

Source: Adapted from Posner et al. (2019).

BOX 8.11   TRANSIENT LOSS OF CONSCIOUSNESS (COLLAPSE) RED FLAGS

Red flags

Refer to the hospital

- Sudden onset or only brief prodromal symptoms
- Sudden onset palpitations followed by collapse
- Family history of sudden adult cardiac death
- TLOC preceded by chest pain, abdominal pain or headache
- History of heart disease
- New breathlessness
- Confusion
- Neurological deficit
- Incontinence
- Lateral tongue biting

Psychogenic Unresponsiveness and Factitious Disorder

It is important to remain calm and compassionate; any antagonising by the HCP, or the police will only serve to prolong the condition. Instead, individuals should be moved to a private area where the spotlight can be taken off them. HCPs should recommend an increased level of observation, make frequent checks and be willing to reconsider their working impression.

SCENARIO 8.2	Transient loss of consciousness

A 35-year-old male with generalised anxiety disorder collapses. Sitting in his cell talking to an officer, he suddenly 'fell' forward to the floor and remained motionless. An officer was with him in his cell because he repeatedly voiced an intent to self-harm. He has been in custody for 2 hours. The HCP notes:

- *A – Own, no tongue biting*
- *B – Breathing well, SpO$_2$ 99%, rate 17 min*
- *C – HR 79 min, normal blood pressure, warm and well perfused, dry*
- *D – Eyes screwed shut, rolls eyes upward when opened. Blood glucose 5.6 mmol/l*
- *E – No evidence of external trauma (no head/facial injury)*

1. *What is the likely cause for this collapse?*
2. *What other causes are likely?*
3. *Outline your management of this scenario.*

COLD AND FLU-LIKE ILLNESSES (INCLUDING COVID-19)

Cold and flu typically occur seasonally during the winter months; the symptoms are similar (Box 8.12) but typically more severe with flu (Box 8.13). In the absence of any significant past medical history, individuals will typically recover well and remain fit to detain. However, some conditions can present as flu-like, including urinary tract infections, sepsis and mastitis. Additionally, HCPs should be mindful of those who may have recently travelled overseas.

COVID-19 (severe acute respiratory syndrome coronavirus 2) caused a worldwide pandemic in 2020. Despite initial lockdowns and restrictions, in May 2023, it was no longer considered a global health emergency. However, there is still a risk from new variants. There is no requirement at present to test or isolate if COVID-19 is suspected. For most, the symptoms will resolve over a few days or weeks. However, as with cold and flu, those most at risk are the pregnant, elderly and immunocompromised or with long-term conditions.

BOX 8.12	SIGNS AND SYMPTOMS

- Blocked or runny nose
- Sore throat
- Cough
- Sneezes
- Headache
- Muscle aches
- Pyrexia
- Pressure in ears and face
- Loss of taste and smell
- Fatigue
- Loss of appetite
- Diarrhoea
- Abdominal pain
- Nausea and vomiting

BOX 8.13	DIFFERENTIATING BETWEEN COLD AND FLU-LIKE ILLNESS

Cold	Flu-like illness
• Gradual onset	• Sudden onset
• Mainly affects nose and throat	• Affects more than just the nose and throat
• Not too unwell to go to work	• Exhaustion, too unwell to go to work

HISTORY

Enquire if they have been around anyone else with a similar illness.

EXAMINATION

Look for any alternative sources of infection (sepsis) or rashes (meningitis).

MANAGEMENT

Unless very unwell, most will be fit to detain (see Box 8.14). Advise individuals to stay hydrated and rest. Paracetamol and ibuprofen can help with fevers and aches and pains. Individuals may bring in their own decongestant medication.

SKIN INFECTIONS

Skin infections are a common complication following any injury breaking the skin surface, caused by bacteria or other microorganisms entering the skin and multiplying, resulting in inflammation and other symptoms.

All individuals are susceptible to skin infections. However, individuals with weakened immune systems, diabetes or who inject drugs are at an increased risk. Skin infections include cellulitis, erysipelas and abscesses (see Box 8.15).

BOX 8.15	WOUND INFECTIONS

Cellulitis	Cellulitis is one of the most common types of skin infections. The skin and subcutaneous tissue become inflamed and infected, usually due to bacteria such as streptococci or staphylococci. Cellulitis can affect any body area but is most common in the legs.
Erysipelas	Erysipelas affects the superficial layers of the skin, the epidermis and the dermis, and is usually caused by streptococci. Erysipelas can overlap with cellulitis; therefore, it is not always possible to differentiate between the two.
Abscess	Abscesses are an encapsulation of pus that occurs within the dermis and subcutaneous layers. They can occur anywhere on the body. However, they most commonly develop on the groin, buttocks, axillae and extremities.

HISTORY

Check the time course. A rapid onset and spreading infection may suggest necrotising fasciitis. Enquire about any recent antibiotics.

EXAMINATION

Look for any signs of sepsis. Cellulitis and erysipelas present as erythema (redness), warmth, swelling and pain around the site. There may be some blistering of the skin, and individuals may complain of malaise, fatigue and fever. Abscesses present similar but will have a painful collection of pus, which may appear as a lump. The lump should be fluctuant, meaning it is wave-like or boggy. Small abscesses may drain naturally, but large abscesses may require surgical drainage.

MANAGEMENT

Good wound care is vital to prevent the spread of infection and promote healing. Wounds should be cleaned and dressed. If necessary, offer analgesia. Mark the affected area with a single-use surgical marker pen to monitor any changes. Occasionally, individuals will require hospital (see Box 8.16).

Consider offering antibiotics, especially to those being held in custody for over 24 hours, or who are unlikely to engage with healthcare services when released. For adults, the first choice is flucloxacillin 500 mg–1 g four times a day for 5–7 days (unless penicillin allergy) (National Institute for Health and Care Excellence 2019). While in custody, review at least daily.

BOX 8.16	SKIN INFECTION RED AND AMBER FLAGS

Red flags

Refer to the hospital

- Facial or orbital cellulitis
- Evidence of sepsis
- Appears unwell
- Confusion or altered mental state
- Necrotising fasciitis
- Osteomyelitis
- Septic arthritis
- Unable to tolerate oral medication

Amber flags

Advise urgent GP follow-up

- Not responding to antibiotics after 2–3 days

CHRONIC LEG ULCERS

An ulcer is a partial or complete loss of the epidermis. Chronic leg ulcers are a break in the skin below the knee persisting for more than 6 weeks. They are believed to affect 1% of the adult population and 3.6% of over 65-year-olds.

Ulceration is differentiated as venous or arterial. Arterial ulcers develop due to reduced arterial flow caused by peripheral arterial disease. Venous leg ulcers develop due to vein incompetence, leading to venous hypertension. People who smoke, inject drugs, are obese, or diabetes, are at increased risk of leg ulcers.

Typically, in custody, chronic leg ulcers are most prevalent among people who inject drugs. People who inject drugs have many risk factors for developing chronic venous insufficiency, due to damage of superficial veins through repeated trauma and thrombophlebitis. Chronic venous insufficiency and subsequent venous hypertension are the main causative factors for developing venous ulceration.

HISTORY

Ascertain how long the patient has had the ulcer and any symptoms of venous insufficiency, such as pain, swelling, pitting oedema, heaviness, aching, itchiness, or skin changes (hyperpigmentation, venous eczema and lipodermatosclerosis). Identify any other causes of ulceration or delayed wound healing, including co-morbidities (diabetes, rheumatoid arthritis, deep vein thrombosis or immobility) or the use of certain medication (nicorandil, corticosteroids, nonsteroidal anti-inflammatory drugs and anticoagulants).

EXAMINATION

Assess the site, size and depth of the ulcer, the appearance of the wound bed and border, and any exudate present.

MANAGEMENT

Chronic leg ulcers rarely require urgent medical attention unless the underlying aetiology is compromised, see Box 8.17. Most leg ulcers are not clinically infected but are colonised with bacteria. Antibiotics are only required where there are signs of infection.

It is important that HCPs working in custody take opportunities to provide wound care and reinforce the importance of regular wound care. While a single dressing in custody will not heal the ulcer, it may help prevent deterioration and further complications.

BOX 8.17   **CHRONIC LEG ULCERS RED AND AMBER FLAGS**

Red flags

Refer to the hospital

- Evidence of sepsis
- Appears unwell
- Necrotising fasciitis
- Limb threatening ischaemia
- Suspected new deep vein thrombosis

Amber flags

Advise urgent GP follow-up

- Suspected skin cancer

SCENARIO 8.3   Leg ulcers

A homeless man, who is known to inject heroin, is brought into custody. They have a large, untreated ulcer on the lower leg, which they have had for many years and is not dressed regularly. The wound has a noticeable foul smell and is discharging pus. They are reluctant to see the HCP and would prefer to go to sleep. The HCP notices they look unwell and feel clammy, although their pulse is 89 minutes and blood pressure 109/67. They look a little drowsy but can report opioid withdrawal symptoms. Their temperature is 35.1°C.

1. *Outline your assessment and management.*

2. *Is the individual fit to detain?*
   a. *What is your rationale?*

3. *What is your clinical impression?*

BACK PAIN

Back pain is a common condition characterised by discomfort or pain in the back, from the neck to the hips and affects up to 80% of adults at some point. Most cases are not serious and can be managed with exercise, physical therapy and analgesia. However, it is important not to miss serious conditions, such as renal colic, abdominal aortic aneurysm, pancreatitis, or cauda equina syndrome (see Box 8.18). The most common cause of back pain is muscle strain or sprain, caused by poor posture, overuse or sudden movements, with pain typically localised to the lower back or lumbar

<table>
<tr><td>

BOX 8.18

</td><td>

BACK PAIN RED AND AMBER FLAGS

</td></tr>
</table>

Red flags

Refer to the hospital

- Altered sensation in the genital area
- Bladder or bowel disturbance
- Severe sudden onset with abdominal pain or leg discolouration
- Severe sudden onset with tenderness over the vertebra
- Recent trauma, such as a fall or motor vehicle accident

Amber flags

Advise GP follow-up

- Severe back pain
- Sciatica not resolving for over 3 weeks
- Aged under 20 years or over 50 years

region, which can be mild to severe. Back pain is often exacerbated by stress and anxiety.

Sciatica is another common cause of back pain characterised by numbness, or tingling in the lower back, buttocks and legs, usually on one side of the body. It is typically caused by compression or irritation of the sciatic nerve, a large nerve running from the lower back down to the feet. Treatment typically involves a combination of rest, physical therapy, stretching and analgesia.

Cauda equina syndrome is a rare but serious condition where the nerves at the bottom of the spinal cord become compressed or damaged. Leading to severe lower back pain, incontinence, numbness or tingling in the buttocks or genital area, and weakness or numbness in one or both legs. It is a medical emergency requiring immediate hospital referral.

HISTORY

Be sure to ask about any recent trauma (i.e. fall or road traffic incident), altered saddle sensation (numbness or tingling around the groin, buttocks and perineum) or bladder or bowel disturbance.

EXAMINATION

Note the individual's gait as they enter the medical room. In the event of trauma, palpate the spinal processes for tenderness.

MANAGEMENT

Non-pharmacological approaches include offering reassurance and encouraging gentle exercise. Where an individual is already prescribed medication for chronic back pain, efforts should be made to continue this. Unless contraindicated, simple analgesia such as paracetamol and ibuprofen should be offered, if necessary, consider additional codeine.

DRUG REACTIONS

Drug reactions involving the skin can range from mild rashes to severe, life-threatening conditions (see Chapter 19 – Emergencies). In custody, recognising these reactions early can be crucial, as individuals may be exposed to a variety of medications, either as part of their pre-existing treatment plans or through substance misuse. Reactions can manifest in various ways, including simple rashes, hives (urticaria), fixed drug eruptions, Stevens–Johnson syndrome and toxic epidermal necrolysis. The severity of these reactions can vary significantly, from minor irritations that resolve with discontinuation of the offending drug to severe conditions requiring immediate medical intervention.

HISTORY

Assess the severity and identify the causative agent, including a thorough history of all medications, including prescription drugs, over-the-counter medications, and any new drugs administered, including those administered while in custody.

<table>
<tr><td>

BOX 8.19

</td><td>

DRUG REACTIONS RED AND AMBER FLAGS

</td></tr>
</table>

Red flags

Refer to the hospital

- Extensive, rapidly progressing rash
- Mucosal involvement
- Severe pain
- Respiratory symptoms or systemic symptoms

Amber flags

Advise GP follow-up

- Mild blistering
- Persistent rash
- Mild systemic symptoms

EXAMINATION

Examine any rashes, inspecting the mouth and mucosal areas. Look for any signs of respiratory distress or shock.

MANAGEMENT

For mild reactions, discontinue the suspected drug, if possible. If the medication is essential, consider the risks and benefits of discontinuing and advise them to see their GP urgently. Provide symptomatic relief, such as antihistamines for itching. Monitor closely for any signs of progression to more severe reactions (see Box 8.19).

CONCLUSION

Managing minor illnesses in custody is a complex task that demands a comprehensive set of skills, knowledge, and experience from HCPs. This chapter underscores the critical importance of being vigilant about "red flags" signalling a condition may not be minor but instead requires immediate medical attention and hospital referral. The key to effective management lies in the ability to differentiate minor ailments from major. Given the range of conditions that can present as minor illnesses, from headaches to abdominal pain HCPs would benefit from ongoing minor illness continuing professional development.

LEARNING ACTIVITIES

1. Write a reflection where you assessed and treated a minor illness.

2. Develop a resource to sign-post patients to local health service resources, such as urgent treatment centres, emergency departments, 111 (or similar) and walk-in centres, along with their opening times.

3. Research, prepare and deliver a presentation to your colleagues about a specific minor illness. Include a background to the condition, the assessment (history and examination) and treatment options.

RESOURCES

Online

- NICE Clinical Knowledge Summaries | www.cks.nice.org.uk
- Syncopedia | www.syncopedia.org

Organisations

- NHS 111 Online (England) | https://111.nhs.uk
- NHS 111 Wales (Wales) | https://111.wales.nhs.uk
- NHS 24 (Scotland) | https://111.wales.nhs.uk
- Health and Social Care (Northern Ireland) | https://online.hscni.net

REFERENCES

Davison, S. (2009). Dizziness. In: *ABC of Emergency Differential Diagnosis* (ed. F. Morris and A. Fletcher), 41–47. Oxford: Blackwell Publishing.

National Institute for Health and Care Excellence (2019). Cellulitis and erysipelas: antimicrobial prescribing. https://www.nice.org.uk/guidance/ng141/resources/visual-summary-pdf-6908401837 (accessed 29 October 2023).

Posner, J.B., Saper, C.B., Schiff, N.D., and Claassen, J. (2019). Psychogenic Unresponsiveness. In: *Plum and Posner's Diagnosis and Treatment of Stupor and Coma* (ed. J.B. Posner, C.B. Saper, N.D. Schiff, and J. Claassen), 291–304. Oxford: Oxford University Press.

FURTHER READING

Morris, F., Wardrope, J., and Ramlakhan, S. (ed.) (2014). *Minor Injury and Minor Illness at a Glance*. Oxford: Wiley-Blackwell.

CHAPTER 9

Minor Injuries

Jennie Smith

Mitie Care and Custody Health Ltd, London, UK & UK Association of Forensic Nurses and Paramedics

---

AIM

This chapter aims to furnish the reader with an overview of the more common minor injuries faced by the custody practitioner. It will provide the knowledge and skills necessary to effectively identify, assess and manage minor injuries in police custody. It will also emphasise the importance of recognising when an individual is not fit for detention.

LEARNING OUTCOMES

By the end of this chapter, readers should be able to:

- Identify minor injuries and recognise what is and is not treatable in the context of police custody

- Apply effective assessment skills to be able to recognise and diagnose a wide range of differing injuries

- Implement an appropriate symptom scale into their practice to ensure that a thorough history is achieved

SELF-ASSESSMENT

1. Outline the different classifications of burns, their different characteristics and management.

2. Outline the Ottawa ankle rules.

3. Review your knowledge around current wound care options in their service and ensure team colleagues are aware.

INTRODUCTION

Whether an injury renders an individual unfit for detention is decided on a case-by-case basis. It is impossible to cover all eventualities in one chapter; however, working from head to toe, we shall endeavour to discuss the most common. A key feature of these assessments is the ability of the healthcare professionals (HCPs) to recognise, assess and manage the clinical picture presented. It is also pertinent to understand the limitations of treatment in custody and understand when a referral to an outside healthcare provider is appropriate.

ASSESSMENT

HISTORY TAKING

It has long been established the diagnosis of most conditions lies in history. This has been covered in other chapters. But it is suffice to state obtaining a clear history is vital. This should include the circumstances around the mechanism of the injury, the involvement of any weapons, any force, or other implements and healthcare input, if any, the individual may have received since sustaining the injury and before arrival

Police Custody Healthcare for Nurses and Paramedics, First Edition. Edited by Matthew Peel, Jennie Smith, Vanessa Webb, and Margaret Bannerman.
© 2025 John Wiley & Sons Ltd. Published 2025 by John Wiley & Sons Ltd.
Companion website: www.wiley.com/go/policecustodyhealthcare

into custody. Once a clear understanding of the history has been obtained, the HCP can move on to examining the patient. Different mnemonics are utilised for history taking, such as SOCRATES, discussed in more detail in Chapter 8 – Minor Illness. These can help gain a comprehensive history and also help characterise the presenting symptoms clearly.

EXAMINATION

The examination will vary depending on the injury presented. It is important HCPs use a range of skills during their examination. Examples would include palpation, assessing power, tone, sensation and range of movement in limb and joint injuries. Looking for other symptoms, including altered vision in head injuries. We shall look at these in more depth throughout the chapter.

SAFETY NETTING

Safety netting provides patients with a clear strategy for managing their injuries post-treatment and post-release from custody. By advising the patient to seek further assessment with any new, worsening or non-resolving symptoms associated with their injury, their responsibilities for their own healthcare are clear. Providing the custody staff with the same safety netting information they are able to understand the risks associated with any detained person in their care.

HEAD INJURY

Head injuries are commonplace in the custody population due to the high level of associated violence. Head injuries are a significant concern in police custody settings due to their potential for severe complications, including traumatic brain injury (TBI). According to the National Institute for Health and Care Excellence (NICE) (2023), over 1 million people attend Emergency Departments (EDs) annually in England and Wales for head injuries. In custody settings, these injuries can occur during arrest, physical restraint, altercations or even accidental falls.

ASSESSMENT

The comprehensive assessment of head injuries is vital in any situation, but more so in the custody environment, given the individual will then potentially be placed in a cell and monitored by non-healthcare detention staff. A thorough and methodical approach to the assessment will benefit the patient, the HCP and the custody staff.

Firstly, a detailed history of the events leading to the head injury should be sought. If the patient is intoxicated or under the influence of a substance, then seek out the arresting officer and see what details they can add. History should include:

1. age of the patient – risk and outcomes change in the over 65-year-olds

2. current medications – particularly anticoagulant medications can be problematic

3. mechanism of injury – was it dangerous? A fall from height, was it caused by a weapon? Has it caused any associated neck pain or loss of consciousness?

A comprehensive assessment is essential for diagnosing the severity and implications of a head injury. Key elements include:

1. **History**: Age, current medications and anticoagulants can be particularly problematic. Any dangerous mechanism of injury and neck pain or loss of consciousness.

2. **Visual inspection**: Look for signs of trauma such as lacerations, bruising, or swelling.

3. **Consciousness level**: Different scales like the Glasgow Coma Scale (GCS), see Box 9.1, or the ACVPU are the obvious choice to assess the individual's level of consciousness.

4. **Pupil reaction**: Check for unequal or non-reactive pupils, which could indicate increased intracranial pressure. Check both pupils are the same size. Ask the patient if they are normally the same size, though they may not know the answer.

5. **Neurological signs**: Assess for focal neurological deficits, such as weakness or numbness in limbs, which could indicate a more severe injury.

6. **Signs of skull fracture**: Look for 'raccoon eyes' (bruising around the eyes) or 'Battle's sign' (bruising behind the ears).

BOX 9.1	GLASGOW COMA SCALE
Eyes (Best eye-opening response)	4 – Open spontaneously 3 – Open to speech 2 – Open to pain 1 – No response
Verbal (Best verbal response)	5 – Orientated to time, place and person 4 – Confused 3 – Inappropriate words 2 – Incomprehensible sounds 1 – No response
Motor (Best motor response)	6 – Obeys commands 5 – Moves to localised pain 4 – Flex to withdraw from pain 3 – Abnormal flexion 2 – Abnormal extension 1 – No response

7. **General symptoms**: Ask the patient about any changes to their vision, blurred or double vision, any nausea or vomiting, any persistent headache, loss of consciousness or seizure activity.

Certain situations in custody pose a higher risk for head injuries; these would include:

1. **Use of force**: Excessive force during arrest or restraint can lead to head injuries.

2. **Altercations**: Physical fights can result in blows to the head.

3. **Intoxication**: Patients under the influence may have impaired judgment and coordination, increasing the risk of accidental injury.

MANAGEMENT

Once a head injury is suspected or confirmed:

1. **Immediate monitoring**: Monitor vital signs and level of consciousness.

2. **Pain management**: Administer analgesics as per your clinical guidelines, avoiding those that could mask neurological symptoms.

3. **Referral**: Any patient with a suspected significant head injury should be immediately referred to the ED for imaging and further assessment.

4. **Documentation**: Thoroughly document your findings, actions, and the patient's condition in both the custody and medical records.

5. **Monitoring in cell**: Recommend at minimum police observation at Level 2 –intermittent observations every 30 minutes.

6. **Safety netting**: Advise the patient to let custody staff know if they have any new, worsening or non-resolving symptoms during their custody stay.

SCENARIO 9.1   Head injury

You are asked to see a 27-year-old with a head injury. He was arrested at 02:37 while he was heavily drunk. He was hit on the head with a bottle of wine. He was not referred to the HCP overnight. It is now 09:02, and he reports a headache and vomited twice. He feels 'terrible' but thinks it is due to a 'hangover'.

1. *Outline how you approach the assessment.*

2. *Outline how you manage this scenario.*

CERVICAL SPINE INJURIES

Cervical spinal injuries, although rare, can have devastating consequences if not promptly identified and managed. In the context of police custody healthcare, these injuries can occur during arrest, restraint, or even in-cell accidents. The stakes are high; failure to diagnose and treat can lead to permanent disability or even death. In a 2008 study of over 200,000 patients looking at the incidence of cervical spine injury following trauma found, only 3.7% had cervical spine damage (Milby et al. 2008). This was even lower in those alert and sober (2.9%) but quite a dramatic increase to 7.7% in those intoxicated or unconscious (Milby et al. 2008). A cohort of patients often encountered in custody.

ASSESSMENT

The initial assessment is crucial and should be conducted as per the NICE (2016) guidelines. The Canadian C-spine rules are a helpful tool to assess cervical spine injury as high, low or no risk, see Box 9.2.

1. **Focal neurological deficits**: Look for any signs of weakness, numbness, or tingling in the arms or legs.

2. **Midline spinal tenderness**: Gently palpate the midline of the neck to check for tenderness, which could indicate a potential fracture or dislocation.

3. **Altered consciousness**: Assess the patient's level of consciousness. Any alteration could be a sign of a more severe injury.

4. **Intoxication**: Always consider the level of intoxication, as it can mask symptoms.

5. **Distracting injuries**: Other injuries can distract from neck pain, making it essential to assess the entire patient.

In a custody setting, it is essential to consider factors like intoxication or agitation, which could mask or mimic symptoms. Always err on the side of caution; if in doubt, immobilise the cervical spine.

High-Risk

Certain situations pose a higher risk for cervical spinal injuries:

1. **Age**: Being over 65 years increases the risk of cervical spine injury.

2. **Dangerous mechanism of injury**: Falls from a height, axial load to the head (e.g. diving into a pool), road traffic accidents, or any form of high-impact trauma require immediate attention.

3. **Use of force**: Any use of force during arrest or restraint that impacts the neck area should raise suspicion.

4. **Pre-existing conditions**: Patients with pre-existing conditions like osteoporosis are at higher risk.

BOX 9.2	CANADIAN C-SPINE RULE

High risk

The person is high risk if there is **ONE** of the following:

- ≥65 years
- A dangerous mechanism
  - Fall from elevation >3 feet (or 5 stairs)
  - Axial load to the head (e.g. diving injury)
  - High-speed motor vehicle collision (e.g. rollover and ejection)
  - Motorised recreational vehicles
  - Bicycle collision
- Paraesthesia in arms or legs

If high-risk immobilise the c-spine and refer to the Emergency Department

↓ If no high-risk features continue ↓

Low risk

The person is low risk if there is **ONE** of the following:

- Simple rear-end motor vehicle collision
  - Excludes being hit by a high-speed vehicle, a large vehicle (e.g. bus), or a rollover
- Able to sit
- Ambulatory at any time since the injury
- Delayed onset of neck pain
- No midline C-spine tenderness

The person remains at **low risk** if they are:

- Unable to actively rotate their neck 45° to the left and right (the range of the neck can only be assessed safely if the person is at low risk and there are no high-risk factors).

The person has **no risk** if they:

- Have **one** of the above low-risk factors **and** are able to actively rotate their neck 45° to the left and right.

If low-risk and unable to rotate neck 45° immobilise the c-spine and refer to the Emergency Department

↓ If no low-risk features continue ↓

No risk

Source: Adapted from NICE (2016).

MANAGEMENT

Management in custody is primarily about stabilisation and referral. If a cervical spinal injury is suspected:

1. **Immediate immobilisation**: According to NICE (2016), if you suspect a cervical spine injury, you must protect the spine with immobilisation and avoid moving the remainder of the spine. Use a cervical collar (if available) or manual in-line spinal immobilisation, especially during any airway intervention.

2. **Pain management**: Administer appropriate analgesics as per your clinical guidelines.

3. **Referral**: Immediate transfer to the ED is mandatory for imaging and further assessment.

4. **Documentation**: Thoroughly document your findings, actions and the patient's condition in both the custody and medical records.

HAND, WRIST AND FINGER INJURIES

Hand, wrist and finger injuries are among the most common complaints in police custody healthcare. These injuries can occur during arrest, restraint, or even altercations between patients. The implications can range from minor discomfort to severe functional impairment.

Hand and wrist injuries account for 10–30% of all ED attendances, a statistic that underscores the importance of proper assessment and management in custody settings (Robinson and O'Brien 2019).

ASSESSMENT

A thorough examination is crucial for diagnosing the type and extent of the injury. Here are some key elements to consider:

1. **Visual inspection**: Look for deformities, swelling, or discolouration. Dinner fork shape which can indicate Colles' fracture or the reverse in a Smiths fracture. Bearing in mind the swelling associated with Colles' can, in rare cases, cause compartment syndrome.

2. **Range of motion**: Ask the patient to flex and extend the fingers and wrist. Limited or painful movement can indicate fractures or ligament injuries (see Figure 9.1).

3. **Sensory and motor function**: Check for numbness, tingling or weakness, which could indicate nerve damage.

4. **Palpation**: Gently palpate the injured area to identify any point tenderness, which could suggest a fracture or dislocation.

High-Risk Injuries

Certain situations pose a higher risk for hand, wrist and finger injuries:

1. **Use of handcuffs**: Incorrect application can lead to nerve compression or fractures.

2. **Altercations**: Physical fights can result in injuries like Boxer's fractures or dislocations.

3. **Pre-existing conditions**: Conditions like rheumatoid arthritis can exacerbate the impact of any new injury.

Boxer's fracture These fractures are characterised by swelling, pain, deformity and bony tenderness over the fifth

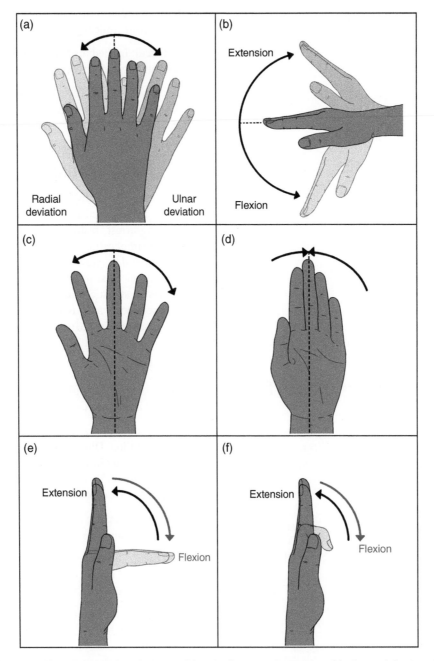

FIGURE 9.1 Range of motion. (a) Radial and ulnar deviation. (b) Wrist flexion and extension. (c) Finger abduction. (d) Finger adduction. (e) Metacarphophalangealflexion and extension. (f) Interphalangeal flexion and extension.

metacarpal. The patient may be unable to fully extend their little finger, there may be a lag in the finger and some rotation on flexion. Make sure a comparison of both hands is conducted and also check if there is any historical injury. Also, be aware of any wounds to the area caused by teeth, as these tend to lead to infections and should be treated with antibiotics prophylactically.

Scaphoid fracture The scaphoid bone is one of the small bones in the hand around the wrist. It is located at the base of the thumb and is often fractured by falling onto an outstretched hand. It is not always immediately obvious on x-ray but can create tenderness on examination of the 'anatomical snuffbox' region at the base of the thumb. As this bone is unlikely to heal on its own and can create future problems, treatment is key. Treatment is usually immobilisation with a cast and a follow-up X-ray or MRI after a couple of weeks. Getting the correct treatment in a timely fashion is important, so it must be considered in custody.

MANAGEMENT

Once an injury is suspected or confirmed:

1. **Immediate immobilisation**: Use splints or bandages to immobilise the injured area.

2. **Pain management**: Administer analgesics as per clinical guidelines.

3. **Wound care**: If there are open wounds, clean and dress them appropriately.

4. **Referral**: For severe injuries, immediate referral to the ED or a hand specialist is crucial.

5. **Documentation**: Thoroughly document your findings, actions, and the patient's condition in both the custody and medical records.

SCENARIO 9.2 Hand injury

You are asked to see a 27-year-old male with a hand injury. He has punched the door in his cell and reports sudden pain. The injury happened only a few minutes ago. There is some minor redness on the right hand, but no obvious deformity or swelling. Some minor abrasions are noted to the knuckles of the right hand. The hand is generally tender all over; there is no specific bony tenderness. They are upset, distressed and report they cannot move their hand or fingers at all.

1. *Outline your approach to this assessment.*

2. *Outline your management.*

JOINT DISLOCATIONS

Joint dislocations are relatively uncommon but can be extremely painful and debilitating when they occur. In police custody settings, these injuries can happen during arrest and the use of handcuffs or other physical restraint, altercations with police or other individuals or even road traffic collisions. The unique environment of police custody makes timely diagnosis and management crucial.

A dislocation is a disturbance from a proper, original or usual place or state. So, this happens when the bones of a joint are knocked out of place. These dislocations can be partial, known as a subluxation or full. Their mechanism can be trauma or the weakening of muscles and tendons in a joint. According to the British Orthopaedic Association, shoulder dislocations are the most common, accounting for over 50% of all major joint dislocations.

Joint dislocations can also be anterior or posterior, but in elbow injuries, lateral and divergent dislocations can also

be seen, though rare. Elbow dislocations are classified using the direction of the dislocation. They can be further categorised as simple or complex, dependent on the associated injuries. This would depend on associated fractures or nerve and other vessel involvement.

ASSESSMENT

A thorough assessment is essential for diagnosing a joint dislocation. Key elements include:

1. **Visual inspection**: Look for obvious deformity, swelling, or bruising around the joint.

2. **Palpation**: Gently palpate the area to identify points of tenderness or irregularity in the joint structure.

3. **Range of motion**: Assess the ability to move the joint. A dislocated joint will typically have a severely limited range of motion and a highly reluctant patient to engage in moving the joint.

4. **Neurovascular examination**: Check for pulse, sensation and motor function distal to the injury to rule out nerve or vascular compromise.

High-Risk Injuries

Certain situations in custody pose a higher risk for joint dislocations:

1. **Use of force**: Excessive force during arrest or restraint can lead to dislocations, particularly of the shoulder or elbow.

2. **Altercations**: Physical fights can result in awkward falls or blows that dislocate joints.

3. **Pre-existing conditions**: Conditions like hypermobility syndrome can predispose patients to dislocations.

MANAGEMENT

Once a joint dislocation is suspected or confirmed:

1. **Immediate immobilisation**: Ideally, a sling or splint, but utilise the available equipment. Review your stock so you are familiar with what is available to you. Stabilise the joint in a position of comfort. But do not manipulate the joint in custody.

2. **Pain management**: Administer analgesics as per your clinical guidelines.

3. **Referral**: All dislocations should be referred to the ED for imaging and further management, including possible surgical intervention.

4. **Documentation**: Thoroughly document your findings, actions, and the patient's condition in both the custody and medical records.

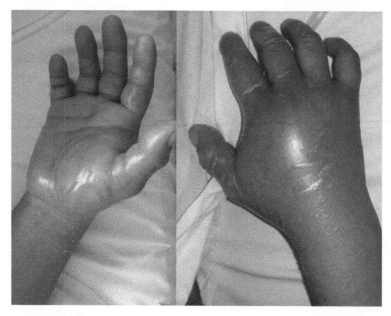

FIGURE 9.2 Compartment syndrome of the hand. *Source:* Rodriguez et al. (2019)/with permission of ELSEVIER.

Possible Complication of Joint Dislocations (Compartment Syndrome)

There appear to be varying risks of compartment syndrome dependent on the type of dislocation presented. Compartment syndrome can be caused by the very mechanism of the dislocation but also by the treatment. For example, causes can include broken bones, crush injuries which cause dislocations and a plaster cast that is too tight, post or repair surgery which treats them. Another cause can be burned, scarred or tight skin.

Compartment syndrome is a very painful and serious condition caused by either bleeding or swelling within an enclosed bundle of muscles known as a 'muscle compartment', see Figure 9.2. Each group of muscles, together with nearby blood vessels and nerves, is contained in a space surrounded by tissue called fascia. Compartment syndrome occurs when the pressure within the compartment increases, restricting the blood flow to the area and potentially damaging the muscles and nerves. It is usually seen in the legs, feet, arms and hands can be acute or chronic. And will cause nerve and tissue damage.

This should not be kept in custody and be transferred to the local ED as soon as possible.

ANKLE INJURIES

Ankle injuries are common in the general population and are no less frequent in police custody settings. These injuries can occur during arrest, physical altercations or even simple missteps within the cell. According to NICE (2020) there are an estimated 354,829 ankle injuries each year.

An ankle injury occurs when the ankle joint is twisted too far from its normal position. Most ankle injuries occur either during sports activities or while walking on an uneven surface. An ankle injury can happen due to tripping, falling, twisting or rotating the ankle or an impact from a road traffic collision.

ASSESSMENT

A comprehensive assessment is essential for diagnosing the type and severity of the ankle injury. Key parts of the ankle assessment include the same as other assessments discussed earlier in this chapter: inspection, palpation, range of motion, plus if the patient is weight bearing. Also, use comparison and look at both ankles. Another diagnostic tool is the use of the Ottawa Ankle Rules.

Ottawa Ankle Rules

Ottawa ankle rules were published in 1992 by the Emergency Department doctors of the Ottawa Civic Hospital, Ottawa, Canada (Stiell et al. 1992). Determining the need for radiograph imaging in ankle injuries, see Figure 9.3. The Ottawa ankle rules have a high sensitivity, making it very effective at identifying almost all fractures.

MANAGEMENT

Once an ankle injury is suspected or confirmed:

1. **Immediate immobilisation**: Use an ankle brace or bandages to stabilise the joint.

2. **Elevation**: Elevate the injured ankle to minimise swelling.

3. **Ice application**: Apply ice packs to reduce inflammation.

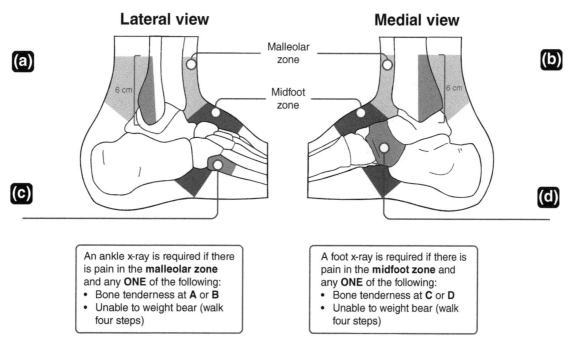

Lateral view

Medial view

Malleolar zone

Midfoot zone

6 cm

6 cm

(a)

(b)

(c)

(d)

An ankle x-ray is required if there is pain in the **malleolar zone** and any **ONE** of the following:
- Bone tenderness at **A** or **B**
- Unable to weight bear (walk four steps)

A foot x-ray is required if there is pain in the **midfoot zone** and any **ONE** of the following:
- Bone tenderness at **C** or **D**
- Unable to weight bear (walk four steps)

FIGURE 9.3   Ottawa ankle rules. (a) Posterior edge or tip of the lateral malleolus. (b) Posterior edge or tip of the lateral malleolus. (c) Base of the fifth metatarsal. (d) Navicular.

4. **Pain management**: Administer appropriate analgesics as per your clinical guidelines.

5. **Referral**: For severe injuries or if a fracture is suspected, immediate referral to the ED is essential.

6. **Documentation**: Thoroughly document your findings, actions, and the patient's condition in both the custody and medical records.

BURNS AND SCALDS

Burns are caused by damage that results from heat, friction, radiation or chemicals. A scald is a burn caused by contact with a hot liquid or steam. Most burns are non-complex and, once assessed, can be managed in primary care. Burns can be classified (see Box 9.3).

Burns and scalds are less common in police custody but can occur due to accidents, self-harm, or even assault. According to the National Burn Care Review Committee (2001), approximately 250,000 people receive burn injuries each year. In a custody setting, timely and appropriate care is crucial to minimise tissue damage and complications.

ASSESSMENT

A comprehensive assessment is essential for determining the severity and extent of the burn or scald. Key elements include some do's and don'ts.

Do remove the heat source if not already, then cool the burn with cool or lukewarm running water for 20 minutes. It is sensible to remove any clothing or jewellery that is near the

| BOX 9.3 | BURN CLASSIFICATION |

Superficial epidermal – a first-degree burn where the epidermis is affected but the dermis is intact. Characterised by red, painful, irritated, dry and slightly swollen skin. The skin should not blister.

Superficial dermal – a second-degree burn where the epidermis and upper layers of the dermis are involved. Characterised by blisters, slough, swelling and weeping raw dermis, which is very painful.

Deep dermal – is a third-degree burn where the epidermis, upper and deeper layers of the dermis are involved, but not the underlying subcutaneous tissues. This can be recognised by dry, blotchy, mottled skin with possible blisters, no capillary refill and associated pain.

Full thickness – is a fourth-degree extending through all the layers of skin to the subcutaneous tissue. The skin can be white, brown or black in colour. Blisters are unlikely, as is capillary refill. The skin will be dry and usually painless, having burned through the nerves.

affected area, then cover the burn with a layer of cling film. Use first-line analgesia. If the face or eyes are affected, ensure that the patient sits up rather than lying down to reduce swelling and send to the ED.

Do not cool the burns with ice or iced water. Do not try and remove anything that might stick to the burn like clothing.

Popping any blisters is advised against as that protects the skin underneath and finally do not de-roof blisters.

ED referrals should be considered in the following circumstances: chemical or electrical burns, any burn larger than a person's hand, burns with deep dermal damage, where you are unsure and finally where there is a possibility of smoke inhalation, coughing, sore throat or difficulty in breathing, whether there are facial injuries burns or not.

To conclude, once a burn or scald is suspected or confirmed, the following checklist will aid in the management of burns:

1. **Immediate cooling**: Use cool running water to cool the area for at least 10 minutes.

2. **Dressing**: Apply a sterile dressing or plastic wrap to protect the wound.

3. **Pain management**: Administer analgesics as per your clinical guidelines.

4. **Hydration**: Ensure the patient is well-hydrated, especially for larger burns.

5. **Referral**: Severe burns, burns on sensitive areas, or burns covering a large surface area should be immediately referred to a burn unit or the ED.

6. **Documentation**: Thoroughly document your findings, actions, and the patient's condition for legal and medical records.

ACID, ALKALINE OR CHEMICAL ATTACKS

Attacks involving acid, alkaline or chemicals are becoming more frequent, and HCPs may be asked to see a patient who may have suffered such burns.

1. **Personal safety:** Full personal protective equipment should be worn; this includes eye protection, apron (ideally long-sleeved), face shield and gloves.

2. **Removal of source:** Carefully remove any contaminated clothing. If chemical is a powder, brush it off the skin. If liquid, rinse the affected areas with copious amounts of clean water. Any contaminated clothing should be placed in hazardous bags.

3. **Treatment:** The affected area(s) should be fully irrigated with cool (but not cold) water for at least 20 minutes, until the burning sensation passes. The area can then be covered with sterile gauze or cling film. If the chemical used is known, ask someone to find out if there are any specific treatment methods. A CBRN[1] officer should be able to give you further information.

4. **Hospital:** All acid, alkaline and chemical burns require assessment at hospital. An ambulance should be arranged so that treatment is ongoing during transport. Ensure the ambulance service is aware that this is an acid, alkaline or chemical burn so any precautions they need to take can be commenced.

TETANUS

Tetanus is an acute disease caused by tetanus neurotoxin. The neurotoxin is produced by bacteria – clostridium tetani. The bacteria create spores, which live in soil and manure. They survive for a long time and get into the body through puncture wounds or even trivial wounds, through intravenous drug use and sometimes through surgery. The incubation period is around 10 days.

This bacterial infection can lead to severe muscle stiffness and spasms. While rare in the United Kingdom due to widespread vaccination, it remains a concern in police custody settings, particularly following puncture wounds or burns. According to Public Health England, there are approximately four cases of tetanus per year in England, but the risk can be higher in specific populations like patients. Another term used for tetanus is 'lockjaw'.

Tetanus-prone wounds are generally puncture or open wounds, where foreign body or bacteria can get access to the body, especially those from the garden or dirty wounds. Compound fractures are prone, as are burns with associated sepsis and the natural defences are removed. Certain animal bites are also prone, but domestic pets should not have tetanus in their saliva, unless they have been rooting in soil.

In the United Kingdom, there is a comprehensive vaccination programme from birth, so most UK-born patients would be covered for tetanus; however, some consideration must be made for others. Those who are immunocompromised, those on immunosuppressants, chemotherapy or are pregnant need further consideration. Those born prior to 1961 when the UK vaccination programme was introduced and those who emigrated to the United Kingdom from a country with no childhood immunisation programme.

ASSESSMENT

A comprehensive assessment is essential for determining the risk of tetanus. Key elements include:

1. **Type of injury**: Puncture wounds, burns, and lacerations are more likely to introduce tetanus bacteria.

2. **Contamination**: Assess the wound for foreign material like soil or rust, which can harbour tetanus spores.

3. **Vaccination status**: Determine the patient's tetanus vaccination history, if possible.

4. **Signs and Symptoms**: While rare, look for early symptoms like muscle stiffness or spasms.

Wounds need to be managed on a case-by-case basis. Wound cleaning is essential to fully understand the

---

[1] Chemical, Biological, Radiological and Nuclear.

underlying wound and its needs. However, wound care in custody is generally limited and many cases will also need antibiotic therapy, which might not be available, so if in any doubt, then referring to the local ED or walk-in centre, may be the most sensible management plan.

BITE INJURIES

Bite injuries are a unique and often complicated type of wound encountered in police custody. These injuries can occur during altercations prior to custody or during arrest and booking into custody, dependent on the heightened state of those involved. The notorious 'fight bite', sustained when a clenched fist strikes the teeth of the other person, causing complex lacerations and probable infection due to oral flora, is not to be underestimated in seriousness. They are associated with some of the worst types of infectious complications, which can lead to permanent joint stiffness and, in worst cases, amputation. Dog bites can arise from police dogs so need careful documentation.

ASSESSMENT

A comprehensive assessment is essential for determining the severity and risk associated with a bite injury. Key elements include:

1. **Visual inspection**: Look for puncture wounds, lacerations, or bruising.

2. **Depth and location**: Assess the depth of the bite and its location, as bites on the hand or face may require more specialised care.

3. **Signs of infection**: Check for redness, swelling, or discharge, which could indicate an infection.

4. **Mechanism of injury**: Determine how the injury occurred, especially if it is a 'fight bite', which typically involves a clenched fist striking an opponent's teeth.

MANAGEMENT

Robust and effective management of bites and particularly fight bite is key. It is these cases, when poorly managed at the time of injury, which will likely produce civil claims at a later point. Once a bite injury is suspected or confirmed:

1. **Immediate cleaning**: Thoroughly irrigate the wound with saline to minimise the risk of infection.

2. **Antibiotic prophylaxis**: Administer antibiotics like co-amoxiclav as per your clinical guidelines to prevent infection.

3. **Tetanus and blood-borne viruses**: Assess the need for tetanus and blood-borne virus prophylaxis, especially if the skin is broken.

4. **Referral**: Bites that are deep, located on the face or hands, or show signs of infection should be immediately referred to the ED or a specialist.

5. **Documentation**: Record all findings, actions, and the patient's condition meticulously for both medical and legal records. Considering recommended specialist photography.

SCENARIO 9.3 Suspected fight bite injury

You are asked to see a 21-year-old, right-handed male who works as a joiner. He has an open wound that had features of a laceration and is bleeding across the surface of the second and third finger below the knuckle. He wants it cleaning a dressing. He reports he got the injury when he punched someone in the mouth.

1. *Outline your approach to this assessment.*

2. *Outline your management.*

3. *The individual is dismissive of the injury, outline the risk associated with such an injury.*

WOUND CARE

The available wound care and treatment will vary depending on each healthcare provider. It is therefore prudent and necessary to understand what is on hand to use, given the variety of minor injuries encountered in the custody environment. However, before tackling any wound or injury care, some basics should be considered.

Where appropriate, don correct PPE for the procedure. If fitting wound cleaning should be next to remove any debris, blood or foreign bodies. Non-woven sterile swabs with either normal saline or tap water are the most suitable for this task, as there is less chance of fibre shed. Then the wound can be re-assessed fully. Then the HCP is able to choose the most suitable options, be that a simple dressing, wound glue or even steri-strips. Due to the lack of a sterile environment and owing to the fact custody should not be seen as a mini-ED, suturing a wound should not take place. This should be married with the required pharmacological adjuncts, simple analgesia or antibiotics dependent on the healthcare service provider protocol.

CONCLUSION

Managing minor injuries in custody is a varied and wide-ranging task that requires skill, knowledge, experience and competence from the HCPs. This chapter outlines the distinguishing features of many common ailments seen in the custody environment and the most suitable treatment plan.

The skill of the HCP lies in the ability to diagnose the injury correctly based on history and clinical picture and then formulating and carrying out fitting care on a case-by-case basis. This should be a constant learning opportunity for all HCPs, one which should be supported with continuous professional development.

LEARNING ACTIVITIES

1. Write a reflective piece on a case where you assessed and treated a minor injury or wound.

2. Research, prepare and deliver a presentation to your colleagues about a specific minor injury. Include background to the condition, the assessment (history and examination) and treatment options.

3. Develop a pathway to signpost patients to the appropriate local service, for example Emergency Department, walk-in centre, GP practice or other.

RESOURCES

Online

- NICE Clinical Knowledge Summaries | https://cks.nice.org.uk/

Organisations

- NHS 111 Online (England) | https://111.nhs.uk

- NHS 111 Wales (Wales) | https://111.wales.nhs.uk

- NHS 24 (Scotland) | https://111.wales.nhs.uk

- Health and Social Care (Northern Ireland) | https://online.hscni.net

REFERENCES

Milby, A.H., Halpern, C.H., Guo, W. et al. (2008). Prevalence of cervical spinal injury in trauma. *Neurosurgical Focus* 25 (5): E10. https://doi.org/10.3171/FOC.2008.25.11.E10.

National Burn Care Review Committee (2001). National burn care review. British Association of Plastic Surgeons. http://79.170.40.160/british burnassociation.org/wp-content/uploads/2017/07/NBCR2001.pdf (accessed 11 January 2024).

National Institute for Health and Care Excellence (2016). Spinal injury: assessment and initial management. https://www.nice.org.uk/guidance/ng41/chapter/Recommendations#assessment-and-management-in-prehospital-settings (accessed 11 January 2024).

National Institute for Health and Care Excellence (2020). How common are sprains and strains? https://cks.nice.org.uk/topics/sprains-strains/background-information/prevalence/ (accessed 15 January 2024).

National Institute for Health and Care Excellence (2023). Head injury: assessment and early management. https://www.nice.org.uk/guidance/qs74/documents/head-injury-briefing-paper2 (accessed 11 January 2024).

Robinson, L.S. and O'Brien, L. (2019). Description and cost-analysis of emergency department attendances for hand and wrist injuries. *Emergency Medicine Australasia* 31 (5): 772–779. https://doi.org/10.1111/1742-6723.13246.

Rodriguez, J., Torres, J., Salinas, V. et al. (2019) Compartment syndrome of the hand after laparoscopic gynecologic surgery. *Journal of Minimally Invasive Gynecology*, 27(1), 220–224. Doi: https://doi.org/10.1016/j.jmig.2019.03.017

Stiell, I.G., Greenberg, G.H., McKnight, R.D., Nair, R.C., McDowell, I., and Worthington, J.R., (1992). A study to develop clinical decision rules for the use of radiography in acute ankle injuries. *Annals of Emergency Medicine*, 21(4), 384–390. https://doi.org/10.1016/s0196-0644(05)82656-3.

FURTHER READING

FFLM | Head injury warning – Advice to custody officers, gaolers & detention officers | https://fflm.ac.uk/wp-content/uploads/2019/12/ A5-HeadInjuryWarning-Prof-J-Payne-James-and-Prof-P-Marks-March-2023.pdf

Substance Use and Misuse

Jennie Smith

Mitie Care and Custody Health Ltd, London, UK & UK Association of Forensic Nurses and Paramedics

CHAPTER 10

AIM

This chapter aims to tackle the broad and diverse topic of substance use and misuse, something healthcare professionals are faced with daily. This will include the definitions of use and misuse, the classifications of drugs, the legislation which governs these substances and how we treat them in the custodial environment.

LEARNING OUTCOMES

Upon completion of this chapter, the reader should be able to:

- Define the difference between substance use and abuse

- Name the different classes of substances

- Identify the signs and symptoms of intoxication and withdrawal across the groups of different substances

SELF-ASSESSMENT

1. Write one example of a drug from each class under the Misuse of Drugs Act 1971, plus the sentence for supply and/or possession

2. List the schedules in the Misuse of Drugs Regulations 2001 and name one drug in each schedule

3. Name the seven categories of drugs included in the Drugs Wheel and the most common drugs under those categories

INTRODUCTION

Many of the individuals who need healthcare intervention in the custody environment use some form of substance. Clearly, this does not apply to every individual, but certainly to a large percentage. Given the potential numbers involved, it is incumbent on the healthcare professional (HCP) to have wide-ranging knowledge and understanding of the substances likely to be encountered, what they look like in intoxication and withdrawal, the treatment regimens associated with each one and the legislation that governs them. This legislative knowledge needs to encompass their classifications, which is linked to the maintenance of law and the corresponding responsibilities of the police and HCP. All of which will be covered in this chapter.

DEFINITIONS

The two main global disease classifications are the International Classification of Diseases, 11th edition (ICD-11), published by the World Health Organisation and the Diagnostic and Statistical Manual of Mental Disorders, edition 5 (DSM-5), published by the American Psychiatric Association. These

Police Custody Healthcare for Nurses and Paramedics, First Edition. Edited by Matthew Peel, Jennie Smith, Vanessa Webb, and Margaret Bannerman.
© 2025 John Wiley & Sons Ltd. Published 2025 by John Wiley & Sons Ltd.
Companion website: www.wiley.com/go/policecustodyhealthcare

documents provide us with the definitions for substance use, abuse, dependence and withdrawal, though slightly different.

Substance use, abuse and misuse are very different things. According to the US Centre for Disease Control and Prevention (CDC) (2023), substance use refers to the use of selected substances, alcohol, tobacco products, drugs and inhalants that can be consumed, inhaled, injected, or otherwise absorbed into the body. Substance use may not be an issue for some people and may not lead to dependency. However, substance abuse and misuse depend on the individual continuing to use the substance despite it causing problems to their health, family, relationships and work. In addition, abuse leads to a reduction and possible discontinuation of recreational, social and occupational activities.

Both ICD-11 and DSM-5 proffer definitions for substance dependence and withdrawal. Pertaining to dependence, both documents describe similar to the CDC that it centres around continued use despite physical and psychological problems caused or exacerbated by the substance. In relation to withdrawal, there are slight variations. Both agree withdrawal includes the development of a substance-specific syndrome due to the cessation of, or reduction in heavy and prolonged use, as well as not being a result of any general medical condition and not accounted for by any other mental disorder. However, DSM-5 states the syndrome should cause clinically significant distress or impairment, something ICD-11 does not include in its criteria.

LEGISLATION

MISUSE OF DRUGS ACT 1971

The Misuse of Drugs Act, enacted in 1971 was brought in to make provisions with respect to dangerous or otherwise harmful drugs, related matters and any associated issues. In tandem with this act, the Advisory Council on the Misuse of Drugs (ACMD) works to keep under review all drugs in the United Kingdom, which might or appear to cause harmful effects, enough to constitute a social problem. It is their role to highlight, advise and make recommendations to Secretaries of State and Ministers of the four nations in relation to these drugs.

The Misuse of Drugs Act 1971 also lays out the classifications of controlled drugs and the rules around importation, exportation, production, possession and supply. These are commonly referred to as the classes, as in class A, B and C drugs, see Box 10.1. These are all under Schedule 2 of the Act, parts I to III. The classification is based on the harm each one can do to society.

MISUSE OF DRUGS REGULATIONS

This regulation, brought about in 2001, allows for the lawful possession and supply of otherwise illegal drugs for legitimate purposes. These regulations also cover prescribing, administration, safe custody, dispensing, record keeping, destruction and disposal of controlled drugs to prevent diversion for misuse. The regulations were updated in 2012 to include other prescribers outside of doctors and dentists, who were the sole groups in the original document.

All drugs controlled under the Misuse of Drugs Act 1971 are placed in Schedules 1–5 of the regulations (see Box 10.2). Allocation to the schedule is dependent on their therapeutic and medicinal usefulness, need for access and the level of harm caused when abused.

These regulations were strengthened in 2005 following the Shipman inquiry. These changes encompassed drug availability and the use of controlled drugs in healthcare settings specifically around audits.

PSYCHOACTIVE SUBSTANCES ACT (2016)

In the 1980s and 1990s, we saw significant increases in drug use across the United Kingdom, which seemed to level out around the turn of the century. This changed in 2006 with the increased interest and availability of a new generation of

---

BOX 10.1	**DRUG CLASSIFICATION**		
Classification	Examples of drug type	Maximum penalty for possession	Maximum penalty for supply
Class A	Cocaine, crack cocaine, ecstasy (3,4-methylenedi oxymethamphetamine (MDMA)), lysergic acid diethylamide (LSD), heroin, methadone, methamphetamine, phencyclidine (PCP), psilocybin (magic mushrooms)	Up to 7 years in prison or an unlimited fine, or both	Up to life in prison or an unlimited fine, or both
Class B	Amphetamines, cannabis, methylphenidate (Ritalin®), codeine, pholcodine	Up to 5 years in prison or an unlimited fine, or both	Up to 14 years in prison or an unlimited, fine or both
Class C	Tranquillisers, some painkillers, gamma-hydroxybutyrate (GHB), ketamine, nitrous oxide	Up to 2 years in prison or an unlimited fine, or both	Up to 14 years in prison or an unlimited, fine or both

<table>
<tr><td colspan="2">BOX 10.2   DRUG SCHEDULES</td></tr>
</table>

Schedule 1	Drugs with no therapeutic value, usually used under Home Office licence for research (e.g. cannabis, MDMA and LSD)
Schedule 2	Drugs with therapeutic value, but associated with high addiction so strictly controlled (e.g. diamorphine and morphine)
Schedule 3	Drugs with therapeutic value that have lighter control associated with their prescription, dispensing, recording and safe custody (e.g. temazepam, midazolam, buprenorphine and tramadol)

Schedule 4	• This comes in two parts. Both have lighter regulation:
	
	  ◦ Part 1 – Mainly benzodiazepines (e.g. diazepam). Possession is an offence without prescription or exemption.
	
	  ◦ Part 2 – Anabolic and androgenic steroids (e.g. testosterone). Possession is not an offence.

Schedule 5	Weaker variants of drugs covered in Schedule 2 that present little risk of abuse and can be sold over the counter as pharmacy medicines (e.g. codeine, medicinal opium or morphine (in less than 0.2% concentration).

drugs known as novel psychoactive substances (NPS). Commonly referred to as 'legal highs'. These were substances developed to mimic the effect of the controlled drugs but designed to fall outside the remits of the Misuse of Drugs Act 1971.

The substances were seen as a bit of a game changer in that they were readily available on the high street from specific shops, known as 'head shops', as well as other retail outlets. Ordering them on the internet was also an option, which was a step away from the historic routes for drug transportation and supply.

The UK government initially tried to combat the issue by outlawing the production of different excipients. However, the manufacturers worked cleverly to change the chemical compounds slightly to bypass the issue. Eventually, on 26 May 2016, the Psychoactive Substances Act came into effect, banning the manufacture, sale and distribution of all psychoactive substances. This act included an exemption list that allows the production of alcohol and tobacco. The ACMD defines NPS as psychoactive drugs not prohibited by the Misuse of Drugs Act 1971 and which are used for their intoxicant properties.

The main drugs within this group are synthetic cannabinoid receptor antagonists (SCRAs), a major issue in the homeless, youth offender institutes and the prison population. The term 'spice' is often used as an umbrella term encompassing SCRAs (DrugWise 2016).

Other groups of NPS include stimulants, for example mephedrone, which mimic amphetamine and MDMA, hallucinogens, opiate-type drugs and lastly tranquillisers. Not all of which have been detected in use in the United Kingdom, but are known to exist.

When we think of substance misuse, we automatically think of illegal substances, those associated with the Misuse of Drugs Act and Regulations, but we must not forget alcohol. There is a strong association between alcohol use, misuse, abuse and the criminal justice system, be it a one-off arrest for drunk and disorderly or many tens of arrests due to domestic violence and abuse exacerbated by someone's drinking. Alcohol and its impacts will be discussed in more detail later in this chapter.

DRUG CLASSIFICATION

Historically psychoactive plants were classified in the pharmacological literature according to their active ingredients; there were three groups, sedatives, stimulants and hallucinogens. But this has changed in recent years due to the development of many new drugs and with it changes to the classification have also been required. Within the field, the sedative group was split into analgesics and depressants. In 2010, a further classification was added due to the influx of NPS as well as the issues surrounding drug like ketamine; the box was just called 'other' but was full quickly.

Move on another year and a further three categories were added, 'other' was replaced with cannabinoids, empathogens and dissociatives, and the replacement of hallucinogens with psychedelics.

The Drugs Wheel was developed due to the increasing number of new psychoactive substances appearing around 2012, which did not fit into the existing classifications (see Figure 10.1). Trying to classify them according to their type proved too complex, hence the addition of the three extra categories, which proved to be much neater and allowed for better harm reduction for the charities and organisations working in the field.

As illustrated earlier, there are hundreds, even thousands of substances available for use and misuse; however, in the custody environment, the most prevalent are alcohol, cannabis, heroin, cocaine, crack cocaine, benzodiazepines, amphetamines and occasionally ecstasy. Each one will be considered in more detail.

INTOXICATION

Intoxication in custody can arise from alcohol, drugs, or a combination of both. It's crucial to understand that mixing substances can lead to different interactions (see Box 10.3). Mixing drugs, including alcohol, significantly increases the risk of adverse reactions. The unpredictable nature of these interactions can lead to fatal outcomes.

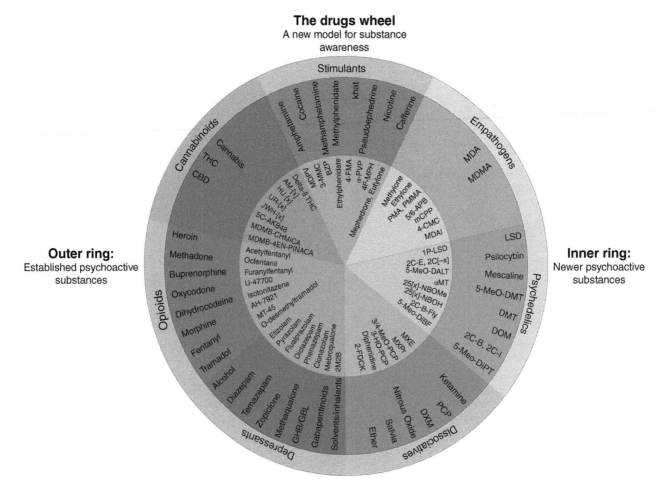

FIGURE 10.1 The Drugs Wheel. *Source:* Adley, Jones, and Measham (2023)/Taylor & Francis/CC BY 4.0.

BOX 10.3	MIXING DRUGS (INCLUDING ALCOHOL)
Additive effects	This occurs when similar substances work together in the body, intensifying their effects. For example combining heroin with methadone can increase the risk of respiratory depression, potentially leading to life-threatening situations.
Antagonistic effects	In some cases, one substance can counteract the effect of another. For instance, a stimulant like cocaine might mask the depressant effects of alcohol, misleadingly suggesting a lower level of intoxication.
Synergistic effects	Certain combinations, like alcohol and benzodiazepines (or any sedating drug), can produce disproportionately severe effects, greatly enhancing risks such as unconsciousness or respiratory failure.

Intoxication can manifest in various ways, ranging from mild euphoria to complete unconsciousness. Upon arrival in custody, individuals might initially seem only slightly intoxicated but could rapidly deteriorate. This uncertainty, whether the level of intoxication is rising or falling, necessitates heightened vigilance. It is also essential to recognise that several conditions can mimic intoxication (see Box 10.4). These might include acute physical health crises or neurological events, as well as mental health emergencies. Careful assessment is required to differentiate these from substance intoxication.

There's always the risk of individuals ingesting or concealing drugs upon arrest to avoid detection. Additionally, they might smuggle substances into the cell and consume them during detention.

ASSESSMENT

When assessing intoxication, HCPs must adhere to the 'walk and talk' rule. Any individual who cannot walk independently **or** speak coherently is not fit for police custody. This principle

BOX 10.4	CONDITIONS MIMICKING INTOXICATION

Medical	Trauma and toxic	Mental health
• Hypoglycaemia	• Head injury	• Bipolar
• Stroke	• Carbon monoxide poisoning	• Psychosis
• Epilepsy or seizures		• Severe depression
• Diabetic ketoacidosis	• Overdose	
• Hypoxia	• Poisoning	
• Infection		
• Dehydration		
• Electrolyte disturbance		
• Liver or renal failure		

is vital as intoxication-related deaths in custody remain a grave concern annually.

Assessments should be carried out as outlined in Chapter 3 – Fitness Assessments, ideally in the medical room. Great care must be taken when asked to see people in a cell because of intoxication. As a minimum, check vital signs (including National Early Warning Score, version 2 if completed locally), pupillary size and response to light. Check for any evidence of head injury (either visible or any history of such). Consider checking a blood glucose in anyone suspected of being intoxicated.

MANAGEMENT

Anyone exhibiting signs of intoxication should be placed under Level 2 – Intermittent Observations, checked at least every 30 minutes as a minimum. Police should be advised to monitor for any signs of worsening condition, such as incontinence or vomiting, and ensure the individual is positioned safely, preferably on their side facing the door. Intoxication should start to resolve and individuals improve over several hours. Anyone not improving as expected should be re-referred to the HCP.

Only advise individuals to be interviewed when they appear sober. This is particularly pertinent for those with alcohol dependency, who might seem sober despite high alcohol levels in their system. HCPs should closely monitor and guide police interactions, ensuring that individuals are fit for interview.

DEPRESSANTS

ALCOHOL

Alcohol, or ethanol, is a legal psychoactive substance present in all alcoholic beverages. Classed as a depressant, it has been referred to as the Jekyll and Hyde of the drug world. In moderation, it is relatively harmless, but misused or abused, it becomes a major physiological, social and public health issue globally (Jones 2016). A survey in 2010 showed alcohol was seen to be more harmful to the individual, their family and society than heroin and crack cocaine (Jones 2016).

Intoxication

There are several categorised stages associated with alcohol intoxication. Each stage has a different clinical and physical presentation and is in tandem with increasing blood and breath alcohol concentration (BrAC). As HCPs are more versed in BrAC levels due to the regular readings provided from intoximeter sampling, these stages have been illustrated with breath alcohol (see Box 10.5). However, individuals may react differently depending on their tolerance (or lack of). Therefore, HCPs must ALWAYS manage the condition they are presented with. For example, someone with a BrAC 67 mcg/100 ml who is slurring their words and unsteady on their feet is at a greater risk than someone who walking and talking normally with a BrAC over 150 mcg/100 ml. HCPs should be mindful that often, alcohol may be mixed with drugs.

Dependence

Dependence is defined by the ingestion of greater than 10 units per day (see Box 10.6), with a tolerance to consistently high levels of blood alcohol. That tolerance occurs at three levels: metabolic, intracellular and behavioural. Dependence eventually creates a narrowing of their repertoire, with most activities focused around drinking, creating a compulsion to continue drinking despite the problems that come along. Sudden cessation will create a withdrawal syndrome. HCPs may see, or have reported, abnormal blood results (such as liver function tests).

Dependence can also cause other neurological disorders, including Wernicke's encephalopathy, a potentially reversible condition (if treated early), created by a lack of thiamine. Alcohol damages the body's ability to absorb thiamine in the intestine, which creates a triad of symptoms. These symptoms include ophthalmoplegia, ataxia or abnormal gait and confusion. Left untreated, this can become Korsakoff's Syndrome, which is irreversible. Korsakoff's has many of the same symptoms as dementia, created by the chronic lack of vitamin B1 needed for brain function. Lastly is alcohol hallucinosis, more recently referred to as alcohol-induced psychotic disorder. Thankfully, this is a rare condition, and usually presents with acoustic verbal hallucinations, delusions and mood disturbances in clear consciousness (Bhat et al. 2012).

BOX 10.5	BREATH ALCOHOL CONCENTRATIONS AND EFFECTS

Degree of intoxication	Breath Alcohol Concentration (BrAC mcg/100ml)	Clinical presentation
Sober	4–25 mcg/100 ml	No obvious effect May feel relaxed

Euphoria	13–60 mcg/100 ml	Mild euphoria
		    More talkative
		    Less inhibitions
		    More self-confidence
		    Impaired fine motor skills

Excitement	39–100 mcg/100 ml	Emotional instability
		    Poor sensory perception
		    Impaired memory
		    Impaired comprehension
		    Loss of balance
		    Impaired coordination

Drunk	66–150 mcg/100 ml	Disorientation
		    Confusion
		    Impaired vision (e.g. double vision)
		    Decreased sense of pain
		    Worsening coordination
		    Staggering gait
		    Slurred speech

HCP should review all those with a BrAC over 150 mcg/100 ml		

Stupor	109–200 mcg/100 ml	General inertia
		    Lack of response to stimulus
		    Unable to walk or stand
		    Vomiting, urinary or faecal incontinence

Coma	153–250 mcg/100 ml	Coma
		    Depressed or absent reflexes
		    Cardiovascular and respiratory depression
		    Potential for death

Death	Over 200 mcg/100 ml	

Source: Adapted from Stark (2020).

Withdrawal

Alcohol withdrawal also happens in stages, as intoxication (see Box 10.7). Any individual who has experienced withdrawal will make it quite clear it is not something they wish to experience again. Aside from the physiological symptoms, it causes high levels of anxiety and distress and requires robust management to prevent alcohol-related seizures or worse. The use of a symptom scale, for example the Clinical Institute Withdrawal Assessment for Alcohol-Revised (CIWA-Ar) or the Glasgow Modified Alcohol Withdrawal Scale (GMAWS), are effective and evidence-based rating scales that can aid the practitioner to diagnose withdrawal, allowing prompt treatment. There is currently no consensus on preferred tools

in custody; however, each provides a measure to monitor severity and track response to treatment.

Treatment Robust management of alcohol withdrawal is required to prevent the deterioration of the patient. Early assessment to establish current alcohol use, level of dependence and history of withdrawal will allow early initiation of treatment and avoid the associated complications, such as seizures and delirium tremens. Clinical management pathways and protocols are essential and should be available to all HCPs working in the custody environment. Symptom-triggered regimens allow for tailored care based on the clinical presentation and the use of symptom rating

BOX 10.6	ALCOHOL UNITS

Beer and lager		Wine		Cider		Spirits	
3.6%	6%	12%		4.5%	7.5%	40%	
1 Pint		Small	Large	Pint		Single	Double
2 units	3.4 units	1.5 units	3 units	2.6 units	4.3 units	1 unit	2 units

BOX 10.7	ALCOHOL WITHDRAWAL STAGES

Stage	Associated symptoms
Stage 1	• Can occur at any point between 6–8 hours after drinking stopped
	• Tremors, sweating, anxiety, insomnia, nausea and vomiting
Stage 2	• Can occur at any point between 8 and 48 hours after drinking stopped
	• Hallucinations
Stage 3	• Can occur at any point between 12 and 48 hours after drinking stopped
	• Seizures
Stage 4	• Usually between 48 and 72 hours
	• Delirium tremens – this is a medical emergency
	• Disorientation, confusion, hyperactivity, auditory and visual hallucinations

SCENARIO 10.1	Alcohol intoxication

You are asked to see a 42-year-old male who has been arrested for drunk driving. He has never been arrested before and little is known about him. On booking in, he appeared drunk and provided a BrAC 161 mcg/100 ml.

1. *How do you approach this assessment?*
   a. *What factors will impact your decision?*

2. *What are the risks of alcohol intoxication?*

3. *How can those risks be mitigated?*

scales. Long-acting benzodiazepines are the treatment of choice, usually diazepam or chlordiazepoxide (Royal College of Psychiatrist [RCP] 2020). But should they be unable to take oral medication then transfer to the Emergency Department should be arranged.

BENZODIAZEPINES

Benzodiazepines also fall under the heading of depressant (see Box 10.8). They are class C drugs as they are prescription-only medications. Benzodiazepines were first manufactured in the 1960s and their harmful effects were not acknowledged until the 1970s. Their effects generally start around 15 minutes after consumption and will last for around six hours without further dosing.

Despite their known addictive properties, they are still the most commonly prescribed mood-altering drugs in the United Kingdom. They have known associations with both tolerance and dependence.

BOX 10.8	COMMON BENZODIAZEPINES

- Diazepam (Valium)
- Lorazepam
- Temazepam
- Clonazepam
- Alprazolam (Xanax)
- Nitrazepam
- Chlordiazepoxide (Librium)
- Clobazam
- Flurazepam

Intoxication

The signs of intoxication are similar to those seen with alcohol and include:

- Psychological
  - Unable to concentrate
  - Calm
  - Euphoria
- Physical
  - Drowsy or sedated
  - Slurred speech
  - Unsteady on feet
  - Dilated pupils
  - Bradycardia or hypotension
- Behavioural
  - In some cases, individuals may experience a paradoxical reaction with agitation, aggression or increased anxiety.
- Other
  - Preoccupation with obtaining and using benzodiazepines

Withdrawal

The abrupt cessation of benzodiazepines is not recommended after prolonged use due to the dangers associated with sudden withdrawal. A slow titrated approach is advisable once dependence is confirmed. Symptoms can be measured and tracked using the Clinical Institute Withdrawal Assessment – Benzodiazepines (CIWA-B); symptoms include:

- Insomnia
- Anxiety
- Agitation
- Depression
- Seizures

Treatment Treatment with long-acting benzodiazepines such as diazepam 10 mg three times a day is recommended, increasing in the presence of severe symptoms (RCP 2020). Benzodiazepine withdrawal is rarely seen in custody due to the long half-life of benzodiazepines abused (i.e. diazepam). However, Xanax (alprazolam) use is becoming more prevalent (either fake or illicit), which has a much shorter half-life.

GHB/GBL

Gamma-hydroxybutyrate (GHB) and gamma-butyrolactone (GBL) are central nervous system depressants known for their use as recreational drugs and, unfortunately, their association with drug-facilitated sexual assault. Often referred to as Liquid Ecstasy, G or Liquid X. It commonly comes in liquid form, sold in small bottles or vials. Given the potency and narrow margin of overdose, individuals sometimes use droppers or syringes for dosing.

Intoxication

GHB/GBL intoxication include:

- Psychological
  - Euphoria
  - Disinhibition
  - Confusion or disorientation
- Physical
  - Drowsiness and sedation
  - Respiratory depression, bradycardia or hypotension
  - Reduced muscle tone (floppy)
  - Seizures
- Behavioural
  - Aggression
  - Sexual disinhibition

Withdrawal

Dependence on GHB/GBL can develop quickly, and withdrawal can be severe and potentially life-threatening; symptoms include:

- Anxiety
- Sweating
- Tachycardiac
- Tremors

Treatment Management involves high-dose benzodiazepines and occasionally baclofen (RCP 2020).

GABAPENTINOIDS

Pregabalin and Gabapentin cause euphoria, relaxation and drowsiness, sedation and respiratory depression. They are sometimes used in combination with opioids to enhance their euphoric effects. Withdrawal symptoms include headache, insomnia, nausea, diarrhoea and convulsions. Continuance of prescribed gabapentinoids should be the aim where possible. Alternatively, benzodiazepines may alleviate some of the acute withdrawal symptoms and in cases where there is a risk of seizures, benzodiazepines can be useful due to their anticonvulsant properties (Department of Health 2017).

OPIOIDS

Opioids are a class of drugs that include both natural and synthetic substances, which act on opioid receptors in the brain to produce pain-relieving and euphoric effects (see Box 10.9). Opiates are a subset of opioids, specifically referred to as natural opioid compounds derived from the opium poppy, such as morphine and codeine. The key difference lies in their origin.

HEROIN

Heroin is an opiate, which comes from opium, a naturally occurring juice extracted from certain poppy seed pods. It is a Class A drug in the United Kingdom and it is a Controlled Drug (CD). It mostly comes as a powder and its colour can be white to brown depending on the purity. It is not water soluble, so it is usually reconstituted with citric acid prior to injection. Citric acid can cause irritation and damage to the vein walls, leading to inflammation and pain upon injection. Repeated use can lead to more severe vascular damage, such as vein sclerosis, thrombosis and an increased risk of infection.

The active chemical in heroin is diamorphine, which the body converts to morphine, a strong painkiller. Morphine alters the natural chemicals in the brain, binding to the opioid receptors that trigger the release of dopamine, one of our feel-good hormones, giving overwhelming feelings of euphoria. However, given morphine is fundamentally a painkiller, it then acts on the nervous system slowing it all down, including breathing and the heart rate, hence why it is so dangerous. This is the same for all opioids, and the intoxication, dependence and withdrawal (including treatment) are the same for all opioids.

BOX 10.9	**COMMON OPIOIDS**

- Buprenorphine
- Codeine
- Diamorphine (heroin)
- Dihydrocodeine
- Fentanyl
- Methadone
- Morphine
- Oxycodone
- Tramadol

Intoxication

Symptoms of opioid use include

- Psychological
  - Euphoria
  - Confused or unable to concentrate
- Physical
  - Small or pin-point pupils
  - Respiratory depression, low blood pressure and low heart rate
  - Dry mouth
  - Drowsiness, sleeping and conscious nodding
  - Slurred speech
  - Slow reflexes
  - Fresh needle track marks or injection sites
- Behavioural
  - Mood swings
- Other
  - Preoccupation with obtaining and using opioids

Dependence

With dependence comes increased tolerance. Tolerance to opioids is a real issue, meaning individuals need to take more and more to get the same feeling of euphoria. This is married to the addictive nature of opioids, constantly chasing that feeling and needing more and more to achieve it. This increase in use is associated with increased risks due to the impact on the nervous system, increasing the risk of overdose and death.

Withdrawal

Opioid withdrawal can come in two stages: early onset, within 6–12 post-last use and after late onset, usually 12 hours or longer after last use. Early onset usually consists of subjective complaints like leg cramps and back and stomach aches. Where late-onset symptoms include:

- Dilated pupils
- Lachrymation (watery eyes)
- Rhinorrhoea (running nose)
- Piloerection (goosebumps)
- Borborygmi (increased bowel sounds)
- Nausea and diarrhoea
- Increased anxiety and agitation

Piloerection and borborygmi are caused by the sympathetic nervous system and therefore more difficult to feign, making them good clinical indicators of withdrawal from opiates. The use of a symptom scale, for example the Clinical Opiate Withdrawal Score (COWS), is often used to assess withdrawal to monitor severity and track response to any treatment.

A major feature of opioid withdrawal is anxiety because opioid-dependent individuals cannot source and use opioids and the fact they know they will develop an uncomfortable withdrawal syndrome. HCPs can play an important role in easing an individuals' anxiety, by listening to their concerns, reflecting those concerns, making detailed assessments and providing reassurance that when treatment is indicated, it will be provided. During these assessments, it is important that HCPs are mindful of their language. Avoid statements such as *'You are not withdrawing'*. Instead, use *'There are no outward signs of withdrawal'*. This approach does not discount what the individual has said; it does not suggest the HCP does not believe them and it is factually correct statement, which is hard to argue with.

Treatment It is often said opioid withdrawal is harmless and not fatal; this is simply not true (Darke et al. 2017). While death from opioid withdrawal is rare, it can occur, especially in protracted cases in frail individuals with other comorbidities. Additionally, Rees (2023) noted custody nurses held negative assumptions about drug-dependent individuals, considering them manipulative and drug-seeking and therefore reluctant to treat. In the absence of clinically objective signs of opioid withdrawal, symptomatic relief such as antiemetics, antispasmodic and simple analgesia may be appropriate. However, in the presence of objective signs, symptomatic relief should not replace treatment as outlined in the following text.

Opioid withdrawal is commonly treated in custody with dihydrocodeine 60–90 mg three or four times a day, despite this being an off-license use of the drug (RCP 2020). It has a short half-life of between 3.5 and 4.5 hours, so it requires

---

SCENARIO 10.2 Opioid withdrawal

You see a 33-year-old male who is arrested for shoplifting. He has a long history of opioid dependence and is complaining he is 'rattling'. He has come to the medical room, but he is very irritable; he responds abruptly to questions and refuses to take the blanket off his head.

1. *How do you approach this assessment?*
    a. *What factors will impact your decision?*

2. *What is the significance of the irritability?*

3. *How can you encourage him to engage in the assessment?*

---

regular dosing (see Figure 10.2), but is perceived to be safer due to this and the decreased risk of overdose. Additionally, there is extensive experience in its use in custody. Once started, dihydrocodeine should be continued at regular intervals and not used 'as required', with individuals bouncing in and out of opioid withdrawal.

Methadone and Buprenorphine

The commencement of opioid substitution therapy (OST), such as methadone or buprenorphine (see Box 10.10), is not recommended in custody. However, it should be continued where possible for those already prescribed whose risk assessment enables the safe continuation. It is important to continue OST when safe, as these long-acting opioids prevent withdrawal, providing a steady state of opioid (see Figure 10.2). Additionally, those who miss three doses of OST are at risk being taken off their OST prescription, which may drive them to seek drugs elsewhere, putting them at risk of overdose and increasing criminality.

OST continuation in custody The process of authorising the continuation of OST in custody varies and HCPs must be familiar with and follow their local policies. OST should only be considered following a thorough clinical assessment as outlined in Chapter 3 – Fitness Assessments. OST should never be given if there is current evidence of intoxication and because of the risk of drugs or alcohol consumed prior to arrest, it is prudent to hold off OST for at least 2 hours following arrival.

Supervised OST should be collected by police from a reliable source (typically the dispensing chemist) with confirmation of recent compliance. If OST cannot be collected or compliance confirmed, then individuals should be treated with dihydrocodeine as outlined earlier.

OST collected from a home address, which is not supervised is at risk of being diverted and not taken by the named individual. Therefore, there is a risk that the administration may cause harm. Practice varies, with some authorising such OST and others treating with dihydrocodeine as outlined earlier.

Because of the long half-lives of OST, individuals may not develop signs of opioid withdrawal. There is no need to withhold OST in the absence of opioid withdrawal signs. However, the presence of opioid withdrawal symptoms should be investigated, as it may indicate they have not taken OST in the previous 72 hours or may indicate the additional use of opioids on top of their OST. If HCPs are suspicious the OST has not been administered in the previous 72 hours, they should not authorise and treat with dihydrocodeine as outlined earlier.

Individuals on prolonged-release buprenorphine injections should not develop opioid withdrawal symptoms in custody.

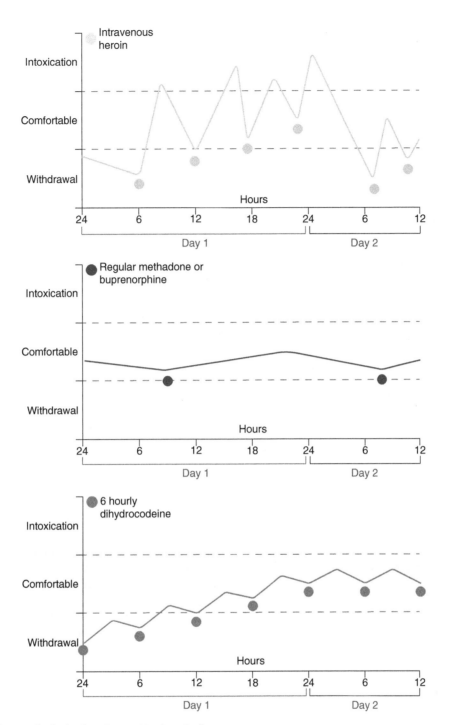

FIGURE 10.2   Opioid use and substitution. *Source:* Matthew Peel.

STIMULANTS

COCAINE AND CRACK COCAINE

Cocaine is the second most used drug in the United Kingdom after cannabis. It comes from the coca plant of South America and is usually a white, odourless powder. Crack cocaine is the end result of mixing cocaine with an alkaline solution, which makes it into small rocks. Cocaine and crack cocaine are Class A drugs and cocaine is a controlled drug. Cocaine can be snorted, taken orally or injected. Crack cocaine can be smoked, heated on foil and vapour inhaled or injected. Cocaine is a stimulant and an anaesthetic. The onset of action depends on the route. It can also be taken alongside heroin, known as 'speed-balling'.

BOX 10.10	METHADONE AND BUPRENORPHINE
Methadone	Methadone is a synthetic opioid with a slow onset, a long half-life (20–37 hours) and peak effect of around 4 hours. A typical maintenance dose is between 60 and 120 mg daily. It is mostly commonly prescribed as a liquid, although it is available in other forms.
Buprenorphine	Buprenorphine, commonly referred to by its original brand name Subutex®, is both a partial opioid agonist and antagonist (blocker) administered sublingually, with a long half-life (on average 38 hours). A typical dose is between 12 and 24 mg daily. At doses above 8 mg, buprenorphine has a high affinity (attachment) to the opioid receptors, reducing the effect of additional opioids (i.e. heroin). Suboxone® is the brand name for a combined buprenorphine/naloxone preparation. More recently, a prolonged-release buprenorphine injection (Buvidal®) has been introduced. It is available as a weekly or monthly injection and avoids the need for daily dosing.

Intoxication

Symptoms include:

- Psychological
  - Euphoria
  - Increased energy and alertness
  - Irritability or agitation
  - Paranoia or anxiety
- Physical
  - Dilated pupils
  - Increased heart rate, blood pressure and temperature
  - Sweating
  - Tremors or muscle twitching
- Behavioural
  - Overconfidence
  - Increased talkativeness
  - Restlessness or hyperactive
  - Impulsive
- Other
  - Runny nose and sniffing

Dependence

Cocaine is a highly addictive drug, mostly due to the brain changes that occur with use increasing dopamine and the associated euphoria. It is generally associated with psychological rather than physical addiction. But some individuals can increase their use to combat the 'come down' feeling after use, creating dependence. Regular use will build up tolerance, requiring higher doses to achieve the same effects. Animal studies showed that even after a significant period of abstinence, one dose reignites the pre-abstinence levels of tolerance, which is thought to give some insight into the reason humans relapse so easily (Fenton 2016).

Whether or not cocaine and crack cause tolerance and subsequently a withdrawal syndrome is hotly debated. This is in part due to the fact that both of these drugs do not cause a physical addiction similar to that of heroin, and based on this, it would be inappropriate and misleading to define and measure any withdrawal with the same classifications as heroin. These, as with all drugs, have their own unique and extremely powerful physical effects on individuals.

Cocaine is very harmful and each year, features as a contributing cause of deaths in police custody. This is because cocaine is particularly dangerous because of its effects on the heart. Anyone complaining of chest pain who uses cocaine (regardless of age) should be treated seriously and promptly because of the risk of coronary artery spasms.

Withdrawal

One of the classic symptoms of chronic cocaine or crack use is, as its description suggests, the stimulation of the user. Which keeps them awake, alert and allows them to function. Remove that stimulant effect and the resulting feeling of the user will include tiredness, exhaustion, an inability to sleep and also a level of associated panic and anxiety, causing emotional and physical distress.

A more comprehensive list of the symptoms is seen below, but sadly, those aware of these symptoms find them too unbearable and, in an attempt to avoid them, will continue to use the substance despite its harmful effects in the long term.

Symptoms include:

- Craving
- Fatigue
- Insomnia
- Depression
- Suicidal ideation
- Self-harm

Treatment No specific medications are approved for cocaine withdrawal. The focus should be on offering reassurance and symptomatic relief.

SCENARIO 10.3 Cocaine intoxication

You are asked to see a 56-year-old male who has been arrested for assault. He reports having consumed several pints of lager and some cocaine. He has asked to see you because of 'heartburn'.

1. *How do you approach this assessment?*
   a. *What factors will impact your decision?*
2. *What is the potential significance of heartburn?*
3. *What condition needs to be ruled out?*

AMPHETAMINE

Originally introduced in the 1930s as nasal decongestants and sold over the counter until the 1970s. It was also used medically to treat obesity and depression, narcolepsy and other disorders. Laws stopped their use as people discovered their potential for abuse and dangerous effects offset the medical advantages.

Pure amphetamine is white, odourless, bitter-tasting crystals. Its colour can range from white – grey – pink. Amphetamine was re-classified in 2007 from Class B to Class A drug.

Intoxication

Signs of intoxication are similar to cocaine use as they are both stimulants and include:

- Psychological
  - Euphoria
  - Anxiety
  - Paranoia
  - Irritable
- Physical
  - Increased heart rate, blood pressure and temperature
- Behavioural
  - Aggression
  - Talkative or fast speech
- Other
  - Insomnia

Withdrawal

Withdrawal from amphetamine is described as the 'come down' and the crash, which can cause symptoms such as prolonged sleeping, irritability, depressed mood, overeating and food cravings.

Treatment Generally, withdrawal from amphetamine is subjective, with no medications demonstrating efficacy in treating withdrawal. However, some medications can help alleviate the symptoms, in the short-term diazepam for anxiety and antidepressants in the longer-term antidepressants for depression.

ECSTASY

Originally classed in the stimulant group, following changes to the Drugs Wheel, it now falls into a category of empathogens. Ecstasy was first made by two German chemists in 1912 and patented in 1914, in case it turned out to be a useful drug. It didn't! During the 1950s, the American military experimented with a whole range of drugs, including ecstasy, for use in chemical warfare, to extract information from prisoners and to immobilise armies. In the 1960s, the drug was rediscovered by an American research chemist Alexander Shulgin, who experimented with it on himself. Then wrote a book about his adventures, 'PIKHAL – A chemical love story'.

As its group, empathogens, suggests, this drug makes people feel in tune with each other, and allows people to build bonds in short periods of time. It was this quality that led to some therapists across history using this with couples whose marriages were failing. Indeed, it is still used in this way in Switzerland. However, this is the exception rather than the rule and owing to some animal trials which showed the potential for brain damage in the subjects, the drug was officially banned in the United States in 1985.

The chemical name is 3,4 methylenedioxymethamphetamine or MDMA for short, carries a possible 7-year prison sentence for possession and a possible 'life' term for supply. It has been most associated with the dance club scene since the 1990s to allow people to dance and party all night. Normally taken in tablet form.

Intoxication

Symptoms include:

- Psychological
  - Marked euphoria
  - Increased sociability and empathy (even with strangers)
  - Energised
- Physical
  - Alert
  - Increased heart rate, blood pressure and temperature
  - Teeth grinding or jaw clenching
- Behavioural
  - Talkative
  - Uninhibited

Withdrawal

This is very similar to amphetamine, featuring depression, anxiety, irritability, paranoia, agitation and cravings, though mostly not physically dangerous. Because the purity of ecstasy is such an unknown and can be mixed with a plethora of other drugs, it can be hard to differentiate true ecstasy symptoms and those associated with the drugs it is cut with. Therefore, a symptom relief approach would be advised.

CANNABINOIDS

CANNABIS

Cannabis is a Class B drug, having been reclassified from a Class C in 2009 and it is the most prevalent illegal drug in the United Kingdom. It is mildly psychotropic and there has been a suggested association with psychoses. In small percentages of people, those who started using cannabis very young and use it every day, addiction can be a problem. But mostly, it creates psychological dependence. It can cause short-term memory loss and attention deficits.

It is most commonly smoked in joints, but it can be eaten in potcakes. Eating cannabis usually intensifies the effects.

Intoxication

Signs include but are not exclusive too:

- Psychological
  - Euphoria
  - Altered perception of time
  - Relaxed or sedate
  - Paranoid or anxiety
- Physical
  - Red eyes (conjunctival injection)
  - Increased heart rate or blood pressure
  - Dry mouth
  - Impaired coordination
  - Dilated pupils
- Behavioural
  - Laughing inappropriately
- Other
  - Distinctive cannabis odour
  - Increased appetite

Withdrawal

The symptoms of withdrawal from cannabis have been likened in severity to those associated with tobacco. As this is generally smoked using tobacco, this also needs consideration as well as its addictive properties. So generally tolerable. They would

include cravings but decreased appetite and associated weight loss. Difficulty in sleeping, anxiety, restlessness, tiredness, anger, irritability, hot and cold flushes and aching muscles.

Treatment It is generally not treated due to its mild presentation and limited duration.

Synthetic cannabinoid receptor antagonists (SCRA's) are the more recent addition to this group. Coined 'legal' highs before the NPS Act came into force in 2016, these were sold as herbal products. Often referred to under the umbrella term of 'spice', their effects start much more rapidly than cannabis and last much longer.

They are responsible for much more severe poisonings, as the constituents of them are rarely known, constantly changed and were often sold as 'unfit for human consumption'. They are also associated with an increased risk of serotonin syndrome, a potentially life-threatening condition that can be caused by taking new drugs.

This chapter has concentrated on the groups of drugs and substances most commonly seen in the criminal justice environment; however, it is pertinent to mention a couple of other drugs that are increasing in use and abuse.

DISSOCIATIVES

KETAMINE

Ketamine is a dissociative anaesthetic with euphoric properties of being dreamlike, detached, confused, nauseated with an altered sense of time and space. It is highly dangerous to use particularly if mixed with other drugs. It makes individuals feel chilled and relaxed with an inability to feel pain, so injury is a real risk. Long-term use can cause irreversible bladder damage, incontinence or having to have their bladder removed. Ketamine is addictive but does not cause physical withdrawal; instead, it is associated with psychological dependence.

NITROUS OXIDE

Nitrous oxide, otherwise known as laughing gas, creates a chilled, giggly person to anyone who inhales it. It may also cause dizziness, distortions of sound and anxiety. Effects last only a few minutes, hence repeated use. It is thought to create psychological dependence but no recognised withdrawal syndrome.

It comes in small cannisters which are often seen on street corners in towns and cities across the United Kingdom. It became a Class C drug in November 2023, making possession (without out a legitimate reason) illegal.

CONCLUSION

This chapter has explored substance use and misuse, the regulation and law behind the different substances seen in the criminal justice populations and how those intoxicated and withdrawing from each substance may present. This is an ever-changing landscape and a key area to ensure up-to-date knowledge to deliver the best care.

LEARNING ACTIVITIES

1. Reflect on a patient you have seen on a regular basis with substance misuse issues. Think about their drug history, how you have managed them and if there is any room for improvement in their care for the next time they present.

2. Prepare a teaching session for your team colleagues on substance use and misuse, including the legislation, classifications of drugs and what intoxication and withdrawal look like for each group.

3. Facilitate a group discussion around the legal and ethical implications of managing opioid withdrawal. Reflect how attitudes, values or beliefs can influence decisions. Following the discussion, present a practice scenario where the group must collaboratively develop a plan for managing a patient's medication regimen, considering all legal, ethical and health-related aspects.

RESOURCES

Online

- Clinical Institute Withdrawal Assessment Scale – Alcohol revised (CIWA-Ar) | https://umem.org/files/uploads/1104212257_CIWA-Ar.pdf

- Clinical Institute Withdrawal Assessment Scale – Benzodiazepines (CIWA-B) | https://www.smartcjs.org.uk/wp-content/uploads/2015/07/CIWA-B.pdf |

- Clinical Opiate Withdrawal Scale (COWS_| https://www.asam.org/docs/default-source/education-docs/cows_induction_flow_sheet.pdf?sfvrsn=b577fc2_2

- Glasgow Modified Alcohol Withdrawal Scale (GMAWS) | https://static1.squarespace.com/static/546e1217e4b093626abfbae7/t/58bfdf5c86e6c0b341fe5603/1488969564512/Glasgow+Modified+Alcohol+Withdrawal+Scale+%28GMAWS%29.pdf

- Royal College of General Practitioners | Resources for secure environments | https://elearning.rcgp.org.uk/mod/book/view.php?id=13151&chapterid=626

Organisations

- DrugWise | https://www.drugwise.org.uk

- Talk to Frank | https://www.talktofrank.com

- The Loop | https://wearetheloop.org

REFERENCES

Adley, M., Jones, G., and Measham, F. (2023). Jump-starting the conversation about harm reduction: making sense of drug effects, drugs: education. *Prevention and Policy* 30 (4): 347–360. https://doi.org/10.1080/09687637.2021.2013774.

Bhat, P.S., Ryali, V., Srivastava, K. et al. (2012). Alcoholic hallucinosis. *Industrial Psychiatric Journal* 21 (2): 155–157. https://doi.org/10.4103/0972-6748.119646.

Centre for Disease Control and Prevention (2023). Substance use. https://www.cdc.gov/nchs/hus/sources-definitions/substance-use.htm#:~:text=Substance%20use-,Substanc (accessed 16 January 2024).

Darke, S., Larney, S., and Farrell, M. (2017). Yes, people can die from opiate withdrawal. *Addiction* 112 (2): 199–200.

Department of Health (2017). Drug misuse and dependence; UK guidelines on clinical management. https://assets.publishing.service.gov.uk/media/5a821e3340f0b62305b92945/clinical_guidelines_2017.pdf (accessed 16 January 2024).

DrugWise (2016). NPS: come of age: a UK overview. https://www.drugwise.org.uk/wp-content/uploads/NPSComeofAge.pdf (accessed 12 February 2024).

Fenton, S. (2016). Scientists discover what cocaine does to the brain to make it so addictive. *Independent* [Online] (3 August). https://www.independent.co.uk/life-style/health-and-families/health-news/cocaine-effects-on-body-brain-why-is-it-so-addictive-scientists-study-addiction-drugs-a7169556.html (accessed 17 August 2024).

Jones, A.W. (2016). Alcohol: acute and chronic use and postmortem findings. *Encyclopedia of Forensic and Legal Medicine* 1: 84–107. https://doi.org/10.1016/B978-0-12-800034-2.00013-6.

Rees, G. (2023). The coproduction work of healthcare professionals in police custody: destabilising the care-custody paradox. *Policing and Society* 33: 51–63.

Royal College of Psychiatrists. (2020). Detainees with substance use disorders in police custody: guidelines for clinical management (fifth edition) [Online]. Royal College of Psychiatrists. https://fflm.ac.uk/wp-content/uploads/2020/12/college-report-cr227.pdf (accessed 3 September 2023).

Stark, M.M. (2020). Substance Misuse. In: *Clinical Forensic Medicine* (ed. M. Stark), 421–468. Cham: Springer.

Use of Force

CHAPTER 11

Matthew Peel[1] and Samantha Holmes[2]

[1] Leeds Community Healthcare NHS Trust, Leeds, UK & UK Association of Forensic Nurses and Paramedics

[2] Leeds Community Healthcare NHS Trust, Leeds, UK

AIM

The chapter will explore the different types of restraints, including physical restraints, leg restraints, spit hoods, handcuffs, batons, irritant sprays, conducted energy device known as taser, dogs and attenuating energy projectiles. In addition, readers will be guided through the complications associated with restraints and advice on how to assess and manage them.

LEARNING OUTCOMES

Upon completion of this chapter, readers should be able to:

- Understand the types of force and restraints used, their purposes and their potential associated complications

- Recognise the signs and symptoms of complications associated with using restraints and develop appropriate strategies for their assessment and management

- Analyse case studies related to restraint-related deaths, understand the potential causes and identify preventive strategies

SELF-ASSESSMENT

1. List the types of force and restraint commonly used on arrest or in custody and their complications

2. What are the potential physical health risks associated with each type of force and restraint?

3. What role do healthcare professionals have in advocating for the rights of restrained individuals and minimising complications?

INTRODUCTION

It is important healthcare professionals (HCPs) understand the use of force options available to officers (see Figure 11.1) and how to monitor individuals for complications, as well as documenting the use of force. Using force can result in injury, serious harm and even death. HCPs are frequently called upon to assess individuals during or following the use of force, either applied on arrest or while in custody. Police officers and custody detention officers are permitted, where necessary, to use reasonable force. That is, it was proportionate to the threat, lawful and necessary. Box 11.1 sets out the legal parameters for the use of force across the United Kingdom.

Any officer using force is accountable for their actions and may be subject to legal or disciplinary proceedings. In 2023, the Supreme Court decided officers facing disciplinary action should have their actions measured against the civil law test, rather than the higher criminal law standard (i.e. on balance of probabilities rather than beyond reasonable doubt).

Police Custody Healthcare for Nurses and Paramedics, First Edition. Edited by Matthew Peel, Jennie Smith, Vanessa Webb, and Margaret Bannerman.
© 2025 John Wiley & Sons Ltd. Published 2025 by John Wiley & Sons Ltd.
Companion website: www.wiley.com/go/policecustodyhealthcare

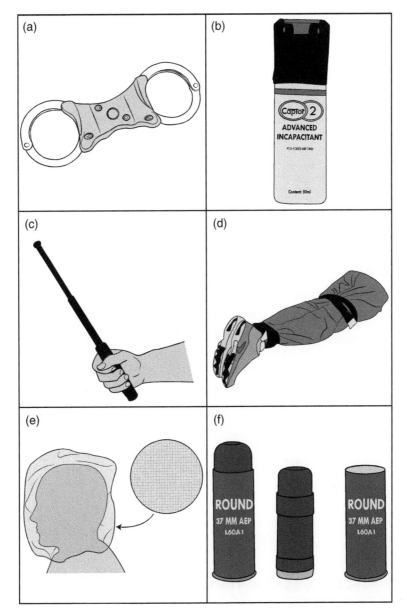

FIGURE 11.1 Use of force options. (a) Handcuffs, (b) irritant sprays, (c) baton, (d) leg restraints, (e) spit hoods and (f) attenuating energy projectiles.

Use of force statistics differs across the United Kingdom (see Box 11.2). The most common tactics are non-compliant handcuffing and ground restraint. Scotland reports significantly less use of force than the rest of the United Kingdom.

PHYSICAL RESTRAINT

Because custody suites are controlled environments, the overriding objective should be containment rather than restraint. Whereas outside of custody, someone offering violence may require restraint to control them and transfer them to custody. In the custody setting, such individuals should be contained in a cell. Restraint for the sole purpose of managing behaviour should be avoided within custody. Restraint should be reserved for specific interventions, such as moving cells, going to the hospital or preventing serious harm.

COMPLICATIONS

Restraint is inherently dangerous. Often situations are unplanned, chaotic and highly charged, involving several officers. Officers have various tactics available to them to gain control and restrain without weapons, so-called unarmed skills (see Box 11.3). Any injuries are typically

BOX 11.1   USE OF FORCE POWERS

Across the UK

- Common law

- Section 3 of the Criminal Law Act 1967

  ○ *A person may use such force as is reasonable in the circumstances in the prevention of crime or in effecting or assisting in the lawful arrest of offenders or suspected offenders or of persons unlawfully at large.*

England Wales

- Section 117 of the Police and Criminal Evidence Act 1984

  ○ *The officer may use reasonable force, if necessary, in the exercise of their power.*

England, Wales and Northern Ireland

- Section 76 of the Criminal Justice and Immigration Act 2008

  ○ *The question of whether the degree of force used by an officer was reasonable in the circumstances is to be decided by reference to the circumstances as the officer believed them to be.*

Scotland

- Section 46 of the Criminal Justice (Scotland) Act 2019

  ○ *A constable may use reasonable force to arrest or take a person in police to any place.*

Source: Crown, 2016 / Public Domain, Criminal Justice and Immigration Act (2008), Criminal Law Act (1967), Police and Criminal Evidence Act (1984).

BOX 11.3   UNARMED TACTICS

- Pain compliance
- Balance displacement
- Pressure points
- Holds
- Strikes
- Takedowns

consistent with blunt force, abrasions, lacerations, bruises, fractures and dislocations. Deaths have been associated with restraint. HCPs should be especially vigilant for any head injuries.

MANAGEMENT

HCPs should maintain an overview of any restraint, liaising closely with the controller to implement the principles of safer restraint (see Box 11.4). If able, the HCP should engage with both the individual and the officers to de-escalate the situation and reduce the need for ongoing restraint. HCPs must consider the reason for the apparent aggression and any evidence of acute behavioural disturbance (see Chapter 19 – Emergencies). HCPs should remind the controller that containment in a cell is preferable to ongoing restraint.

BOX 11.2   USE OF FORCE USE ACROSS THE UK

Method	England and Wales		Scotland		Northern Ireland	
	Number of incidents	% of arrests	Number of incidents	% of arrests	Number of incidents	% of arrests
Non-compliant handcuffing	154,459	23%	4,842	5%	5,397	26%
Limb restraints	43,150	7%	1,332	1%	-	-
Ground restraint/ unarmed tactics	102,370	15%	4,106	4%	10,035	49%
Baton	2,080	0.3%	311	0.3%	118	0.6%
Irritant spray	12,541	2%	238	0.3%	220	1%
Spit hood	8,281	1%	726	1%	123	1%
Taser	3,175	0.5%	138	0.1%	21	0.1%
Attenuating energy projectiles	58	0.01%	-	-	8	0.04%
Police dog	565	0.1%	-	-	146	0.7%

Source: Home Office (2022), Police Scotland (2022), Police Service of Northern Ireland (2022).

SCENARIO 11.1   Restraint

You are called to see a 25-year-old male who is being restrained by the police in the holding cell. He is restrained face down on the floor, with cuffs to the rear, his legs are strapped and he is wearing a spit hood. There are six officers around the individual, who is shouting and screaming. He states the handcuffs are too tight and is shouting for police to get off him.

The police report that he has been like this for some time and think he might have taken something.

1. *Describe your approach and priorities to the assessment of this individual.*

2. *Outline how you differentiate between a substance-induced or psychiatric condition or just a very angry man.*

3. *Outline your advice to the police and further management.*

BOX 11.4   PRINCIPLES OF SAFER RESTRAINT

General

1. Restraint must be necessary, justifiable and proportionate.

2. Recognise that restraint can have a significant emotional and psychological response on anyone involved or witnessing the restraint.

Training

3. Trained and authorised staff may apply approved and taught physical restraint techniques.

Restraint

4. Where three or more officers are involved, one must assume control (the controller). A custody officer not directly involved in the restraint should assume the role as soon as practical.

5. The minimum number of officers necessary should be involved (the likelihood of complications rises with the number of officers involved).

6. Avoid prone restraint or limit to the shortest necessary period.

7. Avoid pressure on the chest, neck, torso or abdomen.

8. Review restraints regularly and remove as soon as able.

Medical

9. Consider any known health risks or known drug or alcohol intoxication.

10. Continuously monitor the Airway – Breathing – Circulation and feed back to the Controller.

11. Seek an HCP review if there are any concerns.

Source: Adapted from Independent Advisory Panel on Deaths in Custody (2013) and College of Policing (2023).

LEG RESTRAINTS

Leg restraints, also known as velcro straps, leg cuffs, leg straps or limb restraints, are carried by most uniformed officers and available in custody suites. They are used to fix both legs together at the ankle and above the knee, restricting movement and preventing kicking out or otherwise injuring officers. They are secured by velcro and should be tight enough to restrict movement but not too tight to cause injury. Officers must not carry individuals using leg restraints.

Officers may temporarily apply restraints to the upper limbs (arms), when taking fingerprints by force and needing to remove handcuffs while still retaining control.

COMPLICATIONS

The prolonged or excessively tight use may lead to deep vein thrombosis, ischaemia, pressure damage, bruising or abrasions.

MANAGEMENT

Ensure straps are placed correctly above the knee and at the ankles and not too tight to impair circulation at the feet and toes (check a capillary refill). Provide some padding between the knees and ankles using a towel or clothing if prolonged use.

SPIT HOODS

Spit hoods are head coverings that prevent individuals from spitting or biting while restrained. They are often used when individuals are threatening or attempting to bite or spit. While spit hoods are controversial, they are often viewed as a necessary tool and prevent the use (or misuse) of alternatives (i.e. towels or clothing placed over the mouth).

COMPLICATIONS

Individuals, particularly those with respiratory or cardiac illnesses, wearing spit hoods, even briefly, may develop physical and psychological reactions including shortness of breath, cough, agitation, disorientation and panic attacks.

MANAGEMENT

Spit hoods are a restrictive intervention and should only be used as a last resort for the least time needed. Make regular assessments of the individual's breathing, circulation and mental state. While evidence suggests spit hoods do not restrict breathing, they can cause the sensation of difficulty in breathing, worsening anxiety and distress (Kroll et al. 2024). So, monitoring the patient's respiratory rate closely is important. If the patient reports difficulty breathing, the hood should be removed immediately. If vomiting, the hood should be removed to prevent aspiration. Equally, the hood should be avoided following the use of irritant spray.

Monitor skin integrity as spit hoods can cause skin irritation. Finally, provide emotional support. The use of a spit hood can be a stressful and traumatic experience. Showing empathy and offering reassurance may be beneficial for de-escalation.

HANDCUFFS

Handcuffs are by far the most used restraint by police. Most compliant and uncompliant arrestees will be handcuffed. Officers are equipped with rigid-style handcuffs, which benefit from easier application, reduced mobility and greater control than the older-style chain-linked handcuffs. The two metal handcuffs are joined by a rigid, fixed ergonomic bar. The handcuffs work on a ratchet system, allowing rotary motion in only one direction. The handcuffs should sit between the hand and the wrist's bony prominence. Hands may be cuffed to the front or rear in the back-to-back or stacked position. Officers can double-lock, preventing them from tightening further. However, this requires the individual's compliance. Handcuffs applied to uncompliant individuals will continue to tighten, increasing the risk of injury. Officers should check the handcuffs are not too tight before double-locking.

Occasionally, officers may use plasticuffs or similar. They work on the same principle as handcuffs, limiting mobility. One study comparing plastic and metal cuffs noted increased injuries and neuropathies with plasticuffs (Kantarci et al. 2013).

COMPLICATIONS

Injuries can range from minor abrasions to fractures and nerve damage.

Soft Tissue

Soft tissue injuries can be caused by excessively tight handcuffs or by moving wrists within the handcuffs. A common blunt-force injury pattern is seen: reddening, swelling, bruising and abrasions. It is not uncommon to see an imprint of the handcuffs. The prolonged use of handcuffs may also lead to pressure ulcers (Haber and O'Brien 2021).

Skeletal

Rarely have fractures been reported with the styloid processes most at risk, particularly the ulnar styloid process (bony prominence on the wrist). Fractures are more likely if handcuffs have been incorrectly placed. Scaphoid fractures have been reported where an individual's entire body mass was supported by rigid handcuffs, such as preventing someone from falling or lifting someone off the floor using the handcuffs (Ball et al. 2008).

Neuropathy

It is not uncommon for individuals to report numbness (paraesthesia) or increased sensitivity (hyperesthesia), below the area the handcuffs were applied. Such neuropathies are typically in the distribution of the more superficial radial nerve (see Figure 11.2). However, they can occur in the medial or ulnar nerve distribution. The risk of neuropathy is increased where handcuffs have been tight, in place for a long time, or there was greater resistance to the handcuffs. Neuropathies typically resolve within several weeks without treatment. However, individuals should be advised to follow up with their general practitioner for nerve conduction studies if symptoms persist. Neuropathies should be sensory only; any loss of motor function warrants further evaluation at the hospital.

MANAGEMENT

Most soft tissue injuries will require simple wound cleaning and dressings if appropriate. Suspected fractures will require further assessment and management at the hospital.

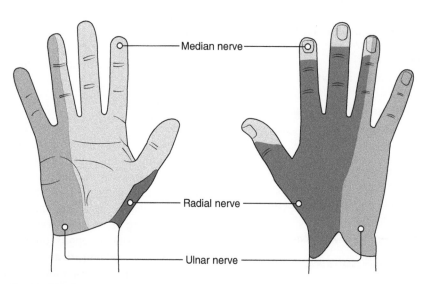

FIGURE 11.2 Nerve distribution (hand).

BATONS

Batons are a type of weapon used by police to defend themselves, subdue suspects or control a situation. Batons are available in various forms, including straight and collapsible, with the latter being more commonly used. Batons have been known to cause severe injuries.

Typically, the care required for baton injuries will vary depending on the location and severity of the injury. HCPs must know the potential risks of baton strikes to provide the best possible care.

COMPLICATIONS

Injuries are in keeping with blunt force injuries, ranging from abrasions, lacerations, bleeding and bruising, including distinct appearance with central clearing to more severe injuries including fractures, nerve or muscle damage and internal bleeding. For management of minor injuries (see Chapter 8 – Minor Injuries). Injury patterns and severity depend on the strike's location and the amount of force used. Some of the most common baton injuries that HCP need to look out for include.

Head Injuries

Head injuries range from mild concussions to serious brain injuries, such as intracerebral haemorrhages and skull fractures.

Fractures

Fractures are relatively common, particularly when striking the arms, legs and ribs. Swelling and deformities may indicate a fracture.

Chest Injuries

Blunt trauma to the chest from batons can result in life-threatening conditions including pneumothorax, haemothorax, pulmonary contusion, flail chest and parenchymal laceration.

Abdominal Injuries

Abdominal pain, distension and vomiting may be symptoms of internal bleeding. Signs of shock, such as pallor, tachycardia and hypotension, should be monitored closely. Be mindful if seeing individuals shortly or immediately following abdominal strikes, they may not have yet demonstrated bruising or evidence of shock.

Psychological Injury

In addition to physical injuries, individuals struck by a baton may also experience psychological trauma. Psychological trauma can manifest in various ways, including anxiety, depression and post-traumatic stress disorder.

MANAGEMENT

A thorough physical examination is required to assess the nature and extent of an individual's injuries. In general, HCPS should:

- Complete a full A-B-C-D-E assessment, including physiological observations, NEWS2, pupillary size and response to light
- Control any bleeding and immobilise any suspected fractures
- Manage minor injuries
- Provide analgesia (as needed)
- Monitor for deterioration
- Provide emotional support
- Document any injuries

IRRITANT SPRAYS

Irritant sprays are non-lethal weapons used to incapacitate individuals. They work quickly, typically causing an intense burning sensation, primarily affecting the eyes, see Box 11.5. Causing the suspect to become disoriented and unable to continue their aggressive behaviour, effectively de-escalating situations and preventing injuries to both officers and suspects. However, they can have negative side effects, such as skin irritation, respiratory problems and eye injuries. The effects last on average almost three hours (Payne-James et al. 2014).

BOX 11.5	IRRITANT EXPOSURE EFFECTS

Symptom	%
Pain full eye	73%
Runny nose (rhinorrhoea)	63%
Red eye (conjunctival injection)	62%
Eyes watering (lacrimation)	59%
Nasal discomfort	56%
Skin irritation	53%
Skin burning	48%
Sore throat	30%
Reduced visual acuity	19%
Photophobia	15%
Shortness of breath	13%
Nausea	13%
Sore chest	12%
Vomiting	3%

Source: Adapted from Payne-James et al. (2014).

BOX 11.6	IRRITANT SPRAYS
CS (CS O-chlorbenzlidene malonitrile 5% solution)	A synthetic compound first developed in the 1920s. It is dissolved using the solvent, methyl Isobutyl Ketone (MIBK) creating a clear, colourless and odourless liquid spray that is propelled using nitrogen.
PAVA (Pelargonic acid vanillylamide 0.3% solution)	A synthetic variant of natural pepper. It is dissolved using a mixture of solvents, Monopropylene glycol, ethanol and water. Creating a yellow liquid spray that is propelled using nitrogen.

There are two forms of irritant sprays (see Box 11.6) with most officers carrying PAVA. Irritant sprays are considered a prohibited weapon under the Firearms Act 1968 and their use is regulated by the Home Office. Trained and authorised officers may use irritant sprays only when it is proportionate and necessary to:

- Protect themselves or others from harm
- Prevent a crime from being committed
- Stop a crime that is being committed
- Make an arrest

The use of irritant sprays remains a controversial issue. Some argue irritant sprays are valuable for officers, while others argue they are too dangerous and should not be used.

COMPLICATIONS

Irritant sprays can cause various complications (see Box 11.7).

The severity of complications depends on the irritant spray used, the distance from which it is sprayed and the individual's sensitivity to the irritant. Those with asthma or other respiratory problems are at an increased risk of developing respiratory complications.

MANAGEMENT

In most cases, symptoms resolve without healthcare intervention; the priority should be removal from contamination (both location and clothing) and ventilation to promote evaporation of the irritant (see Boxes 11.8 and 11.9 for red and amber flags). Symptoms such as chest pain or difficulty in breathing should be managed as outlined in Chapter 19. HCPs should be mindful to wear appropriate PPE to prevent contamination.

SCENARIO 11.2 Irritant sprays

You are asked to see a 28-year-old man who was aggressive in his cell. He was sprayed with PAVA in his cell, five minutes ago. He has a history of asthma, eczema and borderline personality disorder. He is complaining of being unable to breathe or open his eyes. His vitals are HR 120, BP 131/78, RR 21, SpO$_2$ 99% and his chest sounds clear.

1. *Outline your immediate priorities.*

2. *Outline your decontamination advice:*
   a. *To the individual.*
   b. *To the police.*

3. *How might the use of irritant spray impact on the individual's mental health.*

4. *Outline any further management or advice.*

BOX 11.7	IRRITANT SPRAY COMPLICATIONS
Ocular	• Corneal erosion • Corneal abrasion • Periorbital oedema
Respiratory	• Shortness of breath • Wheeze • Sore throat • Chest pain • Bronchospasm • Laryngospasm • Pulmonary oedema
Skin	• Blistering • Skin redness • Chemical burns • Allergic reaction • Exacerbation of skin condition

CONDUCTED ENERGY DEVICE (TASER)

Specially trained and authorised officers can carry a Taser X26™, Taser X2™ or Taser 7™ (see Figure 11.3). While commonly referred to as tasers, they are officially referred to as conducted energy devices (CED). They are designed to cause temporary neuromuscular incapacitation by delivering an electrical current that interferes with the neuromuscular system and produces severe pain (see Box 11.10).

HOW TASERS WORK

Tasers are predominately used in the probe mode. However, they can be used in direct contact mode.

BOX 11.8	IRRITANT SPRAY MANAGEMENT

1. Provide reassurance

2. Remove from contamination (this is critical)
   a. If deployed in a confined space immediately remove
   b. Move to a well-ventilated area and consider the use of a fan directed onto the face
   c. Remove contaminated clothing or bedding and seal in plastic bags (provide clean clothing or bedding)
   d. Clean their hands thoroughly
   e. Remove any contact lenses

3. Advise against touching or rubbing their eyes

4. Washing (after each wash, change clothing and bedding to avoid re-contamination)
   a. Do not use warm water (this will reactivate the irritant)
   b. After 1 hour, if eye symptoms persist, irrigate eyes with normal saline
   c. After two to three hours, if eye symptoms persist, wash eyes/face/head with cool water
   d. For skin reactions (not eyes), if symptoms persist beyond 20 minutes, wash with copious amounts of cool water

Source: Adapted from Faculty of Forensic & Legal Medicine (2021).

BOX 11.9	IRRITANT SPRAY RED AND AMBER FLAGS

RED FLAGS – Refer to hospital
- Cannot open eyes after 30 minutes
- Eye symptoms still present after six hours
- Pulmonary oedema (up to 24 hours post-exposure)
- Wheeze unresponsive to salbutamol (or similar)

AMBER FLAGS – See GP
- Skin conditions still present after 48 hours
- Longer-term respiratory symptoms

Probe Mode

When activated, the taser fires two probes towards an individual, which remain connected via wires. Two probes must connect with the individual (either embedding in the skin or clothing), to create the necessary circuit required for neuromuscular incapacitation.[1] Additionally, probes must be adequately separated (about 23 cm apart), ideally above and below the beltline. This is necessary so that a greater muscle mass is involved. Where only a single probe connects, the taser will not work. Where two probes connect but are not sufficiently separated, the taser may be less effective. When an adequately separated circuit is created, the taser delivers a

	Taser X26	Taser X2	Taser 7
Probe (dart)	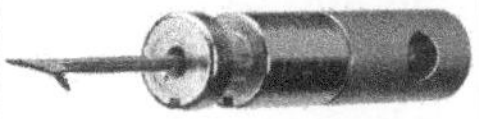 3.8 cm (1 cm dart)	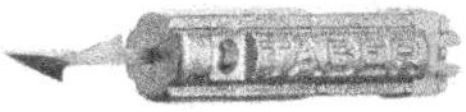 3.4 cm (1.1 cm dart)	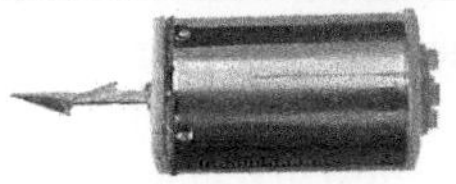 2.2 cm (1 cm dart)
Loaded cartridges	One	Two	Two
Laser sighting	Single red laser	Dual red laser	Dual laser; green (upper) & red (lower)
Range	6.4 meters	7.6 meters	7.6 meters
Pulse rate	19 per second	19 per second	22 per second
Pulse duration	110 microseconds	80 microseconds	45 microseconds

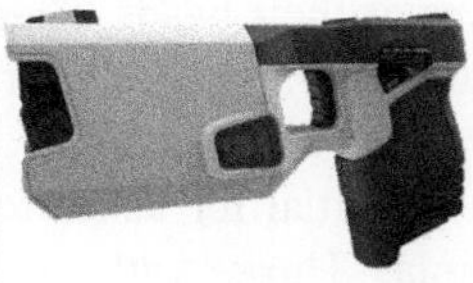

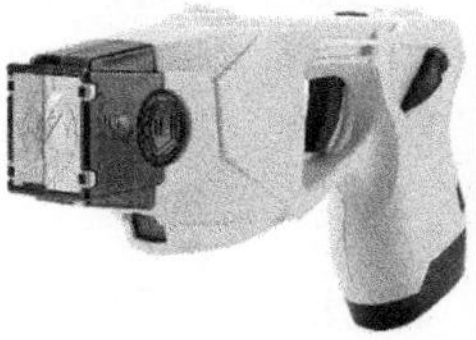

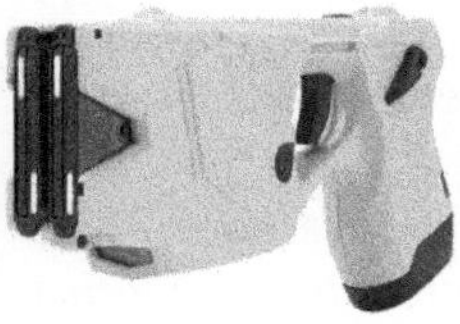

FIGURE 11.3   Taser devices. *Source:* Conducted Energy Device Joint Working Group (2022) / with permission of the UK Association of Forensic Nurses and Paramedics.

[1] The Taser X2 and 7 can fire multiple pairs of probes allowing for a cross-connection between probes from different cartridges within the same device.

BOX 11.10	NEUROMUSCULAR INCAPACITATION

- Inability to control their posture, at risk of an injury from uncontrolled and unprotected fall
- Muscle rigidity
- Convulse, spasm or stiffen
- Intense pain
- Involuntary noises
- Unable to respond to commands
- 'Freeze' on the spot

Source: Adapted with Conducted Energy Device Joint Working Group (2022).

BOX 11.11	TASER COLLATERAL HISTORY

- Evidence of mental health crisis and/or intoxication with alcohol/drugs
- Details of the number and duration of taser discharges
- Effects on the individual
- Any injuries or falls
- Probe sites and removal details
- Any additional use of other force

Source: Adapted from Conducted Energy Device Joint Working Group (2022).

five-second series of rapid and short electrical impulses resulting in neuromuscular incapacitation.

Direct Contact Mode

In direct contact mode, the front of the taser, containing two electrodes, is driven into the individual while electrically charged, causing localised pain only. This mode is less harmful than the probe mode.

COMPLICATIONS

Most complications are minor injuries typically associated with the probes or from falling to the ground. It is important to remember individuals may be unable to break their fall, or protect themselves or their heads. There are reports of barbs penetrating facial bones and causing fractures or embedding in the eye, skull, throat and genitals.

There is a potential for tasers to cause an immediate cardiac arrhythmia. Those with pacemakers or internal cardiac defibrillators, cardiac disease and thinly built individuals with barbs near the heart are at the greatest risk (Roberts and Vilke 2016). Additionally, there are some reports of seizures, strokes and miscarriages. However, caution is needed associating these solely with the taser.

Deaths and Taser

The inquest into Andrew Pimlott's death concluded the taser likely ignited the petrol he had doused himself in, causing him severe burns and death. A further four inquests determined a taser was contributory: all involved additional restraints and two involved recent cocaine use.

Taser Myths

While often claimed tasers deliver 50,000-volt electric shocks, the voltage is much lower. However, it is the electrical charge, not voltage, that risks cardiac complications. A taser's

electrical charge is only 0.1 joules per pulse, compared to 360 joules from automated external defibrillators. Unlike drugs, electricity does not accumulate within the body. Meaning there is no risk of delayed arrhythmia from the taser.

Tasers do not cause heart attacks. Heart attacks or myocardial infarctions are typically caused by the formation and rupture of an atherosclerotic plaque blocking a coronary artery. Tasers have no role in the formation or rupture of atherosclerotic plaques.

ASSESSMENT

The assessment should follow the approach outlined in Chapter 2 – Fitness Assessments. Additional, specific collateral history should be sought from the police and the individual (see Box 11.11). The clinical examination should take a systems approach being mindful of any head injury and the individual's mental state.

MANAGEMENT

Fit and well individuals who are asymptomatic and have no significant injuries do not require hospital. Box 11.12 outlines where an individual may require hospital.

Probe Removal

Probes should be removed as soon as practical, where not embedded in a sensitive area, see Box 11.13.

SCENARIO 11.3   Taser

You are asked to see a 33-year-old male who was tasered on arrest. The police reported he was behaving aggressively and had assaulted a police officer. He was tasered once with a Taser 7, with immediate neuromuscular incapacitation. He fell backwards onto concrete and was immediately cooperative afterwards. Both barbs were embedded in his clothing and did not penetrate his skin, one in the right leg and one in the centre of the abdomen.

It is over an hour since he was tasered and you have been asked to assess his fitness to detain. He is normally well, taking no medication. His vital signs are all normal. He reports some aches and pains.

1. *Outline your approach to assessing his fitness to detain.*

2. *What is the greatest risk to the individual?*

3. *How do you manage his aches and pains?*

4. *After the assessment, he asks if he needs an ECG because he was electrocuted. How do you respond?*

BOX 11.12	TASER RED AND AMBER FLAGS

RED FLAGS – Immediate hospital referral

- Suspected Acute Behavioural Disturbance
- Probe penetrated and remains embedded in a sensitive area
  - Face, neck, genitals, spine, hands, feet, joints or near major cardiovascular structures

- Any implanted device, such as:
  - Pacemaker
  - Defibrillator
  - Vagus nerve stimulator

- Pregnancy
- Chest pain, palpitations or irregular pulse
- Any Airway – Breathing – Circulation concerns
- Any head injury appearing intoxicated or meeting the National Institute for Health and Care Excellence 'Head injury: assessment and early management' guideline
- 'Drunk and incapable'

AMBER FLAGS – Consider hospital

- Significant burn
- Probe penetrated but is no longer embedded, in a sensitive area
- <18 years
- Previous spinal or neurosurgery
- Injuries outside the scope of custody healthcare

Source: Adapted with Conducted Energy Device Joint Working Group (2022).

DOG BITES

Police dogs are trained to assist the police by tracking, searching and capturing individuals. Dogs may 'catch and hold' individuals using their teeth, often biting limbs until instructed to release by their handler.

COMPLICATIONS

Common injuries associated with dog bites include puncture wounds, lacerations and abrasions. Depending on the location, they may also damage the nerve, vascular or tendon

BOX 11.13	REMOVING PROBES

1. Wear personal protective equipment (gloves and apron).

2. Cut the wires (if not already) approximately 5 cm from the probe.

3. Warn the individual they will feel some discomfort.

4. Support and stretch the skin around the probe (careful to avoid accidental sharp injury).

5. Grasping the probe, apply firm rapid traction (see Figure 11.4 for Taser 7 probe removal).

6. Inspect the probe (if retained fragments are suspected refer to the hospital).

7. Clean the area and apply a simple dressing.

structures. Because of their exceptional strength, bites may also cause crush injuries, bruises and fractures. Finally, if left untreated, there is a risk of infection.

MANAGEMENT

Initially, encourage the wound to bleed and irrigate thoroughly with warm running water. Box 11.14 outlines when referral to hospital is indicated; otherwise, clean and dress with a simple self-adhesive absorbent dressing. Wounds should not be closed. Check their tetanus status. Any bite where the skin has been punctured and drawn blood should be treated with prophylactic antibiotics, see Box 11.15.

ATTENUATING ENERGY PROJECTILES (BATON ROUNDS)

Attenuating energy projectiles (AEPs) are rarely used compared to other methods (see Figure 11.2). They are intended to be less than lethal firearms restricted to authorised and trained police officers. Soft-nosed projectiles are fired from a specially designed gun towards an individual, resulting in a blunt-force impact, causing localised severe pain either to dissuade an individual from continuing to present a serious risk to self or others, or providing an opportunity to gain control and subdue the individual. AEPs should be aimed at the torso or limbs, but there are reports of AEPs striking the head and face.

COMPLICATIONS

AEPs are designed not to penetrate the skin. Injuries are likely to be in line with blunt force injuries, bruises, lacerations and fractures, depending on the injury site. Skull and rib fractures have been documented. Serious ocular injuries have also been reported when AEPs have struck an eye. Finally, there is the risk of internal damage to organs such as the liver and spleen from AEPs striking the abdomen.

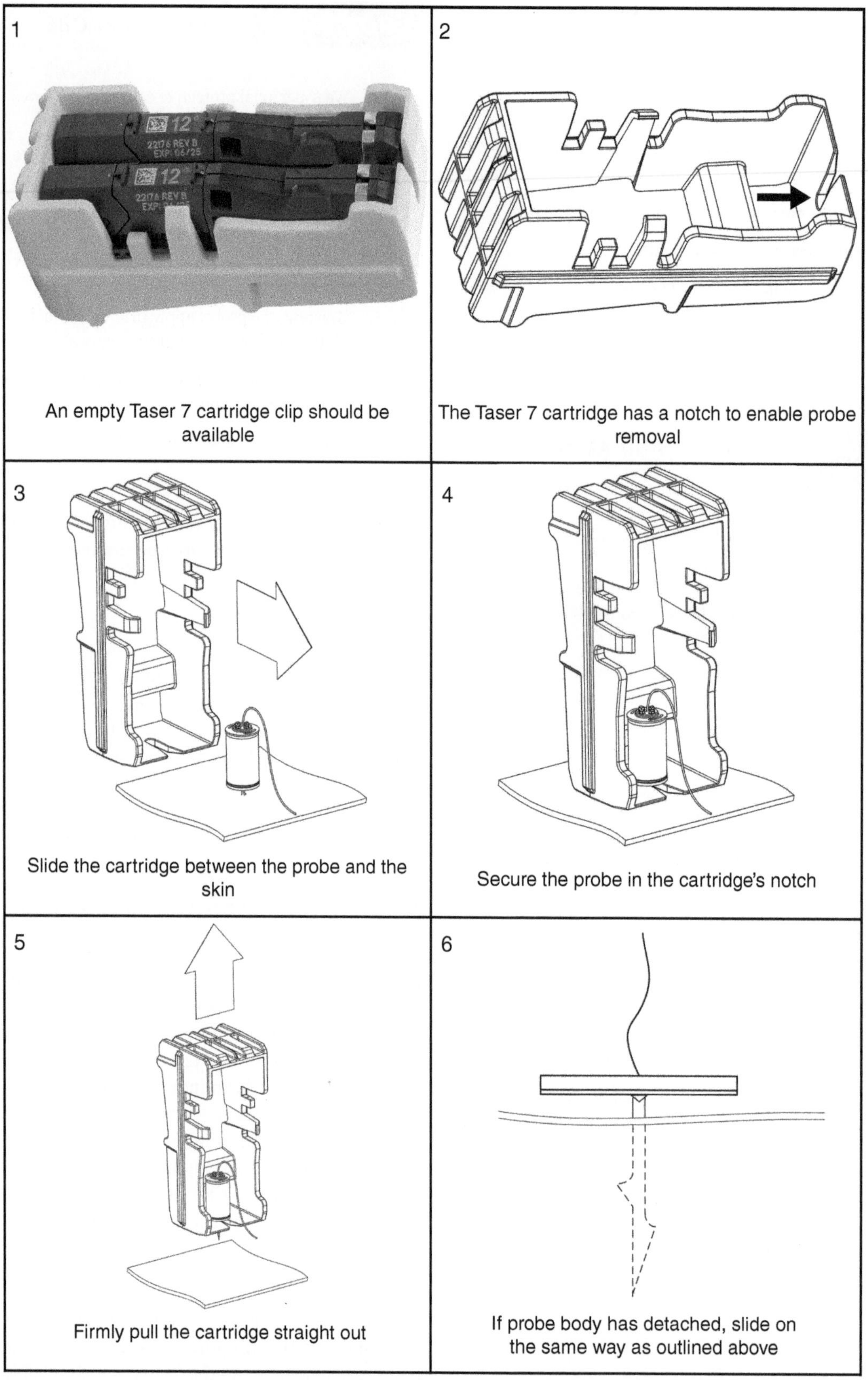

1 An empty Taser 7 cartridge clip should be available

2 The Taser 7 cartridge has a notch to enable probe removal

3 Slide the cartridge between the probe and the skin

4 Secure the probe in the cartridge's notch

5 Firmly pull the cartridge straight out

6 If probe body has detached, slide on the same way as outlined above

FIGURE 11.4 Taser 7 probe removal. *Source:* Conducted Energy Device Joint Working Group (2022) / with permission of the UK Association of Forensic Nurses and Paramedic.

BOX 11.14   DOG BITE RED FLAGS

RED FLAGS – Immediate hospital referral

- Heavy bleeding
- Wounds involving
  - Hands, face, feet, muscles, nerves, tendons or arteries
- Crush injuries
- Foreign body
- Heavy bleeding
- Wounds involving
  - Hanes, face, feet, muscles, nerves, tendons or arteries
- Crush injuries
- Foreign body

BOX 11.15   PROPHYLACTIC ANTIBIOTICS (ADULTS)

- Co-amoxiclav 250/125 mg or 500/125 mg tablets. One tablet three times a day for three days.

If penicillin allergy:

- Metronidazole 400 mg tablets. Take one tablet three times a day for three days.
- Doxycycline 200 mg tablets. Take two tablets on the first day and then one tablet for a further two days.

Source: Adapted from National Institute for Health and Care Excellence (2023).

MANAGEMENT

Assess and manage any associated blunt force injuries and look for any signs of shock. Examine the abdomen for injury, tenderness, swelling or bruising. The presence of Cullen's[2] or Grey Turner's[3] signs may indicate intraabdominal bleeding.

RESTRAINT-RELATED DEATHS

Any form of restraint can result in death; Box 11.16 outlines characteristics that may increase the risk of death. Restraint-related deaths are mostly likely to occur during the arrest or detention phase. It is important to note the use of force did not necessarily contribute to those deaths. While official statistics suggest black people are twice as likely to die than white people, in or following custody, according to INQUEST, black people[4] are seven times more likely (Inquest 2023a).

BOX 11.16   RISK FACTORS

- Mental illness (i.e. schizophrenia)
- Overweight
- Drug or alcohol intoxication/withdrawal
- Heart disease or significant past medical history
- Acute behavioural disturbance
- Prone restraint
- Neck holds
- Prolonged restraint (over 15 minutes)
- The greater the number of officers involved

ILLUSTRATIVE CASES

Sean Rigg

Sean was a 40-year-old musician and music producer who suffered from schizophrenia. After missing his depot, he developed a mental health crisis and behaved erratically. The police arrested Sean, placing him in handcuffs in the prone position for eight minutes. When he arrived at custody, he was left unattended for 10 minutes in the van before being moved inside, where he was left for a further 35 minutes, unresponsive on the floor. He was eventually noted to be in cardiac arrest and was taken to hospital by ambulance.

At his inquest, the jury concluded the police's use of force was *'unsuitable and unnecessary . . . [and] more than minimally contributed to his death'* (Casale 2013).

Thomas Orchard

Thomas was a 32-year-old caretaker who suffered from schizophrenia. Following interruptions to his medication, he relapsed, causing him to appear bizarre. The police were called, and seven officers restrained Thomas, handcuffing him to the rear and applying leg restraints. When he arrived at custody, an Emergency Response Belt[5] (ERB) was put around his face and he was carried to a cell. After 12 minutes of lying motionless, officers entered the cell and Thomas was in cardiac arrest.

A Home Office pathologist determined Thomas's death resulted from restraint, including prolonged prone positioning and the use of an ERB, leading to asphyxia (Inquest 2017). In 2023, 11 years after Thomas's death the jury at his inquest found police failures around the use of an ERB as a spit guard may have contributed to his death (Inquest 2023b). The jury also highlighted the impact of prolonged restraint, including the use and manner of use of the ERB was not necessary or reasonable.

---

[2] Bruising and swelling around the umbilicus.
[3] Bruising to the flanks, between the last rib and the top of the hip.
[4] African, African Caribbean and mixed African, African Caribbean.

[5] A fabric belt with handles intended to be used on the legs and arms.

CONCLUSION

Using force and restraints can pose significant physical challenges for the police, individual and HCPs. As we have explored in this chapter, the various types of restraints used, including physical restraints, handcuffs, spit hoods, batons, irritant sprays, CED, dogs and attenuating energy projectiles, each carry their own health risks and complications. It is crucial for HCPs in this environment to be well-versed in recognising and managing these complications, while also advocating for the rights and welfare of individuals. This involves a comprehensive understanding of the ethical and legal parameters surrounding using force and restraints and applying best practice guidelines to ensure optimal care.

LEARNING ACTIVITIES

1. Write a reflection where you were asked to see someone who was being restrained. Consider how your attitudes, values and beliefs may have impacted your approach to the assessment, advice and ability to communicate with officers and the individual.

2. Participate in joint simulated situations with the police, involving the use of restraints and practice assessing individuals, identifying potential risks and managing complications related to the use of force and restraints.

3. Conduct a group discussion on the ethical and legal considerations related to the use of force and restraints. How can HCPs advocate for the rights of individuals and ensure their welfare?

RESOURCES

Online

- College of Policing | Authorised Professional practice | Use of force, firearms and less lethal weapons | https://www.college.police.uk/app/armed-policing/use-force-firearms-and-less-lethal-weapons
- UK Association of Forensic Nurses and Paramedics | Conducted energy device (taser) information hub | www.ukafnp.org/ced

Organisations

- INQUEST | www.inquest.org
- Restraint Reduction Network | Resources | https://restraintreductionnetwork.org/resources/?_sft_resource-category=models-of-restraint-reduction#results

REFERENCES

Ball, L., Ferran, N., and Barton, C. (2008). Scaphoid fracture due to rigid handcuffs. *The Journal of Hand Surgery* 33E (4): 484–487.

Casale, S. (2013). Report of the independent external review of the IPCC investigation into the death of Sean Rigg. https://webarchive.nationalarchives.gov.uk/ukgwa/20131004165058/http://www.ipcc.gov.uk/investigations/sean-rigg-metropolitan-police-service (accessed 13 July 2023).

College of Policing (2023). Principles of using force in custody. https://www.college.police.uk/app/detention-and-custody/control-restraint-and-searches (accessed 13 July 2023).

Conducted Energy Device Joint Working Group (2022) *Healthcare Assessment in Police Custody After Conducted Energy Device (CED) Discharge; Full Guideline*. London: UK Association of Forensic Nurses and Paramedics. https://ukafn.org/wp-content/uploads/2022/09/Healthcare-assessment-in-police-custody-after-conducted-energy-device-CED-discharge-Aug-2022.pdf (accessed 29 July 2023).

Criminal Justice (Scotland) Act (2016). Criminal Justice (Scotland) Act 2016 https://www.legislation.gov.uk/asp/2016/1/section/45/enacted (accessed 10 July 2023).

Criminal Justice and Immigration Act (2008). Criminal Justice and Immigration Act 2008 https://www.legislation.gov.uk/ukpga/2008/4/section/76 (accessed 10 July 2023).

Criminal Law Act. (1967). Criminal Law Act 1967. https://www.legislation.gov.uk/ukpga/1967/58/section/3 (accessed 10 July 2023).

Faculty of Forensic & Legal Medicine (2021). Irritant sprays: clinical effects and management. https://fflm.ac.uk/wp-content/uploads/2021/02/Irritant-sprays-clinical-effects-and-management-Dr-J-McGorrigan-Prof-J-Payne-James-Jan-2021.pdf (accessed 16 October 2023).

Haber, L.A. and O'Brien, M. (2021). Shackling ulcer: an upper extremity ulcer secondary to handcuffs. *Journal of General Internal Medicine* 36 (7): 2146.

Home Office (2022). Police use of force statistics, England and Wales: April 2021 to March 2022. https://www.gov.uk/government/statistics/police-use-of-force-statistics-england-and-wales-april-2021-to-march-2022/police-use-of-force-statistics-england-and-wales-april-2021-to-march-2022#ced-conducted-energy-device-use (accessed 29 June 2023).

Independent Advisory Panel on Deaths in Custody (2013). Common principles of safer restraint. https://static1.squarespace.com/static/5c5ae65ed86cc93b6c1e19a3/t/60520a7e1497e117dcf65795/1615989374834/IAP+common+principles+for+safer+restraint.pdf (accessed 10 July 2023).

Inquest (2017). Not-guilty jury verdict in the manslaughter trial of police sergeant and two detention officers following death of Thomas Orchard. https://www.inquest.org.uk/thomas-orchard-police-manslaughter-trial

Inquest (2023a). I can't breath; Race, death & British policing. https://www.inquest.org.uk/Handlers/Download.ashx?IDMF=edfc7c01-e7bb-4a17-9c33-8628905460e6 (accessed 13 July 2023).

Inquest (2023b). Thomas Orchard: inquest finds police failures may have contributed to death following prolonged restraint. https://www.inquest.org.uk/thomas-orchard-inquest-concludes (accessed 22 December 2023).

Kantarci, M.N., Kandemir, E., Berber, G. et al. (2013). Evaluation of plastic and metal handcuff-related injuries under custody in medical examinations. *Turkiye Klinikleri Journal of Medical Sciences* 33 (2): 360–365.

Kroll, M.W., Hail, S.L., and Brave, M.A. (2024). Do saliva-saturated spit hoods interfere with ventilation? *American Journal of Forensic Medicine and Pathology* 45 (1): 10–14.

National Institute for Health and Care Excellence (2023). Bites - human and animal. https://cks.nice.org.uk/topics/bites-human-animal/ (accessed 10 July 2023).

Payne-James, J.J., Smith, G., Rivers, E. et al. (2014). Effects of incapacitant spray deployed in the restraint and arrest of detainees in the Metropolitan Police Service area, London, UK: a prospective study. *Forensic Science, Medicine and Pathology* 10 (1): 62–68.

Police and Criminal Evidence Act. (1984). Police and Criminal Evidence Act 1984 https://www.legislation.gov.uk/ukpga/1984/60/section/117 (accessed 10 March 2023).

Police Scotland (2022). Operation safety use of force; Quarter 4 performance reports April 2021 to March 2022. https://www.scotland.police.uk/spa-media/3fnhurfk/use-of-force-external-performance-report-q4-2021-22.docx (accessed 10 July 2023).

Police Service of Northern Ireland (2022). Use of force by the police in Northern Ireland; 1 April 2021 to 31 March 2022. https://www.psni.police.uk/sites/default/files/2022-09/PSNI%20Use%20of%20Force%20Statistical%20Report%201%20Apr%202021%20-%2031%20Mar%202022v2.pdf (accessed 10 July 2023).

Roberts, E. and Vilke, G.M. (2016). Restraint techniques, injuries, and death: conducted energy devices. In: *Encyclopedia of Forensic and Legal Medicine*, Seconde, vol. 4 (ed. J. Payne-James and R.W. Byard), 118–126. Oxford: Elsevier.

FURTHER READING

Conducted Energy Device Joint Working Group. Healthcare assessment in custody conducted energy device – full guideline. https://irp.cdn-website.com/552775eb/files/uploaded/Healthcare-assessment-in-police-custody-after-conducted-energy-device-CED-discharge-Aug-2022.pdf.

Peel M, Tremlett D (2022) Assessing and managing people exposed to conducted energy device (Taser) discharge. *Emergency Nurse* 30 (4): 16–23. doi: https://doi.org/10.7748/en.2022.e2125

Road Traffic Law and Procedures

CHAPTER 12

Alex Guymer

Mitie Care and Custody Health Ltd, London, UK

AIM

This chapter aims to enhance healthcare professionals' (HCPs) understanding of road traffic legislation and alleviate some of the common misconceptions and anxieties surrounding such legislation, its wording and the procedures regularly requested of HCPs. The chapter will also explore legal and ethical principles.

LEARNING OUTCOMES

Upon completion of this chapter, readers should be able to:

- Understand the relevant sections of the road traffic legislation

- Understand a constable's powers to request samples

- Obtain knowledge of prescribed limits under the road traffic legislation in the United Kingdom (UK)

- Understand the procedures requested of HCPs

SELF-ASSESSMENT

1. What are the common anxieties and misconceptions surrounding procedures undertaken as part of road traffic legislation?

2. Outline one case that has provided case law in relation to the Road Traffic Act and how it has impacted our practice.

3. Consider the advantages and disadvantages of including the field impairment test in a medical assessment as part of the Road Traffic Act Section 4 (Section 15 Northern Ireland) process.

INTRODUCTION

Road traffic procedures form a large percentage of work healthcare professionals (HCPs) undertake. Despite this, there are often anxieties and misconceptions surrounding the procedures and legislation, which can be reduced by having a good foundation of understanding of the relevant legislation. In addition to the HCP's role under road traffic legislation, HCPs have a clinical responsibility and should complete a full assessment as outlined in Chapter 3 – Fitness Assessments, including fitness to be detained (especially if they appear under the influence, or have been involved in a road traffic collision). This was reinforced by the Independent Office for Police Conduct (2023) in their 2022/23 review of deaths in custody, where two individuals died after becoming ill from injuries[1] sustained in a collision. Additionally, some individuals will require an interview. Finally, it may also provide an opportunity to offer a brief intervention for those suffering from drug or alcohol misuse.

It is vital that HCPs understand the relevant legislation:

- Road Traffic Act 1988 (England, Scotland and Wales)

- The Road Traffic Act 1988 (Prescribed Limit) (Scotland) Regulations 2014

- The Road Traffic (Northern Ireland) Order 1995

---

[1] One suffered a subdural haematoma and the other an intra-abdominal haemorrhage.

Police Custody Healthcare for Nurses and Paramedics, First Edition. Edited by Matthew Peel, Jennie Smith, Vanessa Webb, and Margaret Bannerman.
© 2025 John Wiley & Sons Ltd. Published 2025 by John Wiley & Sons Ltd.
Companion website: www.wiley.com/go/policecustodyhealthcare

It is important to also understand the case law in relation to road traffic procedures, as this forms the evidence base for why we do or do not follow certain processes.

To assist officers with meeting the legislative requirements, the devolved nations have developed a series of forms (see Box 12.1). While these forms are completed by the officer, it is important HCPs are familiar with and have a good understanding of the relevant forms.

The Road Traffic Act 1988 was enacted partly to prosecute offences relating to driving under the influence of alcohol and, or drugs within England, Scotland and Wales. Northern Ireland enacted their own version in 1995 and while similar, there are some variations (e.g. careless driving does not have to result in death; it also includes grievous bodily injury).

Comprehensive documentation is critical in all aspects of forensic and healthcare procedures. But perhaps more so with road traffic, as these are the most common reasons HCPs provide statements and attend court. Comprehensive documentation makes statement writing and court attendance easier.

BOX 12.1	**ROAD TRAFFIC FORMS**

England and Wales

- MG DD/A: Drink/drugs station procedure
- MG DD/B: Drink/drugs procedure general (police station only)
- MG DD/C: Drink/drugs hospital procedure
- MG DD/F: Roadside impairment testing

Scotland

- DD1: Section 5 (alcohol) Station procedure where approved breath specimen device available
- DD2: Section 5 (alcohol) Station procedure where approved breath specimen device not used or procedure not concluded
- DD3: Section 4 (unfit through drink/drugs) Station procedure where approved breath specimen device is available
- DD4: Section 4 or 5 Station procedure where approved breath specimen device not used or procedure not concluded
- DD5: Section 3A, 4, 5 or 5A Hospital procedure
- DD5A: Hospital procedure driver incapable of giving consent
- DD6: Preliminary impairment test

Northern Ireland

- PSNI DD/A: Drink/drugs station procedure
- PSNI DD/B: Drug/drugs procedure general
- PSNI DD/C: Drink/drugs hospital procedure

ROAD TRAFFIC LEGISLATION

To aid in understanding the relevant sections, an exploration of wording and terminology is important. While Northern Ireland's sections differ, the wording is similar or identical (see Box 12.2).

CAUSING DEATH BY CARELESS DRIVING WHILST UNDER THE INFLUENCE OF DRINK OR DRUGS

An individual commits an offence if they cause the death[2] of another by driving a mechanically propelled vehicle (see Box 12.3) at the time of the incident, with either the presence of alcohol above the prescribed limit in breath, blood or urine or with a specified drug level above the prescribed limit in blood or urine. An evidential sample can be requested within 18 hours of the offence, individuals failing to provide a sample may be liable to prosecution.

DRIVING, OR BEING IN CHARGE, WHEN UNDER THE INFLUENCE OF DRINK OR DRUGS

It is an offence to drive or be in charge of, a mechanically propelled vehicle when unfit through drink or drugs. 'In charge' includes, sitting in or on the vehicle with the key in the ignition while on a road or public place. Individuals can challenge their 'being in charge' but this will be for the court to decide and should not delay procedures. Officers can request a sample of blood or urine once the HCP has assessed the individual and determined the presence of a condition, which might be due to a drug[3] (*see 'Assessing for a condition which might be due to a drug'*).

DRIVING, OR BEING IN CHARGE OF A MOTOR VEHICLE WITH ALCOHOL CONCENTRATION ABOVE PRESCRIBED LIMIT

It is an offence to drive, attempt to drive or be in charge of, a motor vehicle on a road or public place with a proportion of alcohol above the prescribed limit in breath, blood or urine (see Box 12.4). Importantly, the offence only applies to motor vehicles. Officers often chose to sample breath using an approved evidential devise, HCPs are largely uninvolved.

---

[2] Or grievous bodily injury (Northern Ireland).

[3] There are some exceptions, in Scotland the DD4 allows officers to request a sample of blood or urine for section 4 without the HCP's opinion if there is a positive preliminary drugs test. In England and Wales, the MG DD/B allows officers investigating both section 4 and 5A to request a sample of blood if there is a positive preliminary drugs test. In Northern Ireland where a subject has provided a positive preliminary drug test on a device of a type approved for the purpose, officers may request a sample of blood or urine.

BOX 12.2	ROAD TRAFFIC LEGISLATION ACROSS THE UK

Road Traffic Act 1988 (England, Wales and Scotland)	The Road Traffic (Northern Ireland) Order 1995	Offence wording
Section 3A	Section 14	Causing death[4] by careless driving when under influence of drink or drugs
Section 4	Section 15	Driving, or being in charge, when under influence of drink or drugs
Section 5	Section 16	Driving or being in charge of a motor vehicle with alcohol concentration above prescribed limit
Section 5A		Driving or being in charge of a motor vehicle with concentration of specified controlled drug above specified limit
Section 7	Section 18	Provision of specimens for analysis
Section 7A	Section 18A	Specimens of blood taken from persons incapable of consenting
Section 9	Section 20	Protection for hospital patients
Section 10	Section 21	Detention of persons affected by alcohol or a drug

BOX 12.3	VEHICLE DEFINITIONS

Motor vehicle	A mechanically propelled vehicle intended or adapted for use on roads (i.e. cars, motorcycles and lorries. The key aspect is the vehicle is designed or adapted to be used on public roads and is mechanically propelled.
Mechanically propelled vehicle	A broader term, including all mechanically propelled vehicles, including combustion and electric motors/engines. It does not have to be intended for road use.

BOX 12.4	PRESCRIBED LIMITS OF ALCOHOL

	England, Wales and Northern Ireland	Scotland
Breath	35 mcg/100ml	22 mcg/100ml
Blood	80 mcg/100ml	50 mcg/100ml
Urine	107 mcg/100ml	67 mcg/100ml

Source: Crown / Public Domain.

[4] or grievous bodily injury (Northern Ireland).

Refusing to Provide a Sample of Breath

Individuals refusing to provide a breath sample without a reasonable excuse are liable to prosecution for 'failure to provide' under section 7 (Section 18 Northern Ireland). According to case law, no excuse is reasonable unless the person is physically or mentally unable to provide it, or the provision would entail a substantial risk to health (*R v Lennard* 1973). It is solely for the officer to decide if the excuse provided is reasonable. If they decide the excuse to be reasonable, they may request a blood sample. The case law around this issue is complex; as in *DPP v Kinnersley* [1993], Kinnersley refused to provide a sample and did not cite a reason at the police station. However, he advised the court he believed providing a sample would risk exposure to HIV. The court found Kinnersley not guilty. Other reasonable excuses have included failure to understand the procedure (due to limited English), too distressed and panic attacks. It is not for HCPs to determine, or confirm the presence of a reasonable excuse. However, if asked they should advise whether any sample is preferrable and the best route to securing a prosecution (Stark and Brener 2000).

DRIVING, OR BEING IN CHARGE OF A MOTOR VEHICLE WITH CONCENTRATION OF SPECIFIED DRUG ABOVE SPECIFIED LIMIT

Across England, Wales and Scotland, Section 5A came into force in 2015. Demonstrating the government's zero tolerance on drug driving, with limits set lower than initially recommended. Currently, Northern Ireland has no comparable offence. This offence is similar to aforementioned

BOX 12.5	SPECIFIED LIMITS OF DRUGS

Controlled drug	England and Wales limits (mcg/l)	Scotland limits (mcg/l)
Amphetamine	–	250
Benzoylecgonine (Cocaine)	50	50
Clonazepam	50	50
Cocaine	10	10
Delta-9-Tetrahydrocannabinol (Cannabis)	2	2
Diazepam	550	550
Flunitrazepam	300	300
Ketamine	20	20
Lorazepam	100	100
Lysergic acid diethylamide (LSD)	1	1
Methadone	500	500
Methylamphetamine	10	10
Methylenedioxymethamphetamine (MDMA)	10	10
6-Monoacetylmorphine (Heroin)	5	5
Morphine	80	80
Oxazepam	300	300
Temazepam	1000	1000

Source: Crown / Public Domain.

drunk-driving, requiring an individual to drive, attempt to drive or be in charge of a motor vehicle on a road or public place, with a drug level above the specified limit (see Box 12.5). Officers typically perform a roadside drug test, the DrugWipe®. If positive, officers can request a blood sample to analyse for the presence of up to 17 drugs. While preliminary tests are typically done at the roadside, officers may perform them in custody. Drug limits are specified for blood only; therefore, urine samples cannot be taken.

DrugWipe Refusal

Individuals refusing a DrugWipe are liable for four points on their licence and a driving ban (discretionary). However, officers investigating section 5A, can request the HCP assess the individual for the presence of a condition which might be due to a drug (*see 'Assessing for a condition which might be due to a drug'*). If such a condition is found, officers can request a blood sample under section 5A. There is an inconsistent approach to individuals who refuse a DrugWipe by police. However, the decision rests with the police as to how they proceed.

PROVISION OF SPECIMENS FOR ANALYSIS

This is the officer's power to request evidential samples of breath, blood or urine, depending on the offence, at a police station or hospital. Breath samples are taken by the officers, blood is always taken by HCPs and depending on local agreements, officers or HCPs may take urine samples. Individuals refusing to provide a sample without a reasonable excuse may be liable to prosecution.

SPECIMENS OF BLOOD TAKEN FROM PERSONS INCAPABLE OF CONSENTING

Officers can request a blood sample from someone incapable of consenting (i.e. unconscious) for any of the above offences in certain circumstances (*see 'Incapacitated drivers'*).

PROTECTION FOR HOSPITAL PATIENTS

Preliminary or evidential samples can only be taken if the medical practitioner in immediate charge of their care has been notified and does not object (*see 'Hospital procedure'*).

DETENTION OF PERSONS AFFECTED BY ALCOHOL OR A DRUG

It is the Custody Officer's responsibility to decide when to release a drunk or drug driver. However, rarely, where they believe a released individual may commit further offences under Section 4, 5 or 5A (Section 15 or 16 Northern Ireland), they are required to consult with a medical practitioner. Nurses and paramedics cannot provide advice in such circumstances.

AVIATION, TRAIN AND MARITIME OFFENCES

HCPs may occasionally be asked to take samples for aviation, train or maritime offences, each with its separately defined limits (see Box 12.6). While different offences, the sampling procedure remains the same.

BOX 12.6	PRESCRIBED LIMITS OF ALCOHOL (AVIATION, TRAIN AND MARITIME)

	Aviation (pilot and aircrew)	Train	Maritime
Breath	9 mcg/100 ml	9 mcg/100 ml	25 mcg/100 ml
Blood	20 mcg/100 ml	20 mcg/100 ml	50 mcg/100 ml
Urine	27 mcg/100 ml	27 mcg/100 ml	67 mcg/100 ml

Source: Crown / Public Domain.

THE HEALTHCARE PROFESSIONAL'S ROLE

When officers request evidential samples, they first obtain 'consent' while completing the necessary forms (see Box 12.1), before seeing the HCP. This process may be recorded through body-worn cameras or custody suite video systems. Afterwards, the individual is asked by the officer to reconfirm their 'consent' in the presence of the HCP. It is common practice for HCPs to request written consent using specific forms.

As the HCP, it is important to fully explain the process to individuals, ensuring they can decide to either agree to have phlebotomy and the subsequent evidential blood samples, or refuse and this is carefully documented. Where a person removes their arm or undertakes behaviours that make taking blood safely impossible, this should be discussed with the individual that this will be recorded as a refusal and the procedure abandoned.

Officers may proceed with 'failure to provide' as in *DPP v Beech* (1992) and *DPP v Camp* (2017), where both cases clarified being too intoxicated to understand or comply is not a valid defence (see Box 12.7). In such cases, officers may also consider Section 4 (Section 15 Northern Ireland) in addition to 'failing to provide' a specimen. This ensures the court hears all pertinent details, which might not otherwise be the case.

ROAD TRAFFIC PROCEDURES AND SAMPLING

Most commonly, there are two procedures that will be asked of an HCP. These are taking blood samples and, less commonly, completing an assessment to determine the presence of any condition that might be due to drugs under Section 4 (Section 15 Northern Ireland). Most procedures are undertaken within custody, however, on occasions, it may be necessary to attend hospital.

BOX 12.7	*DPP V BEECH* (1992) AND *DPP V CAMP* (2017)

The defendants were both charged with failing to provide a specimen for analysis. The primary issue revolved around the defendants' claims they could not understand the instructions due to being intoxicated.

The court held their inability to understand instructions or the consequences of non-compliance, even if caused by intoxication, was not a valid defence. In essence, the court ruled being too intoxicated to understand the requirement to provide a specimen did not exempt an individual from the legal obligation to do so.

These cases established a significant legal precedent, clarifying intoxication cannot be used as a defence for failing to provide a specimen when required under road traffic legislation.

CUSTODY BLOOD PROCEDURE

Blood samples are most frequently undertaken for section 5 or 5A offences (except in Northern Ireland). However, blood can be requested in all drinking and drug-driving offences. Ultimately, the procedure does not alter and is straightforward, but there are vital steps that should not be omitted (see Box 12.8 and Figure 12.1). There is no legal requirement to wait for an appropriate adult (AA) for children or vulnerable adults before taking blood if they consent. However, if they refuse, an AA should be called to assist the individual in deciding before police move to 'failure to provide' (*Miller v DDP* 2018). How this is applied varies from county to county and is a police decision.

Practice may vary, but there is no limit to the number of attempts HCPs can take blood, if they reasonably expect to be successful and the individual agrees. However, case law has determined a suspect can cite a lack of confidence in the HCP's ability after three unsuccessful attempts (*R v Harling* 1970).

HOSPITAL PROCEDURE

Individuals in hospital are not required to provide a positive preliminary breath or saliva test, nor are they required to be assessed for the presence of a condition that might be due to drugs. Officers suspecting a hospitalised individual of a road traffic offence can request a blood sample (or urine, depending on the offence). Before securing the HCP's attendance, officers should confirm the medical practitioner directly responsible for the individual's care has no objections (i.e. the procedure would not interfere with their care and treatment). The wording requires a medical practitioner, which does not include advanced clinical practitioners or similar.

The blood procedure follows the principles outlined in Box 12.8. However, HCPs should avoid taking blood from a limb with an infusion. HCPs can take blood from intravenous cannulas, central lines and arterial lines[5] with permission, if competent, ensuring ports are cleaned using the alcohol-free cleansing wipe and 10 ml of blood is withdrawn and wasted before the evidential sample. Alternatively, a hospital clinician may assist under the HCPs direct supervision. However, the sample remains the HCPs evidence. Hospital clinicians are under no duty to assist with this procedure.

Incapacitated Drivers

Occasionally HCPs may be required to obtain blood or urine samples from an incapacitated driver who cannot consent (i.e. unconscious). HCPs are legally permitted to take blood from incapacitated drivers in the circumstances outlined below, under the Police Reform Act 2002, or The Criminal Justice (Northern Ireland) Order 2005. The Faculty of Forensic & Legal Medicine (2023b) supports this arrangement in principle but warns HCPs cannot use force or restraint to take the sample, where a patient refuses or resists.

---

[5] Mark sample as 'Arterial blood'.

| BOX 12.8 | AN EXAMPLE OF A BLOOD PROCEDURE (THERE IS NO CONSISTENCY OF PRACTICE) |

1. Ensure the officer has the necessary authority to request blood.

2. Obtain agreement from the individual.

3. Ask about any allergies.

4. Using a specific '**RTA Blood Sampling Kit**' demonstrate its integrity, highlighting the expiry date and seal before opening it in front of them.

5. Demonstrate the blood vials to the individual, noting the white powder is a preservative agent.

6. Apply a disposable tourniquet and identify the most suitable site for venepuncture.

7. Clean the skin using the alcohol-free cleansing wipe included in the kit.

8. Insert the needle[6] and withdraw approximately 8 ml of blood using a syringe.
   a. Document the time the sample is taken.
   b. The legislation requires **ONE** sample of blood, which is divided into **TWO** (*Dear v DPP* 1988). This means HCPs cannot use vacutainer hubs to collect samples directly, nor can they combine separate attempts (i.e. cannot use 2 ml from one attempt and 6 ml from second attempt to make up 8 ml. They can only use either 2 ml or 6 ml sample).

9. Divide the sample equally between the two vials in view of the individual (maximum 4 ml each vial).

10. Agitate both samples for a minimum of 30 seconds, ensuring the preservative is well mixed.

11. Label the vials and attach a traceability barcode (see Figure 12.2).

12. Place each vial in the provided securitainer, package with cotton wool and seal lid, in front of the individual.
    a. Document the time the sample is sealed.

13. Hand both samples to the officer.
    a. Document the time the samples are handed over, and the officer's details (name and collar number).

14. The officer will offer the individual the opportunity to keep one of the vials to be tested independently by the police (at their own cost).

15. The officer seals the samples in their individual evidence bags.

16. Complete a HO/RT5 (Home Office/Road Traffic 5) document and provide a copy to the officer.

Officers can request a sample in an 'incapacitated' patient; But the individual **must** have been involved in an accident and incapable of consenting for **medical reasons**. It is for the officer to determine whether the person is incapacitated. However, if circumstances arise where the HCP believes the person has the capacity, then blood should be requested under Section 7 (Section 18 Northern Ireland) (and vice versa).

Samples are taken as outlined earlier. However, the legislation does not allow the officer to analyse the samples. Instead, they are both stored until the individual's condition improves, the officer will then revisit the suspect once their condition has improved, where they will then obtain 'consent' to testing (or not[7]). The suspect will then be offered one-half of the sample by the officer at that time as with a standard procedure under Section 7.

---

[6] HCPs may use butterfly needles to assist if needed, note the use, batch number and expiry date.
[7] Refusing to have the sample analysed will likely result in a 'failure to provide' prosecution.

| SCENARIO 12.1 | Unconscious OPL |

You have been called to the hospital where a 33-year-old male has been involved in a collision. He is currently in the Resuscitation Room, intubated and ventilated. The police have sought the permission of the doctor in charge of his care and there are no objections to taking the sample. He is currently stable; the clinical team is awaiting his CT Head results and, if nothing surgical, intends to attempt to wake him up. Also present are the man's partner and mother. He currently has a single intravenous cannula, with sedation running through.

1. *Describe how you outline your role and the procedure to the man's mother and partner.*

2. *The mother asks if she can refuse on his behalf. How do you respond to this?*

3. *In the event venepuncture is unsuccessful, outline your options.*

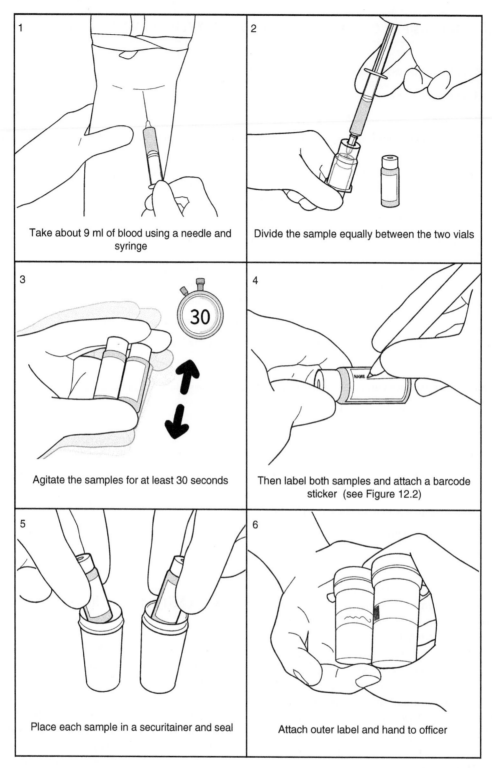

1. Take about 9 ml of blood using a needle and syringe

2. Divide the sample equally between the two vials

3. Agitate the samples for at least 30 seconds

4. Then label both samples and attach a barcode sticker (see Figure 12.2)

5. Place each sample in a securitainer and seal

6. Attach outer label and hand to officer

FIGURE 12.1 Blood procedure.

Needle Phobia

Individuals may state they have needle phobia as a medical reason not to provide a blood sample; in these circumstances, the HCP may be asked to assess the individual (see Box 12.9). A phobia is a visceral response to a specific stimulus creating a systemic response resulting in altered physiology (i.e. sweating, nausea, vomiting, panic attacks, tachycardia, hypertension or syncope [or near-syncope]). It is not a dislike or repugnance of needles. It can be very difficult to assess the veracity of such claims. Both Sections 4 and 5 (15 and 16 Northern Ireland)

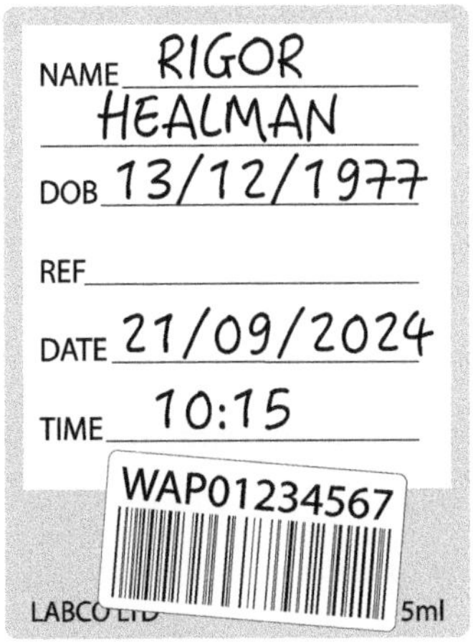

NAME RIGOR

HEALMAN

DOB 13/12/1977

REF

DATE 21/09/2024

TIME 10:15

WAP01234567

LABCO LTD 5ml

FIGURE 12.2 Labelled sample.

BOX 12.9   **NEEDLE PHOBIA ASSESSMENT**

History	• When did you first notice your fear of needles?
	• Was there any specific event triggering this fear?
	• On a scale from 1 to 10, how would you rate your fear of needles?
	• How does this fear affect your life and medical care?
	• What symptoms do you experience when you think about or are exposed to needles?
	• Have you ever avoided medical (including dental) treatment or check-ups due to your fear of needles?
	○ Can you tell me about any specific instances where this happened?
Examination	• Note behaviour and mental state.
	• Check vital signs.
	• Feel hands for tremor or sweating.
	• Inspect dentition, look for evidence of dental treatment or lack of (ask date of any dental treatment).
	• Note any surgical scars or evidence of cosmetic treatment (i.e. fillers and Botox) (ask date of any such treatment).

allow urine to be analysed and as outlined earlier, any sample is the best means of securing a prosecution (Stark and Brener 2000).

Section 5a does not prescribe limits in urine; therefore, only blood is suitable. However, officers may be able to

---

BOX 12.10   ***CUNS R V HAMMERSMITH MAGISTRATES' COURT*, 2016**

Cuns was arrested for a drink-drive offence but failed to provide a sample of blood, stating he was needle-phobic. Cuns was found guilty of failing to provide a sample but appealed. The High Court confirmed a genuine phobia of needles could be a reasonable excuse. However, the prosecution only has to disprove a reasonable excuse (i.e. needle phobia) if the defendant provides some evidential basis, so the issue is in play.

Simply declaring a needle phobia is not enough, as it would be easy or a person to assert during the course of specimen taking and it would be a large task for the prosecution to disprove. As such, it is the defendant's responsibility to prove beyond all reasonable doubt their needle phobia claim is founded.

In a similar case at Swindon Magistrates' Court in January 2020, a tattooed defendant claimed he was scared of needles; magistrates threw out the needle phobia defence, stating he had not provided enough medical evidence.

---

investigate a Section 4 offence and obtain urine. This is ultimately up to them. If for Section 5a an individual cites a needle phobia as a medical reason why a sample should not be taken the matter will be for the HCP to determine if the excuse is reasonable. If the HCP is satisfied, their excuse is reasonable, unless another offence is investigated, the investigation ends. However, if the HCP is not satisfied or unable to determine (i.e. individual not willing to engage), officers may then decide to consider failure to provide, where the individual will be required to provide the court with evidence of their needle phobia (see Box 12.10).

HCPs should document their observations, including behaviours and where appropriate, record responses verbatim. Note the presence (or absence) of any procedures requiring needles. Finally, note any evidence of recent blood tests or immunisations.

SCENARIO 12.2   Needle phobia

A 27-year-old male is brought to the medical room by police. He provided a positive DrugWipe for cannabis and was arrested for driving a motor vehicle with concentration of specified controlled drug above specified limit (Section 5a). On sitting down, he immediately indicates he is needle phobic and is unable to provide a sample of blood. He does agree to providing a sample of urine.

1. *Outline your response to him regarding the offer of providing a urine sample.*

2. *Outline your assessment of his needle phobia.*

ASSESSING FOR A CONDITION WHICH MIGHT BE DUE TO A DRUG

The other common procedure is a medical assessment following an arrest under Section 4 (14 Northern Ireland) *'driving, or being in charge, when under influence of drink or drugs'*. However, in Northern Ireland, the law still restricts this to medical practitioners. While historically known as an 'impairment test', this is both incorrect and misleading. It is not necessary to give an opinion about impairment or 'unfitness to drive'. Furthermore, HCPs would require additional permission as this element is not covered by the officer's request[8].

Impairment Test

The so-called impairment test, also known as the Field Impairment Test (FIT), is a series of five tests assessing an individual's ability to understand and follow instructions, balance and perception. Some officers may complete this at the roadside (or in custody), or it may not be performed at all. However, regardless of the officer's impression as to whether the individual is impaired or not[9], the officer still requires the HCP to identify whether there is a condition that might be due to a drug. Different areas vary in their approach to the FIT test although HCPs are not required to undertake a FIT, as it has not been scientifically or statistically calibrated (Faculty of Forensic & Legal Medicine 2019), there may be some advantages to its application when completing an assessment under Section 4 of the RTA, but there should also be consideration of the disadvantages.

The Assessment

The purpose of the medical assessment is twofold; firstly, to identify the presence of a condition which might be due to a drug and secondly, to be satisfied there is no acute medical condition mimicking intoxication. The assessment follows the scheme outlined in Chapter 3 – Fitness Assessments and HCPs should consider if any information provided by the officer, the history or examination might be due to a drug. This includes their observations of driving or behaviour. Importantly, this is not an assessment to determine if the individual is 'under the influence', it is an assessment to determine if there is any condition which might be due to a drug , whether that drug is prescribed, over-the-counter or illicit. The threshold to state a condition might be due to drugs is low, and if there is any chance (even 1%), then the threshold is met.

Often, individuals do not present as 'under the influence', appearing sober with no signs of drug use, when seen by the HCP. As such, HCPs often rely on the officer's observations, who may describe the individual as appearing

---

> ### BOX 12.11   CONDITIONS MIMICKING INTOXICATION (NOT EXHAUSTIVE)
>
> - Head injury
> - Neurological condition
>   - Epilepsy (post-ictal state)
>   - Stroke or transient ischaemic attack
>   - Brain tumour
> - Hypoglycaemia (or other metabolic disturbances)
> - Liver or renal failure
> - Mental illness
>   - Mania
>   - Hypomania
>   - Psychosis
>   - Major depression

intoxicated and the improvement therefore becomes a condition that might be due to a drug. HCPs can base their opinion solely on the information from the officer, as established in *Angel v Chief Constable South Yorkshire* (2010).

HCPs are not required to identify a specific drug or type of drug and officers should not request this information.

It would be unlikely to suggest a condition present is not due to a drug, unless there is evidence of an acute medical condition mimicking intoxication (see Box 12.11). In such circumstances, the condition could still be due to drugs, the individual should be transferred to hospital and officers advised to follow the relevant hospital procedure. Alternatively, if an ambulance has been called and taking the sample would not delay or interfere with care or treatment, the HCP may consider it more appropriate to take the sample at that time.

Documentation

The Faculty of Forensic & Legal Medicine (2023a) *'Pro Forma – Assessments (alcohol & drugs) under the RTA'* can be used as an aide memoir and support documentation. As outlined above, comprehensive documentation is essential, clearly indicating the HCP's thoughts regarding which conditions might be due to drugs. A proforma is also available for those who complete the FIT and this should be completed.

Refusal to be Examined

Individuals may refuse to be examined and this is not an offence. However, the HCP can still observe their behaviour and take information from the officer to reach an opinion on

---

[8] Any HCP examining a person for this purpose should obtain the individuals' permission since this is not covered by the request at B18 [MG DD/B].
[9] Not a 'pass' or 'fail'.

whether there could be a condition that might be due to a drug (*DPP v Gibbons* 2001). If the HCP believes there is such a condition, the officer can then request a sample of blood, which, if the individual refuses without a reasonable excuse, will be liable for prosecution (failure to provide).

CONCLUSION

In conclusion, road traffic procedures form a significant part of an HCPs role. The process of obtaining samples is relatively straightforward and when using a systematic approach, can be completed in other settings such as hospitals. It is important those carrying out procedures should have a solid knowledge of the legislation and case law, as this allows HCPs to execute their role within the road traffic act to the highest ability.

Throughout this chapter, we have explored the legislation governing the role of a healthcare practitioner under the Road Traffic Act and analysed the relevant sections of the act that often create doubt and anxieties around road traffic law. By understanding the information provisioned within this chapter, it will allow forensic healthcare practitioners to obtain a solid foundation of understanding around the Road Traffic Act and associated processes.

SCENARIO 12.3	Section 4 (Section 15 Northern Ireland) assessment

You are asked to assess a 36-year-old male who has been arrested for driving when under the influence of drink or drugs (Section 4 (Section 15 Northern Ireland)). The officers have not performed a DrugWipe. The officers ask you to examine him to see if there is a condition that might be due to drugs/alcohol.

1. *Outline how you approach the assessment.*

2. *The officer states that on arrest, the individual appeared sleepy and they had to wake him several times en route to the police station. He replies he has a newborn baby, is not getting much sleep and it is 4 am. He appears alert currently and other than a little bit irritated, there is nothing else to note.*
   a. *Is there a condition that might be due to drugs/alcohol?*
   b. *Outline your rationale.*

3. *Describe what may constitute a condition that might be due to drugs/alcohol.*

LEARNING ACTIVITIES

1. Write a reflective piece where you have been involved in a road traffic procedure that has challenged your knowledge around the act and consider how this has developed your practice.

2. Critically appraise a time where you have obtained evidential samples in an alternative location such as a hospital blood procedure and consider your feelings as a result of completing the procedure.

3. Analyse a statement you have written in relation to a road traffic procedure or prepare a scenario-based statement relating to the road traffic act procedures. Now consider the strengths and weaknesses of your statement and the potential cross-examination questions that could be posed and how you would respond.

RESOURCES

Online

- College of Policing | Authorised Professional practice | https://www.college.police.uk/app
- Police National Legal Database | Road Traffic Act | https://www.pnld.co.uk/

Organisations

- UK Association of Forensic Nurses and Paramedics (www.ukafnp.org)
- Faculty of Forensic and Legal Medicine (www.fflm.ac.uk)
- Royal College of Nursing | Nursing in Justice and Forensic Health CareForum(https://www.rcn.org.uk/Get-Involved/Forums/Nursing-in-Justice-and-Forensic-Health-Care-Forum)

REFERENCES

Angel v Chief Constable South Yorkshire (2010).

Cuns R (on the application of) v Hammersmith Magistrates' Court (2016).

Dear v DPP (1988) RTR 148, Crim LR 316, 20th Nov 1987, QBD DC.

Director of Public Prosecutions v Camp (2017) EWHC 3119 (Admin)

DPP v Beech (1992) RTR 239; [1992] Crim.L.R. 64, DC.

DPP v Gibbons [2001] EWHC Admin 385.

DPP v Kinnersley [1993] RTR 105.

Faculty of Forensic & Legal Medicine (2019). Assessments (alcohol & drugs) under the RTA. https://fflm.ac.uk/forensic-practitioners/assessments-alcohol-drugs-under-the-rta/#:~:text=The%20major%20change%20has%20been,result%20in%20complex%20drug%20interactions (accessed 14 August 2023).

Faculty of Forensic & Legal Medicine (2023a). *Pro Forma – Assessments (Alcohol & Drugs) Under the RTA*. London: Faculty of Forensic & Legal Medicine https://fflm.ac.uk/wp-content/uploads/2023/07/Assessments-alcohol-drugs-under-the-RTA-Prof-M-Stark-and-Prof-I-Wall-Aug-2023.pdf (accessed 14 September 2023).

Faculty of Forensic & Legal Medicine (2023b). *Taking Blood Samples from Incapacitated Drivers*. London: Faculty of Forensic and Legal Medicine https://fflm.ac.uk/wp-content/uploads/2023/04/FFLM-BMA-Guidance-on-taking-blood-from-incapacitated-drivers-April-2023.pdf (accessed 15 August 2023).

Independent Office for Police Conduct (2023). *Annual Deaths During or Following Police Conduct*. London: Independent Office for Police Conduct https://www.policeconduct.gov.uk/publications/annual-deaths-during-or-following-police-contact-report-202223 (accessed 11 August 2023).

Miller v DPP [2018] EWHC 262 (Admin).

Police Reform Act. (2002). Police Reform Act 2002. https://www.legislation.gov.uk/ukpga/2002/30/contents (accessed 15 August 2023).

R v Harling (1970) RTR 441.

R v Lennard [1973] 2 All ER 831.

Railways and Transport Safety Act (2003). Railways and Transport Safety Act 2003. https://www.legislation.gov.uk/ukpga/2003/20/introduction (accessed 14 August 2023).

Road Traffic Act (1988). Road Traffic Act 1988. https://www.legislation.gov.uk/ukpga/1988/52/contents (accessed 14 August 2023).

Stark, M.M. and Brener, N. (2000). Needle phobia. *Journal of Clinical Forensic Medicine* 7 (1): 35–38.

The Criminal Justice (Northern Ireland) Order (2005). The Criminal Justice (Northern Ireland) Order 2005. https://www.legislation.gov.uk/nisi/2005/1965/contents (accessed 15 August 2024).

The Road Traffic (Northern Ireland) Order (1995). The Road Traffic (Northern Ireland) Order 1995. https://www.legislation.gov.uk/nisi/1995/2994/contents (accessed 14 August 2023).

The Road Traffic Act 1988 (Prescribed Limit) (Scotland) Regulations (2014). The Road Traffic Act 1988 (Prescribed Limit) (Scotland) Regulations 2014. https://www.legislation.gov.uk/sdsi/2014/9780111024478 (accessed 14 August 2023).

FURTHER READING

Faculty of Forensic & Legal Medicine | Drug-driving competencies | https://fflm.ac.uk/wp-content/uploads/2021/10/FFLM-Drug-Driving-Competencies-Prof-M-Stark-Dr-A-Gorton-Oct-2021.pdf

Evidence Collection (Documenting Injuries and Samples)

Esther McPhail

Mitie Care and Custody Health Ltd, London, UK

CHAPTER 13

AIM

The aim of this chapter is to provide healthcare professionals with a comprehensive understanding of the principles and practices involved in evidence collection in forensic healthcare settings, focusing on documenting injuries and the collection of various types of samples.

LEARNING OUTCOMES

Upon completion of this chapter, readers should be able to:

- Understand the different types of injuries and how to document them accurately

- Discuss the factors affecting wound healing and the appearance of injuries over time

- Identify and describe the various types of forensic samples and the appropriate methods for their collection

- Explain the importance of maintaining the chain of custody and its implications for legal proceedings

---

SELF-ASSESSMENT

1. What are the anatomical layers of the skin? Outline the key features of skin.

2. Can you list the physiological differences between incision and laceration, including the mechanisms of injury and potential legal consequences of misinterpretation.

3. List five types of evidence and the best-suited collection method.

4. Explain the evidential chain of custody and the consequences if it is not maintained.

INTRODUCTION

The role of the healthcare professional (HCP) encompasses many wide and varied tasks. Some of these have therapeutic benefits for the patients, and others do not and are considered part of the evidential and legal processes. These evidential tasks include the collection of forensic samples and documenting physical injuries, in relation to a plethora of offences. Both forensic sampling and documenting injuries can be labour intensive, yet their forensic importance cannot be underestimated.

The four-way linkage theory postulates there are four key components in any investigation: suspect, victim, scene and evidence, see Figure 13.1. Solving a case reliably and objectively requires linking these four components, thereby increasing the probability of a successful resolution.

Successful recognition, documentation, collection and preservation of evidence from a crime scene are key in

Police Custody Healthcare for Nurses and Paramedics, First Edition. Edited by Matthew Peel, Jennie Smith, Vanessa Webb, and Margaret Bannerman.
© 2025 John Wiley & Sons Ltd. Published 2025 by John Wiley & Sons Ltd.
Companion website: www.wiley.com/go/policecustodyhealthcare

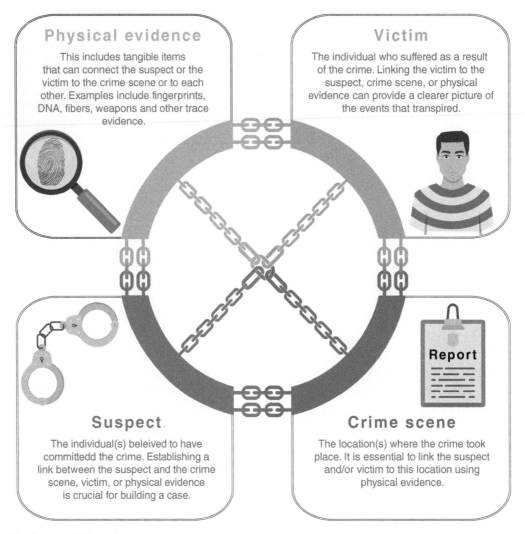

Physical evidence

This includes tangible items that can connect the suspect or the victim to the crime scene or to each other. Examples include fingerprints, DNA, fibers, weapons and other trace evidence.

Victim

The individual who suffered as a result of the crime. Linking the victim to the suspect, crime scene, or physical evidence can provide a clearer picture of the events that transpired.

Suspect

The individual(s) beleived to have committedd the crime. Establishing a link between the suspect and the crime scene, victim, or physical evidence is crucial for building a case.

Crime scene

The location(s) where the crime took place. It is essential to link the suspect and/or victim to this location using physical evidence.

FIGURE 13.1   The four-way linkage theory.

investigations. In the forensic healthcare arena, the crime scene will be the victim or suspect. It is in the best interests of the injured party, those alleged to have caused the injury and the criminal justice systems to ensure there is as much information available as possible.

When asked to document injuries, the HCPs are being asked to consider physical evidence. That physical evidence must be recorded in a manner that will preserve its integrity and evidentiary value, given it is highly likely to be scrutinised by the courts, its agents and other parties. Due to this potential review of documented injuries, the legibility, accuracy, relevance and use of appropriate body mapping templates are all considerations for the HCP in practice. All of which will be discussed further in this chapter.

DOCUMENTING INJURIES

Injuries are typically illustrated using body diagrams supplemented with a narrative description. Figure 13.2 outlines the body in the anatomical position and associated descriptions.

When documenting injuries, it is important to record wound details as outlined in Box 13.1.

SCENARIO 13.1   Documenting injuries

You have been asked to document the injuries of someone arrested for assault. They are frustrated after being detained for 17 hours. They are fully dressed and just show you a bruise on the left side of their face. They refuse to allow you to examine any further, stating they have no other injuries.

1. *How do you approach this request?*

When documenting injuries, we need to consider several factors, which can be grouped into physical, kinetic and biological, see Box 13.2. These factors alter the anatomy and physiology of the skin and therefore, warrant serious consideration.

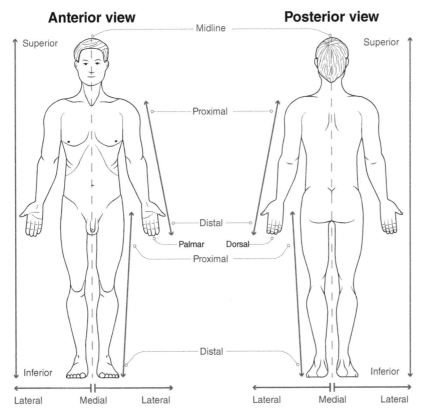
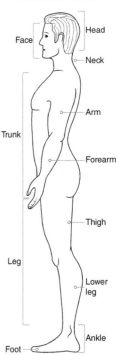

FIGURE 13.2 Anatomical position and description.

BOX 13.1 **DOCUMENTING INJURIES**

For each injury, include the following details:

- **Type:** Describe the type of injury (i.e. bruise, abrasion and laceration).

- **Site**: Describe the exact location. If the injury is considered significant, measure the distance from fixed anatomical landmarks.

- **Size**: Measure and record dimensions (length, width, depth).

- **Colour:** Note the colour(s) of the injury and the surrounding area.

- **Shape**: Describe the shape or pattern (e.g. linear, circular, irregular, patterned).

- **Margins**: Observe and record the characteristics of the injury edges.

- **Surrounding area**: Note any swelling, bruising, abrasions or other changes around the injury.

- **Associated features**: Note any additional findings like discharge, scarring or tissue damage.

- **Pain and function**: Record any pain or functional impairment reported by the patient.

BOX 13.2 **PHYSICAL, KINETIC AND BIOLOGICAL FACTORS**

Physical and kinetic factors	Biological factors
• Degree of force – the kinetic energy applied	• Age
• Area over which force applied	• Gender
• Duration of force application	• Nutritional state
• Mobility of the body part – fixed body part absorbs all the energy whilst a moving part will convert the energy to movement	• Coagulopathy
	• Biochemical tissue properties
• Anticipation/co-ordination[1]	• Disease
	• Medication

Source: Adapted from Wilkinson and Hardman (2020).

DEFINITIONS

It is common to see the words 'injury' and 'wound' used interchangeably in these cases, so it is pertinent to define

---

[1] The body's ability to effectively prepare and adjust its muscle activity and posture in anticipation of or in response to physical forces, aiming to minimise injury. It involves synchronized actions of different body parts to distribute impact forces more evenly or to execute movements that reduce the risk of harm.

Wound	Damage to the integrity of biological tissues, including skin, mucous membranes and organ tissues.
Injury	Damage to living tissue but the addition of an external causation. External causation could include blunt force trauma, penetrating trauma, burns, toxic exposure, asphyxiation or overexertion.

both (see Box 13.3). The legal system defines 'injury' as harm suffered by a person due to some act or omission done by another.

SKIN: ANATOMY AND PHYSIOLOGY

To comprehensively report and document injuries, an underlying knowledge and understanding of their anatomy is essential see Figure 13.3. Here are a few skin facts:

- It is the body's largest organ
- Accounts for up to 15% of body weight
- An average adult has 21 square feet of skin
- It contains 11 miles of blood vessels
- Every square inch has about 300 sweat glands
- Renews itself every 28 days
- Sheds 9 lbs of dead skin annually

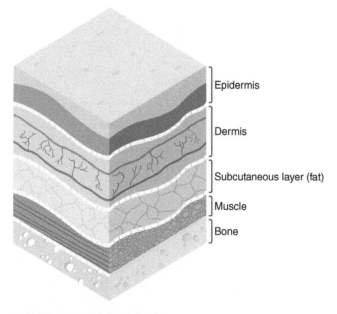

FIGURE 13.3   Skin anatomy.

- The thickest skin is the soles of the feet, and the thinnest is the eyelids.

Wound Healing

Wounds heal through four phases: haemostasis, inflammation, proliferation and remodelling. For successful healing, all four phases must occur in the proper sequence and time frame. Wound healing is complex and will vary depending on the size and location of the wound. Wound healing can also be delayed with diabetes, venous or arterial disease, infection or ageing. It is important to include whether a wound is bleeding, whether granular tissue is present or other features and may involve the description of scars.

Primary intention Wounds that heal by primary intention (where the edges are brought together and closed with sutures, staples or adhesive tapes) demonstrate a streamlined and efficient healing process due to minimal tissue loss, see Box 13.4. Minimising the wound defect and reducing clot formation, facilitating quicker epithelialisation and minimal scarring.

Secondary intention Secondary intention healing occurs where the edges are not brought together, such as ulcers, large abrasions or significant tissue loss. The wound heals from the bottom up as granulation tissue gradually fills the wound, see Box 13.5. This process can be slower and more complex due to the larger wound area and the potential for infection. There is often more significant scarring compared to primary intention healing.

Time frame	Pathophysiology	Appearance
0 h	Wound filled with clots and inflammatory cells arrive	Fresh wound with clot, edges apposed
3–24 h	Neutrophils infiltrate, epithelial closure begins	Redness, slight swelling, early closure visible
Day 3	Macrophages and granulation tissue formation	Pink, granular tissue, reduced swelling
Day 5	Granulation tissue and collagen deposition	Less inflammation, granulation and early scarring
Week 2	Collagen remodels, scar formation	Scar more evident, wound contracted and firmer
2 months	Connective tissue matures, reduced inflammation	Mature, flat and lighter scar

Source: Kumar et al. (2021)/with permission of Elsevier.

BOX 13.5   WOUND HEALING (SECONDARY INTENTION)

Time frame	Pathophysiology	Appearance
0 h	Formation of blood clot and initiation of inflammatory response	Open wound with blood clot, possible debris
1–3 d	Inflammatory cells clean the wound; granulation tissue begins to form	Red, inflamed, possibly swollen, with some exudate
3–7 d	Proliferation of granulation tissue; collagen deposition begins	Red or pink, granular tissue; decreased inflammation; evidence of tissue growth
1–2 wk	Rapid growth of granulation tissue; collagen continues to build	Moist, beefy-red tissue; granulation tissue fills the wound bed
2–6 wk	Wound contraction; epithelialization progresses from wound edges	Wound size reduces; edges contract; new, thin layer of epithelial tissue visible
6 wk – several months	Maturation of collagen; continued wound contraction and strengthening	Wound contracts further; scar tissue forms, becoming firmer and paler

CLASSIFICATION OF INJURIES

In forensic healthcare, the classification of injuries is most commonly linked to the mechanism of the injury. So, there are several categories that encompass the injuries we can and are likely to encounter (see Figure 13.4).

Erythema

Erythema is not bruising; it is a redness of the skin or mucous membranes caused by dilatation of the underlying capillaries, which normally subsides with time. Possible causes include acute trauma, 'flushing', pressure, sunlight, infection, dermatological conditions, allergies and reactions to chemicals, to name a few. Erythema can be differentiated from bruising by applying finger pressure – erythema blanches to pressure, whereas bruises do not.

Bruises

Bruises are typically caused by blunt force trauma,[2] causing damage to the underlying blood vessels (capillaries, veins and arterioles) (see Figure 13.4a). As there is no break in the

---

[2] Bruising following needles or injections is a 'puncture wound'.

epidermis, the blood leaks into the surrounding tissue, migrating along the fascial planes between the skin layers. Gravity may affect the direction and nature of leakage. In addition, other factors affect bruising (i.e. age, nutritional state, bleeding disorders and medications). The result of migration is bruises may not reflect the size or the shape of the causative object. HCPs should be mindful of conditions mimicking bruising (see Box 13.6).

The colour of bruises is important to note but is **NOT** an accurate indicator of age. The time course of colour change is very variable and dependent on multiple factors such as; lymphatic and venous drainage, site, size and depth of the bruise, age, gender, obesity, general nutritional state, medical history, medication and coagulation factors. Bruising typically starts as a dark red mark caused by haemoglobin and then typically progresses to purple/blue, through to yellow, green and brown as macrophages break down the haemoglobin and bile pigments are released (bilirubin). As the debris at the bruise site clears, the colours will fade and eventually disappear. A yellow discolouration may indicate an injury is at least 18 hours old (Langlois and Gresham 1991). The reverse, a lack of yellow, does not and cannot be accepted as a bruise being under 18 hours old. However, there is wider evidence that any ageing based on colour is unreliable (Maguire et al. 2005), complicated further by skin colour, and the ability to recognise yellow differs amongst individuals and declines over time (Hughes et al. 2004).

Intradermal bruising As outlined above, often, the shape of a bruise and the relationship between the causative object is unreliable. There is one exception, which is the superficial bruise caused by moderate 90° force, where the leakage of the blood is confined to intra-dermal bruises (upper surface of the skin) and these marks reproduce the nature of the object that caused them (e.g. footwear pattern, tyre tread marks) and is more significant forensically.

Fingertip Fingertip bruises are clusters of round or oval bruises measuring between 1 and 2 cm, sometimes seen on the inner aspect of the upper arm(s) or thigh(s), although they can appear anywhere. There may be a larger single bruise visible on the opposite side of the limb from a thumb.

Bruising with central sparing Doughnut bruises occur when a spherical object (i.e. a ball) forcibly connects with the skin – causing blunt force trauma, compressing the central zone suddenly with the increase of pressure occurring at the edge, bursting blood vessels, yet dragging at the main margins causing a 'doughnut' shaped bruise, see Figure 13.5a.

Tramline bruises are caused by cylindrical objects (i.e. sticks or batons), forcibly coming into contact with the skin. Again, this causes blunt force trauma, which breaks down the tissues at the edges as it strikes the skin but spares the central compressed area. Similar injuries may be seen when

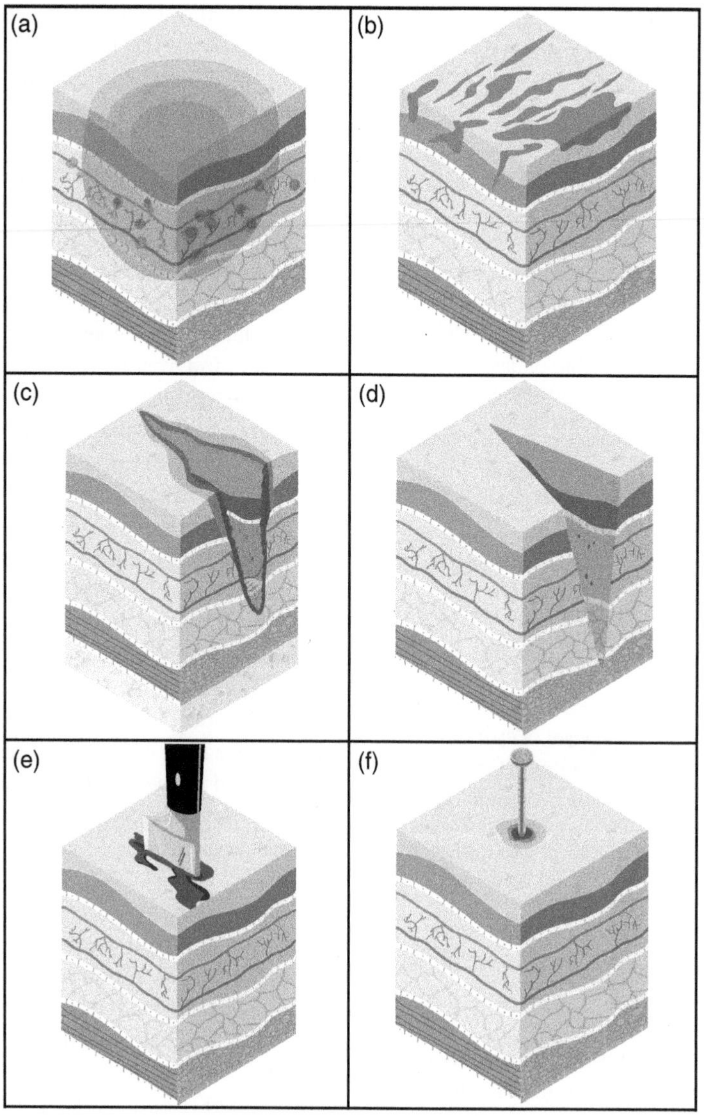

FIGURE 13.4   Category of injuries. (a) bruise, (b) abrasion, (c) laceration, (d) incision, (e) stab and (f) puncture.

BOX 13.6	CONDITIONS MIMICKING BRUISING

- Natural skin appearance
- Meningococcal septicaemia
- Coagulation disorder
- Connective tissue disorder
- Medication (anticoagulants, antiplatelets and NSAIDs)
- Birthmarks
- Cultural practices
- Photosensitive/contact dermatitis
- Cellulitis

individuals are hit with thick rope, or similar items at high pressure and speed, see Figure 13.5b.

Petechial bruising Petechial bruising, where small pinpoint purple marks are seen, is often associated with a sudden rise in pressure, leading to blood vessels bursting or can be associated with health conditions that lead to 'leaky' blood vessels through inflammation or infection, see Figure 13.5c. A 'love bite' forms due to the suction and pressure of tissues compressed against the palate and teeth. This negative pressure results in leakage of blood vessels, leading to small pinpoint (petechial haemorrhages) or larger bruises. The 'classic love bite' tends to have the same colour due to the uniformity of pressure.

Haematoma Haematomas are a distinct type of bruise characterised by blood forming a palpable fluctuant collection under the skin. Haematomas can be drained like an abscess.

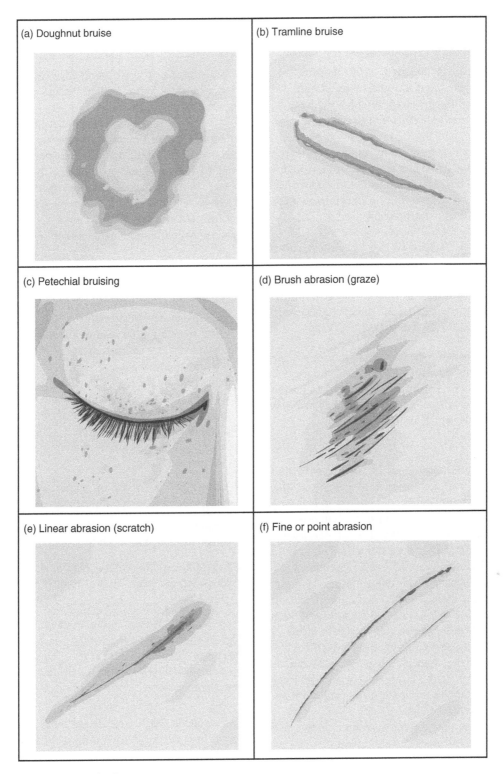

FIGURE 13.5 Examples of injuries (a–f).

Abrasions

Abrasion is the technical term for what are commonly referred to as grazes or scratches, see Figure 13.4b. These are limited to the epidermis therefore often are moist or healing. However, they can bleed a small amount when the vessels of the convoluted papillary dermis are damaged. Although abrasions are typically clinically trivial, they have significant forensic importance:

- Always reflect the site of impact
- Can indicate the shape and surface pattern of the causative object
- Can indicate the direction of travel
- May contain debris or foreign bodies of forensic importance

Abrasions are normally caused by a tangential or glancing impact across the skin, pulling or dragging the epidermis towards the distal end of the injury. This causes ragged edges and ragged tags along the length of the abrasion and a heaping up of keratin at the distal end of the lesion. This makes it possible to tell the direction in which the force has been applied and this may be useful forensic evidence.

Brush abrasion (graze) Brush abrasions occur when there is friction between the skin and a broad, rough surface, such as a wall or road, see Figure 13.5d. The depth and extent of the abrasion will depend on the irregularity of the surface, the speed or force and the area of the body involved.

Linear abrasion (scratch) Fingernails may leave small, curved abrasions and if dragged across the skin, they may leave linear abrasions of approximately a centimetre in width, see Figure 13.5e. Linear abrasion may be seen in isolation, in a parallel pattern or multiple patterns and directions. They may be associated with wheals, which disappear over time.

Fine or point linear abrasion Fine or point abrasions are very narrow linear abrasions caused by objects with a narrow or fine pointed edge, like a broken fingernail, a metal nail, a pinhead or a blunt knife, see Figure 13.5f. Point abrasions may be accompanied by wheals, which disappear over time.

Lacerations

Lacerations are the splitting or tearing of the skin caused by blunt force trauma, typically over bony areas, see Figure 13.4c. They can also be caused by rolling/grinding motion (e.g. being run over by a vehicle). Lacerations are most likely to occur over areas such as the knees, scalp, elbows and face. They are less likely to occur in fleshy body parts, such as the abdomen or buttocks.

The edges of lacerations are ALWAYS ragged due to the tearing mechanism associated with these injuries. However, lacerations close to the bone, such as the forehead, can initially appear to have clean edges and require close inspection. Lacerations may involve the superficial or deeper layers, so they can bleed profusely, depending upon their depth and the damage to the underlying vessels. 'Tissue bridges', may be visible within the depth of the injury, as not all layers may have been torn apart. On the surface, bruising, abrasions and skin flaps may be present (see Figure 13.6g).

The incorrect use of the term 'laceration' is the most common mistake made when documenting injuries. It is not just a technical error but has wider implications. For example, if a knife cuts an individual and the wound is described as a laceration, the offender may escape the punishment associated with knife crime, as lacerations are a result of blunt and not sharp force.

Sharp force wounds

Sharp force wound is an umbrella term for incised, stab and slash wounds.

Incision Incisions are made by a sharp cutting edge (i.e. glass, razors, metal edges and knives) (see Figure 13.4d). The wound edges should be clean and straight, with no surface abrasion or bruising. Because a cutting edge causes incised wounds, they sever these more resilient tissues and no tissue bridges are seen (see Figure 13.6h).

Multiple and typically parallel incised wounds to the anterior aspect of the wrist and forearm are typically associated with a self-inflicted injury. They may be associated with a similar pattern of injuries on other parts of the body. Incised wounds to the neck are rarely seen in accidents. The presence of any 'tentative' or 'hesitation' wounds, may suggest self-inflicted wounds. Blunt knives or objects may create a mixed injury with elements of incision, abrasion and laceration.

Stab wound Stab wounds are deeper than they are long (see Figure 13.4e). They penetrate tissue more deeply and have a greater potential for harm. Any stab wound should be referred to the Emergency Department as the potential for internal injuries that cannot be seen will require further assessment. Stab wounds are characteristically slit-like and may gape slightly to become almond or oval-shaped, also known as elliptical, see Figure 13.6i. The wound rarely reflects the exact shape and measurement of the blade. If the knife/blade is plunged and then withdrawn directly, the skin stretches as the implement is introduced and retracts slightly after the blade is withdrawn. The wound is, therefore, slightly shorter and wider than the blade.

- If the blade is 'rocked' on withdrawal, the wound may be longer than the width of the blade.

- Change of angle on withdrawal can lead to a 'notching' effect; twisting can result in a crescentic wound.

- The shape of the wound may mirror the cross-sectional shape of the blade (e.g. fishtail/triangular wound for a single blade).

Handles of weapons may cause bruising around the edge of the stab wound, resulting in a mixed wound. Most resistance to stab wounds is offered by clothing; once penetrated, it takes comparatively lower force to penetrate underlying tissue.

Slash wounds Slash wounds are longer than they are deep. This is because the sharp (cutting) object is drawn across the skin rather than into the skin, causing an injury that may follow the curvature of the body and vary in depth (see Figure 13.6j).

Puncture Wounds

A puncture wound causes a small round wound (with or without bruising) much deeper than it is wide. They can vary in size depending on cause, such as needles, ice-picks or nails, see Figure 13.4f.

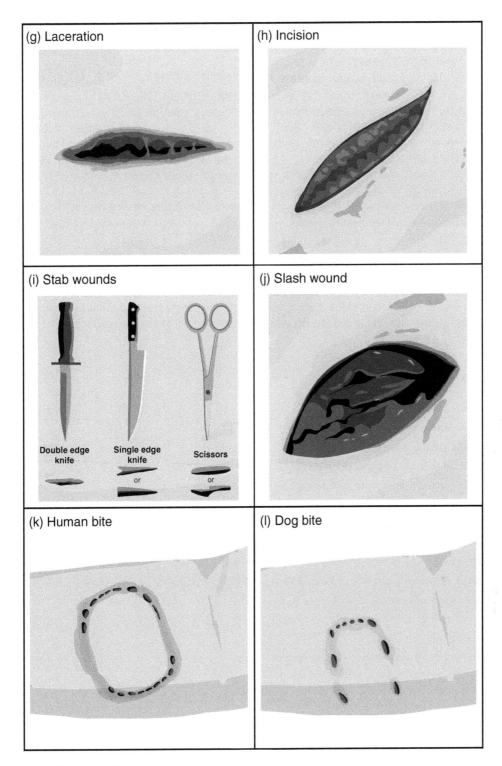

FIGURE 13.6 Examples of injuries (g–l).

Mixed Wounds

On occasion, there may be features of more than one type of injury such as being hit by a glass bottle, where the force of contact tears some of the tissues, but the glass also creates incisions, and bruising may be present, so describe what can be seen if there are features that are difficult to classify.

Bites

A bite mark is caused by a biting injury, either animal or human. There is no classical bite mark injury, as they can present wildly different, depending on the location, if over clothing and how they react (i.e. pulling away).

Human bites Human bites may appear round or oval, consisting of two opposing U-sharped arches from the upper and lower teeth, with the central area bruised or free from injury, see Figure 13.6k. However, it is not uncommon for there to be only a single U-shaped arch. Additionally, there may be a combination of avulsion, bruising, abrasions, lacerations or dental indentation (or impression). Bite injuries over muscle or bone are generally more defined than those in soft areas, such as the abdomen, breast or buttocks.

Bite marks can be of major forensic significance as they can accurately reflect the dentition of an assailant. Forensic sampling (swabbing) of the area may be required. If necessary, a forensic odontologist may be involved to take dental impressions.

Animal bites The shape and size of the wound will depend on the type and size of the animal. A characteristic of animal bites is puncture wounds, caused by their narrower and sharper teeth than humans, see Figure 13.6l. Often, when dogs bite, they attempt to shear and tear the tissue. This can cause a mix of lacerations, abrasions, bruising or even fractures. In addition, dogs can exert high pressure using their jaws.

Restraint Injuries

Handcuff injuries The use of handcuffs can result in a mix of reddening, swelling, bruising and abrasions to the wrist. These may extend partially or fully circumflex around the wrist. It is important to document injuries and any areas of paraesthesia in the event of a complaint against the Police. For further information, see Chapter 11 – Use of Force.

Taser barbs Barbs can leave a very small puncture mark following the barb removal. For further information, see Chapter 11 – Use of Force.

OTHER TERMS

There is a vast array of terms associated with injuries, all used in varying ways. It is important to use the correct terminology. See Box 13.7 for other terms used.

BOX 13.7   OTHER INJURY TERMS

Avulsion	Forcible detachment of an area of skin
Blast injury	A type of wounds caused by explosions.
Blister	Fluid-filled pocket in the upper skin layers.
Burn	Skin or tissue damage from heat, chemicals, electricity or radiation.
Concussion	Brain injury from a blow or jolt to the head or body.
Contusion	Another term for a bruise, no longer recommended.
Cut	A skin wound from a sharp object. Avoid, instead use incision, stab, puncture or slash wound.
De-gloving	An injury where the skin is completely torn off from the underlying tissue, often resembling the removal of a glove.
Defence injury	A group of injuries consistent with defending oneself. Typically seen on the hands and arms.
Dislocation	Displacement of a joint.
Ecchymosis	Another term for a bruise, no longer recommended.
Fracture	A bone break.
Gunshot wounds	A term used to group wounds caused by firearms.
Haemo-serous fluid	A mixture of blood and serum, often seen in wound healing.
Keloid scaring	Thick, puckered, itchy clusters of scar tissue that grow beyond the edges of the wound or incision. They are often red or darker in colour than the surrounding skin.
Penetrating trauma	Open wound from an object entering the body.
Reddening	Another term for 'erythema'.
Scab	A crust that forms over a wound during healing.
Scald	Burn from hot liquids or gases.
Scarring	The process of wound healing that results in fibrous tissue replacing normal skin. This can vary in severity and appearance, with initial red or purple scars often becoming flatter and paler (silver/white scars) over time.
Ulcer	Sore on the skin or mucous membrane with tissue breakdown.

FORENSIC SAMPLES

Forensic samples taken from suspects are primarily used to collect trace evidence that could be relevant to an investigation (see Box 13.8). Trace evidence is small, often microscopic or nearly invisible, materials found at a crime scene or on a person or object. For example fibres, hair or skin cells help establish connections between a suspect, victim and the crime scene. However, some larger pieces may be visible without magnification.

TIMING

The best practice is for forensic samples to be taken as soon as possible as forensic evidence is fragile; it can get lost or degenerate over time. However, in reality, this is only sometimes possible. Most samples can be recovered up to three days (72 hours) post-event (see 'Resources') and whilst the guidelines refer to specific timespans for these, a case-by-case discussion is recommended as some extenuating factors might need to be taken into consideration (i.e. if the suspect has had access to washing facilities). Any samples taken outside the timeframe are less likely to provide positive results. When asked to take samples outside the recommended timeframe, they can still be done, but it may require a discussion with the investigation or forensic team. It's essential to consider the information from other sources regarding the circumstances, which could offer further relevance, assist with decisions and direct the forensic strategy of the case.

SCENARIO 13.2   Forensic samples

You have been asked to take some intimate samples (penile shaft, coronal sulcus and glans) swabs from someone suspected of rape. The offence occurred five days ago. The suspect is agreeable to having the samples taken. However, the recommended timeframe for such samples is three days or 72 hours.

1. *How do you approach this request?*

INTIMATE AND NON-INTIMATE SAMPLES

Forensic samples collected in custody are defined as intimate and non-intimate, see Box 13.9. Only HCPs can take intimate samples. Non-intimate samples can be taken by police officers (or other police staff). The provision of services differs nationally. Some HCPs may be expected to take all intimate and non-intimate samples; some may only take intimate samples.

Across the United Kingdom, the relevant legislation allows non-intimate samples to be taken without consent, using force. However, HCPs work within their professional guidance, and for forensic examination outside the Road Traffic Act, they should have valid consent and therefore cannot be compelled to take such samples. In Scotland, intimate samples can be

---

BOX 13.8   TYPES OF TRACE EVIDENCE

Biological material	This includes bodily fluids like blood, saliva, semen or sweat, which can contain DNA.
Chemical residues	In cases of suspected poisoning or drug use, swabs can detect chemical residues on the skin. Swabs should not be used for collection of gunshot residue or accelerants.
Fibres and hair	The presence of fibres or hair not belonging to the individual can link them to a crime scene or a victim, particularly in assault or sexual offence cases.
Microscopic particles	This can include anything from dust and pollen to specific types of particles that might link an individual to a particular location or activity.

BOX 13.9   INTIMATE AND NON-INTIMATE SAMPLES

Intimate samples	Non-intimate samples
• Dental impression[3]	• Head hair
• Sample of blood, urine,[4] semen or any other tissue fluid	• Mouth
	• Hand swabs
• Pubic hair	• Fingernails
• Swabs from any part of the genitals[5]	
• Any bodily orifice other than the mouth[6]	

Source: Immigration and Asylum Act 1999, Department of Justice (2015), Home Office (2016).

---

lawfully taken without consent under the authority of a sheriff's warrant. However, the HCP's ethical and professional obligations apply.

The samples most requested within custody are:

- Intimate penile swabs

- Pubic hair combing

---

[3] Taken by a registered dentist (typically a forensic odontologist).
[4] Urine samples can be taken by police officers (England, Wales and Northern Ireland).
[5] In Scotland, swabs of the genitals are not considered an intimate sample (Immigration and Asylum Act 1999).
[6] Nostrils, ear canals, anus, vagina or navel (not exhaustive).

- Hand and nail swabs
- Blood samples for toxicology

CONTAMINATION

Contamination is the introduction of DNA or other trace evidence to a sample before, during or after recovery from a suspect (Forensic Science Regulator 2024). Contamination, particularly from DNA, is a critical concern. DNA analysis is highly sensitive and can be easily contaminated through simple actions such as sneezing, coughing or speaking over the samples, as well as through the transfer of DNA from one item or individual to another.

Contamination compromises the integrity of the evidence and can potentially mislead investigations, impacting outcomes. Therefore, strict adherence to anti-contamination principles (see Box 13.10), including personal protective equipment, meticulous handling of evidence and proper storage and transportation methods, is imperative. Ensuring the evidence remains reliable and accurate. Unfortunately, most custody suites do not have specific forensic examination rooms. Instead, HCPs will often use the medical room, for which there is a wide range of standards.

Gloves

HCPs should always wear double, non-latex powder-free gloves (i.e. nitrile gloves) during the entire process, including handling, preparing, sampling and sealing the exhibits. When taking gloves from the box, discard the top glove in case of contamination; in addition, the first and last gloves of a box should be discarded (Forensic Capability Network 2023).

The outer gloves are changed between different sample sites before handling equipment or touching any other surface. Double gloving avoids skin shedding during glove changes (Faculty of Forensic & Legal Medicine 2023). There is no need to exhibit gloves unless there is obvious material on them.

Multiples Suspects

Wherever possible, police should be encouraged to separate suspects needing forensic samples between different suites. If multiple suspects from the same offence are in custody simultaneously, HCPs should manage these case-by-case to ensure they minimise contamination (Forensic Science Regulator 2024). For example, siblings may have different considerations than multiple unrelated individuals. In exceptional circumstances, where necessary to use the same HCP, document the reason, rationale and steps taken to reduce the risk of contamination.

EVIDENTIAL CHAIN OF CUSTODY

The evidential chain of custody is a critical concept in forensic science and criminal investigations. It refers to the chronological documentation or paper trail showing the collection, custody, control, transfer and analysis of evidence. This documentation typically includes details about who handled the evidence, when it was handled, the purpose of handling it and any changes to the evidence (like opening a sealed bag for analysis). The importance of maintaining the continuity of the chain of evidence cannot be overstated. It assures the court the evidence has not been tampered with or contaminated.

BOX 13.10	ANTI-CONTAMINATION PRINCIPLES

Prevention
- Use a forensic examination room specifically designed and used for forensic sampling, which is maintained to prevent contamination between individuals.
- Suspects are conveyed to the forensic examination room in a manner that limits contamination opportunities.
- HCPs working practices reduce the opportunity for contamination
- Equipment is appropriately cleaned,[7] and DNA-grade[8] consumables are used.
- All personal items, stationery and unnecessary equipment should be stored away – work surfaces should be clear and free from clutter.

Measures
- Restrict those present to only those critical and wearing barrier clothing (see Figure 13.7) (except for the suspect).
- Double gloving (non-latex powder-free) – changing the top gloves when handling different sample sites, before handling equipment or after touching any other surface.
- Restrict access to the forensic store room.
- Appropriately clean surfaces and equipment before and after use.
- Use specific forensic collection kits.
- Use recovery, sampling and packaging techniques that avoid contact with areas that are not part of the material of interest.

Detection
- Compare DNA profiles generated against an elimination database of reference DNA profiles.

Source: Adapted from Forensic Science Regulator (2024).

---

[7] Examples of cleaning agents include 10% sodium hypochlorite (bleach, Presept™) solution, 1% Solution Rely+On™ Virkon®, Microsol (10 %) and Distel (1%) (Trigene Advance) and Activ8™ (non-corrosive).
[8] Manufactured in a way to be free of detectable DNA.

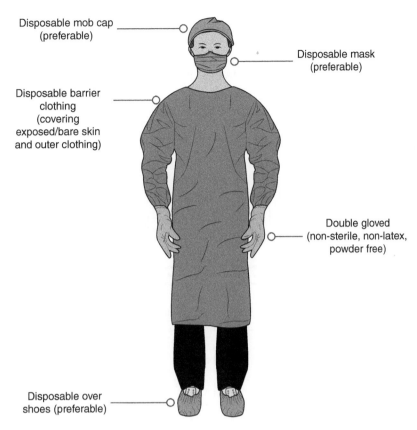

FIGURE 13.7   Barrier clothing.

Evidence Bags

Polythene evidence tamper-evident bags are used to securely and safely transport and store forensic samples. Their design ensures that once sealed, any unauthorised access to the contents is evident, maintaining the integrity of the evidence.

Each bag has a designated area for labelling, see Box 13.11 It is crucial to fill out all the required fields accurately to maintain the chain of custody and ensure the evidence can be correctly identified and linked to the specific case, see Figure 13.8.

BOX 13.11	LABELLING EVIDENCE BAGS (MAY VARY BETWEEN FORCE AREAS)

- Force details

- Exhibit reference number

- Suspect's name

- Date and time sample taken

- Description of sample site and type (i.e. right hand swabs – wet and dry)

- HCP's details and signature

The sample (i.e. swabs, scissors and comb) is placed inside the bag; care is taken to ensure the sample does not compromise the bag's integrity or sealing mechanism. Once the bag is filled and labelled, the protective strip covering the adhesive is removed and the bag is sealed by pressing the adhesive area closed. Once sealed, the bag cannot be opened without leaving visible signs of tampering.

Exhibit Reference Numbers

Exhibit reference numbers are a critical component. Providing a unique identifier for each piece of evidence, linking it to the person who collected it and ensuring it can be accurately traced from scene to court. A three-letter exhibit reference number is preferred over two letters to reduce the chance of duplication (although regional differences exist). HCPs can create their exhibit reference using the first letter of their first, middle and surname. Alternatively, they can use the first letter of their first name and the first two letters of their second name. For example, Nora Tracewell uses 'NTR'.

Transfer to Police

Once the samples are taken and sealed in the evidence bags, they are handed to the police officer. The officer takes custody of the samples and completes their details on the reverse of the evidence bag, maintaining the chain of custody.

TO CLOSE, PEEL OFF BLUE TAPE TO EXPOSE GLUE AND PRESS ORANGE TAPE DOWN FIRMLY.

EVIDENCE BAG

BIOHAZARD

A12345678

PLEASE ENSURE THAT ALL BOXES IN BOLD ARE COMPLETED AT THE SCENE OF THE EXHIBIT RECOVERY

Organisation: WESTSHIRE CONST.

Exhibit No: NTR / 01 / A + B

Case Ref No:

Property Ref No:

Description of Exhibit: RIGHT HAND SWABS - WET AND DRY

Recovered/Obtained from: RIGOR HEALMAN

Recovered/Obtained by: HCP

Name: NORA TRACEWELL

Rank/Title:

No: **Signed:**

Time/Date Recovered/Obtained: 21 / 08 / 2024 11:10

Operation Name:

Incident/HOLMES No:

Major Incident Exhibit No:

Sample/Reference No:

Lab Ref No:

Court Exhibit No:

R-V

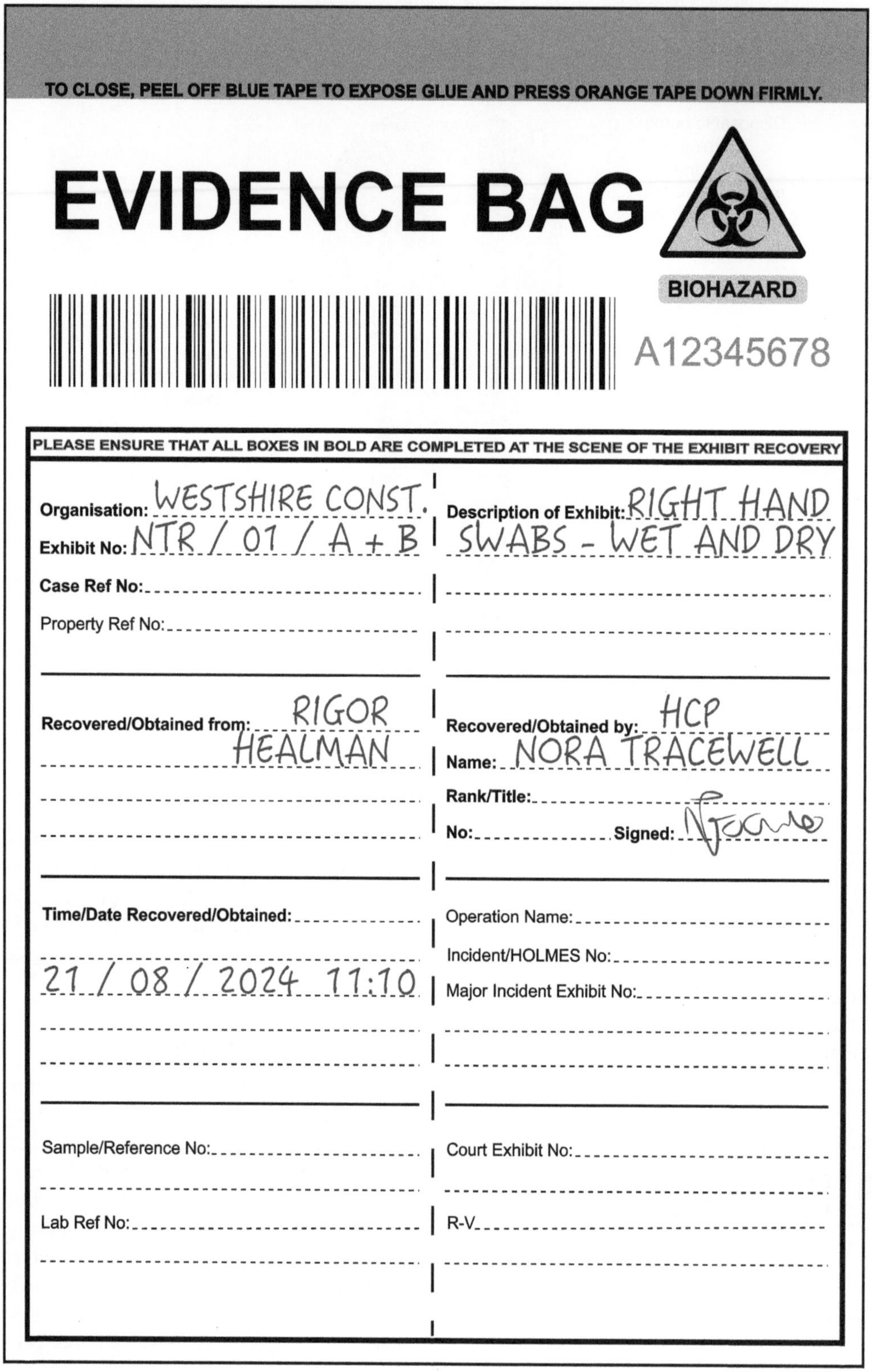

FIGURE 13.8 Labelled evidence bag (may vary between force areas).

Documentation

Contemporaneous documentation of the procedure is essential, and the HCP should include the timing and persons present in their clinical notes. The documentation should chronologically include all the details of the samples in order of time taken, including the tracking details/barcodes of the evidence bags. Comprehensive documentation, including a summary of the incident at the time, will assist in writing your statement later when it is requested, as the statement should reflect the clinical notes recorded.

FORENSIC SWABS

Forensic swabs are taken using specific forensic DNA-grade swabs. These are distinct from the sterile swabs HCPs are familiar with in clinical settings. While they are sterile, they are treated or manufactured in a way that the swabs are free from detectable DNA.

Take care when handling the sterile water ampule. Open using fresh, clean gloves and waste the initial first drops to flush the nozzle before applying three to four drops onto the swab, in case of contamination (Forensic Science Regulator 2024). Refrain from over-moistening the swab; it should not be so wet that it drips. The nozzle should not touch the swab and should be discarded if it makes contact with any contaminated surface.

A wet swab followed by a dry swab in forensic evidence collection is designed to maximise the amount and variety of material collected (Hedman et al. 2020). The first swab is moistened with several drops of sterile water to help pick up trace materials that might be more easily transferred to a wet surface. This is particularly effective for absorbing biological materials like body fluids (blood, saliva, semen) or skin cells. The water in the swab can help to loosen and lift cells and substances that might not adhere as well to a dry swab. Following the wet swab with a dry one, ensures any residual material not picked up by the wet swab is collected. The dry swab can absorb any moisture left from the wet swab, which may contain additional trace evidence. It also collects particles that might adhere better to a dry surface.

When taking swabs, it is essential to follow a methodical approach to ensure the collection of adequate and uncontaminated evidence. The swab should be rolled across the skin surface with a moderately firm pressure. This rolling action helps in picking up trace materials from the entire area of contact. Avoid using a back-and-forth motion as it might redeposit material back onto the skin. Too much pressure collects the suspect's DNA and can miss the surface material, or may damage the swab, while too little might not collect enough material. The pressure should be enough to ensure good contact with the skin without causing discomfort or harm. Finally, ensure the entire swab comes into contact with the skin. This maximises the area from which evidence is collected.

Labelling Swabs

Proper labelling of forensic swabs is a crucial step in the chain of custody and the overall forensic process, see Box 13.12. Accurate and comprehensive labelling ensures each swab can be correctly identified and linked to the specific case, location and individual from which it was collected (see Figure 13.9).

BOX 13.12 LABELLING SWABS (VARIES BETWEEN FORCE AREAS)

- Name of the suspect
- Description of sample site
- Type of swab (wet or dry)
- Date and time sample taken
- Exhibit reference number

Source: Adapted from Forensic Science Regulator (2024).

SAMPLE SITE: RIGHT HAND (WET SWAB)
NAME: RIGOR HEALMAN
DATE: 21/08/24 **TIME:** 11:10
EXHIBIT NO: NTR / 01 / A
BIOHAZARD

FIGURE 13.9 Example of labelled swab (varies between force areas).

This is vital for maintaining the integrity of the evidence and for its admissibility in court.

Hand Swabs

The technique for swabbing hands involves rolling a moistened swab over the surface of the hands (palmar and dorsal) and between the fingers, followed by a dry swab, see Figure 13.10. Each hand is swabbed and exhibited separately. HCPs should develop a standard routine, such as always swabbing the dorsal aspect between the fingers and the palmar aspect in order. This is helpful if there are any questions in court regarding their process.

Nail Swabs

Using a moistened swab, scrape underneath and swab around all the fingernails gently, followed by a dry swab. Each hand is swabbed and exhibited separately (see Figure 13.11).

Penile Swabs

Penile swabs are divided into two separate sets. Initially, swab the shaft of the penis and external foreskin (if present); this involves using a wet swab followed by a dry swab (see Figure 13.12). A second set of swabs is taken from the internal foreskin (if present), the coronal sulcus (the groove behind the glans), and the glans (head) of the penis (see Figure 13.13). This area is particularly important as it is more likely to retain biological material following sexual contact. Gentle rolling and dabbing motions are typically used to maximise evidence collection without causing discomfort.

Given the invasive nature of penile swabs, they must be conducted with sensitivity and respect for the individual's dignity and privacy.

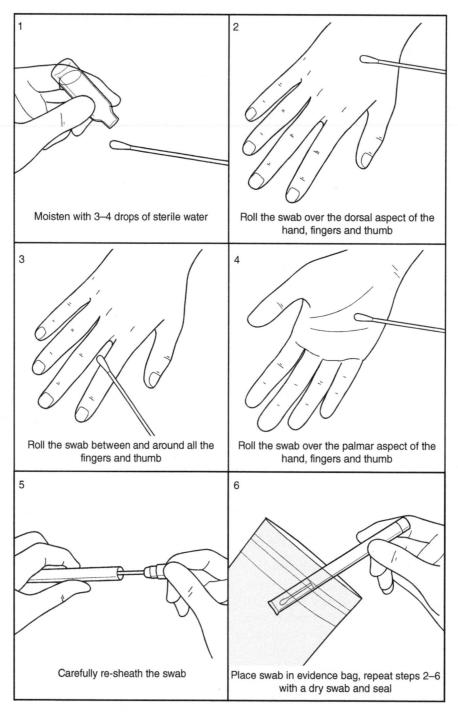

1 Moisten with 3–4 drops of sterile water

2 Roll the swab over the dorsal aspect of the hand, fingers and thumb

3 Roll the swab between and around all the fingers and thumb

4 Roll the swab over the palmar aspect of the hand, fingers and thumb

5 Carefully re-sheath the swab

6 Place swab in evidence bag, repeat steps 2–6 with a dry swab and seal

FIGURE 13.10   Hand swabs.

Mouth Swabs

Because the mouth is moist, there is no need for a wet swab; both swabs are dry. The first swab remains swab A and the second swab remains swab B. The swab should be thoroughly rubbed around the entire mouth, including under and over the tongue, all sides of the teeth and gums, inside cheeks and any dentures, dental fixtures or oral piercings. This should be repeated with the second dry swab.

Other Skin Swabs

When there appears to be blood or another substance on a person's skin – for instance, on the face, arm or chest – a skin swab is used to collect this material for analysis. The swab is taken as outlined above. However, an additional control skin swab is an essential part of this process. This involves taking a wet and dry swab from an area of skin to serve as a baseline or control sample. The area chosen for the control swab should

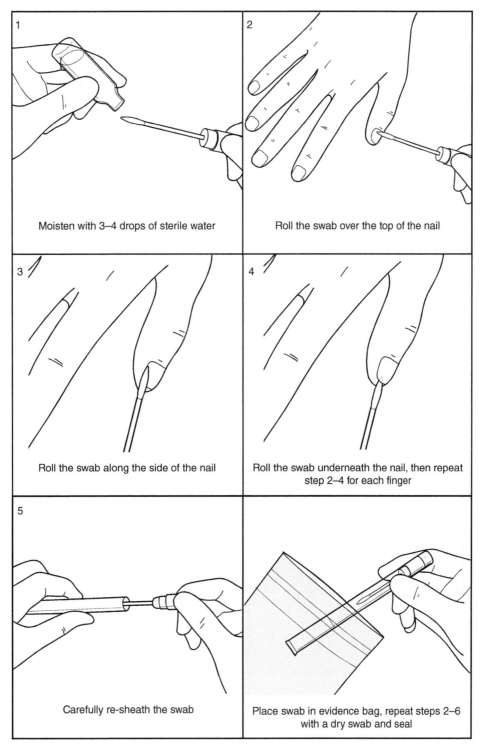

1 Moisten with 3–4 drops of sterile water

2 Roll the swab over the top of the nail

3 Roll the swab along the side of the nail

4 Roll the swab underneath the nail, then repeat step 2–4 for each finger

5 Carefully re-sheath the swab

Place swab in evidence bag, repeat steps 2–6 with a dry swab and seal

FIGURE 13.11 Nail swabs.

be as similar as possible to the sampled area but unaffected by the visible substance.

Consider skin sites such as peri-oral, as often sexual offences include oral contact, hand swabs as sexual offences can include digital penetration by the suspect and based on a first account, wider areas if appropriate.

OTHER FORENSIC SAMPLES

Nail Clippings

Nails should only be clipped if there is visible material seen. Otherwise, nail swabs are satisfactory. Nails are clipped as

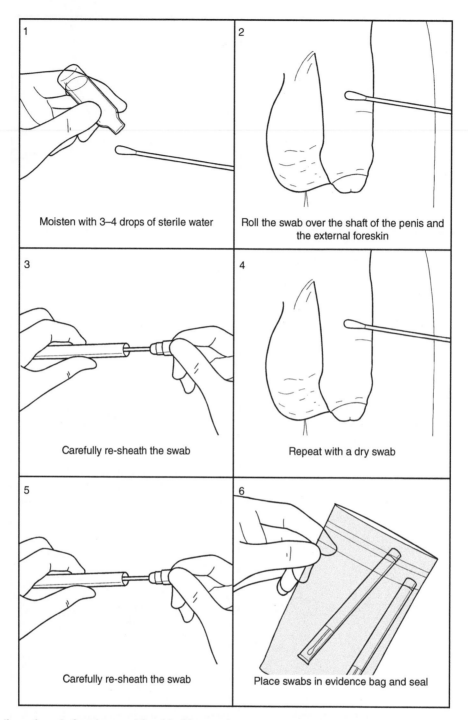

FIGURE 13.12 Penile swabs – shaft and external foreskin (if present).

close to the nail bed as possible to collect any material lodged underneath while over a sterile sheet, see Figure 13.14. The sterile sheet is then carefully folded and placed in an evidence bag.

Hair (Combing and Cutting)

Head hair and pubic hair combing and cutting are used to collect trace evidence in various investigations. These procedures are designed to recover hairs, fibres and other potential trace or biological evidence that may be critical in linking a suspect to a crime scene or another individual.

Head hair The individual's head hair is systematically combed using a clean, sterile comb while the individual leans over a sterile sheet. The combing dislodges any loose hairs and foreign particles. The material collected in the sterile sheet is carefully folded to avoid losing any material before being placed in an evidence bag. A hair sample is then cut close to

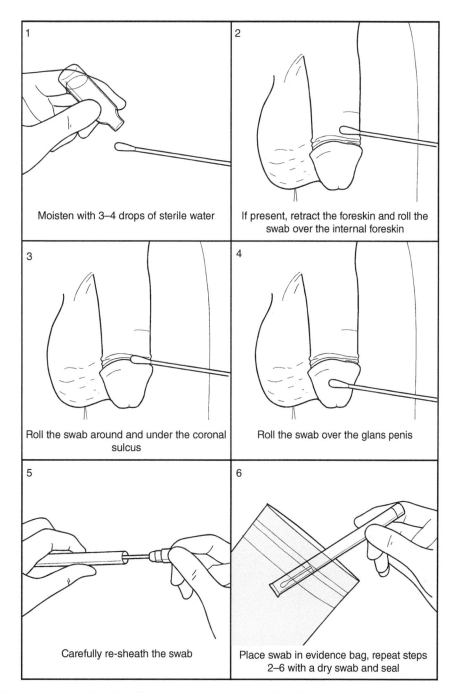

1 Moisten with 3–4 drops of sterile water

2 If present, retract the foreskin and roll the swab over the internal foreskin

3 Roll the swab around and under the coronal sulcus

4 Roll the swab over the glans penis

5 Carefully re-sheath the swab

6 Place swab in evidence bag, repeat steps 2–6 with a dry swab and seal

FIGURE 13.13 Penile swabs – Internal foreskin (if present), coronal sulcus and penile glans.

the root and secured within a sterile sheet, folded and placed in a separate evidence bag for comparison.

Pubic hair The individual's pubic hair is systematically combed using a sterile comb towards a sterile sheet between their legs or just under the buttocks. Any material collected in the comb and sterile sheet is then carefully folded to avoid losing any material before this is placed in an evidence bag (see Figure 13.15). Routine pubic hair cutting is no longer recommended. Pubic hair only needs cutting if there is matting with

biological material (or other forensically significant material) (see Figure 13.16).

TOXICOLOGY SAMPLES

Police may request toxicology samples to be collected to determine if drugs or alcohol played a role in a violent or serious crime, murder or in situations where drug facilitation is suspected, such as in cases of sexual assault or robbery. Forensic toxicology heavily relies on the analysis of blood, urine, hair

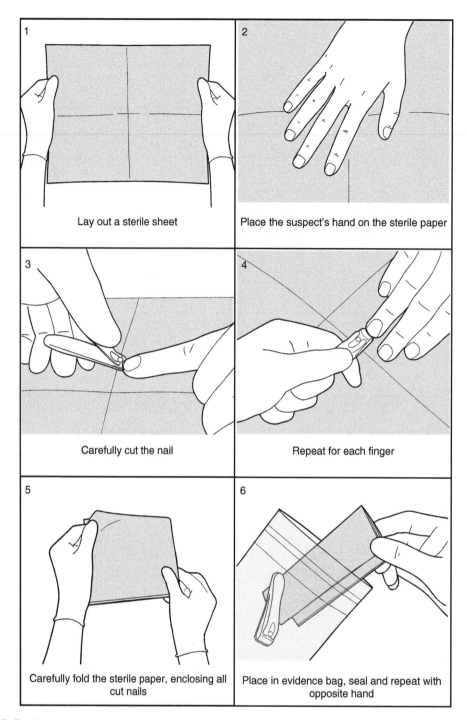

1 Lay out a sterile sheet	2 Place the suspect's hand on the sterile paper
3 Carefully cut the nail	4 Repeat for each finger
5 Carefully fold the sterile paper, enclosing all cut nails	6 Place in evidence bag, seal and repeat with opposite hand

FIGURE 13.14 Nail clippings.

or nail samples, each offering unique insights into an individual's exposure to drugs, alcohol and toxins.

Blood Samples

Blood samples are particularly valuable for their ability to provide a direct measurement of substances in the bloodstream at the time of sampling. They are recommended to be taken within 72 hours of the offence. Blood tests are known for their accuracy and can detect a broad range of substances. Depending on the kit, HCPs may have one 10 ml vial or two 5 ml vials. Each vial should be filled at most three-quarters to prevent the vials from breaking when frozen. Unlike road traffic procedures, the suspect is not provided with a sample for independent testing.

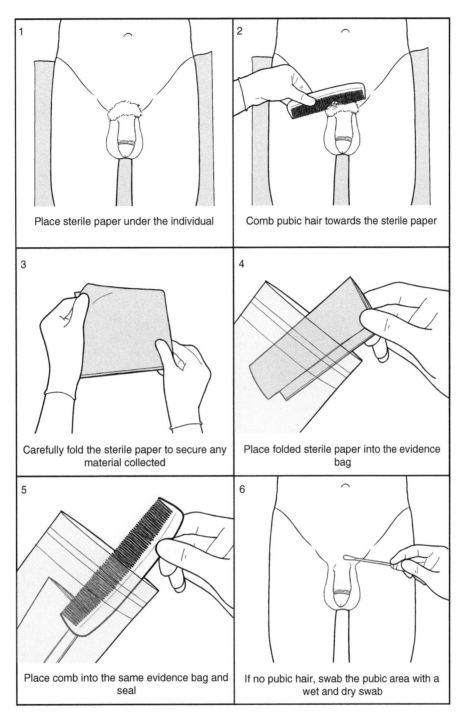

1. Place sterile paper under the individual
2. Comb pubic hair towards the sterile paper
3. Carefully fold the sterile paper to secure any material collected
4. Place folded sterile paper into the evidence bag
5. Place comb into the same evidence bag and seal
6. If no pubic hair, swab the pubic area with a wet and dry swab

FIGURE 13.15   Pubic hair combing.

Volatile substances Volatile substances such as solvents, aerosols, gases (i.e. nitrous oxide) or nitrites (i.e. amyl nitrite) are rapidly metabolised and eliminated from the body. Samples should be collected as soon as possible after exposure, as gases and aerosols dissipate from the bloodstream within hours or even minutes. A double sample (two 10 ml vials or four 5 ml) should be taken and frozen within an hour of sampling and remain frozen until analysed (including in transit).

Urine Samples

Urine samples offer a wider detection window than blood, making them useful for ascertaining substance use or exposure. They are particularly effective in detecting metabolites, the breakdown products of various substances after the drug's effects have diminished.

In cases occurring within the last 24 hours, collect two separate urine samples. Each sample should ideally contain

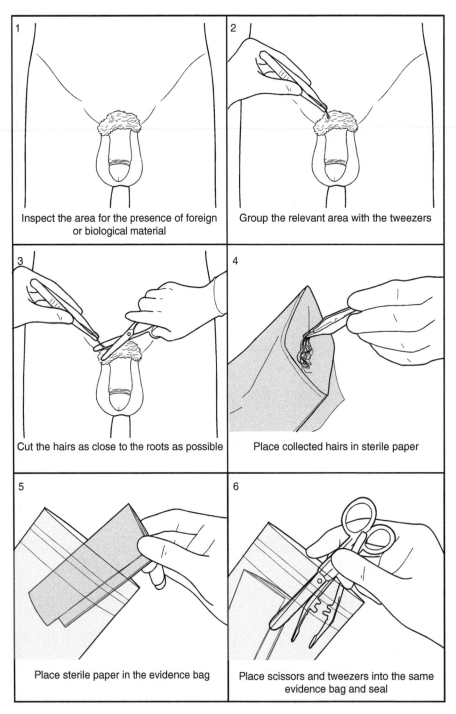

FIGURE 13.16 Pubic hair cutting.

about 20 ml of urine, decanted into a glass tube with a capacity of at least 25 ml, filling the tube just over three-quarters full. The first should be taken as soon as practical. The second should ideally be obtained within an hour of the initial, although it should still be collected even if this timeframe is exceeded.

Head Hair

Hair samples add another dimension to forensic toxicology. They provide a timeline of substance use or exposure, as drugs and their metabolites are deposited in the hair shaft. Analysis of hair can reveal a history of drug use over a more extended period, often covering months, and can be crucial in building a case where long-term substance use is relevant. Head hair for toxicology should only be taken a minimum of four to six weeks after the date of interest due to the requirement for the hair to grow out of the hair shaft where is exposed to the substance.

Nail Samples

Nail samples are increasingly being utilised due to their ability to provide a historical record of substance use or exposure. They can be particularly useful in those with little or no hair. Nails are clipped as outlined above. However, the sample should be stored at room temperature.

OTHER FORENSIC SAMPLING CONSIDERATIONS

Very Rare Intimate Samples (Female Intimate, Transgender or Male Anal or Rectal)

There are rare instances where other intimate samples (such as vaginal samples in females or anal/rectal samples in males and transgender individuals) are necessary. Handling suspects of any gender who require such intimate examinations and sample collection presents unique challenges due to limited common exposure to these procedures. HCPs must adhere to established protocols while considering several crucial principles:

1. **Appropriate environment**: The examination should be conducted in a private setting equipped with a proper examination couch, adequate lighting and necessary equipment. This setup is vital to preserve the dignity of the individual being examined.

2. **Qualified HCPs**: The HCP performing the examination must have comprehensive theoretical knowledge and practical competencies. This includes proficiency in documenting injuries. The use of self-swabs, though a contentious issue, may be an option under certain circumstances.

3. **Preventing cross-contamination**: Strict procedures must be in place to prevent any cross-contamination during the collection and handling of samples.

Each of these principles is fundamental in ensuring the process is conducted with the utmost respect, professionalism and adherence to legal and ethical standards.

Children

Children and samples are considered in Chapter 16 – Special Circumstances.

Lack of Capacity

Sampling those who lack capacity or cannot give valid consent is challenging outside the road traffic legislation, so each area will have policies to manage these cases as there is no consensus in practice. However, Section 63 of both the Police and Criminal Evidence Act 1984 and Police and Criminal Evidence (Northern Ireland) Order 1989 allows a constable to take a non-intimate sample without consent with the authorisation of an Inspector. Section 19B Criminal Procedure (Scotland) Act 1995 allows a constable to use reasonable force to take a sample, with the authority of an inspector (as a minimum).

Off-site Examinations

Off-site examinations may also be requested, and each area will have policies to manage these cases as there is no consensus in practice.

STORAGE OF SAMPLES

It is the police's responsibility to store the sample. The storage of samples can either be in the fridge, the freezer or at room temperature. This information can be found in the FFLM FSSC guidance; see 'Resources'.

CONCLUSION

This chapter has outlined the critical role of HCPs in evidence collection within forensic settings. By understanding the intricacies of documenting injuries and collecting samples, practitioners can ensure the integrity and admissibility of evidence in legal proceedings. The chapter emphasises the importance of meticulous documentation, adherence to protocols and awareness of legal implications, equipping HCPs with the knowledge and skills necessary to contribute effectively to the justice system.

LEARNING ACTIVITIES

1. Write a reflection on a case where the quality of your injury documentation could have been better and how you changed your practice as a result.

2. Write a reflection on a case where taking samples was made difficult because of the behaviour of the suspect. For example, they were uncooperative, very angry or aggressive. Examine how that impacted your interaction, the sampling procedure and your attitude. Explore strategies to cope with such a scenario again.

3. Reflect on a situation where you took samples outside of the recommendations. Outline your rationale, decision-making and the actual sampling process taken. Consider how you might write this for a statement or explain in court.

RESOURCES

Online

- FFLM | Recommendations for the collection of forensic specimens from complainant and suspects | https://fflm.ac.uk/resources/publications/recommendations-for-the-collection-of-forensic-specimens-from-complainants-and-suspects/

- Forensic Medicine for Medical Students| https://www.forensicmed.co.uk

Organisations

- Forensic Capability Network | https://www.fcn.police.uk/

- Forensic Regulator | https://www.gov.uk/government/organisations/forensic-science-regulator

REFERENCES

Department of Justice (2015). Police and criminal evidence (Northern Ireland) order 1989 (PACE) - Code D revised code of practice for the identification of persons by police officers. https://www.justice-ni.gov.uk/sites/default/files/publications/doj/pace-code-d-2015-final-version.pdf (accessed 11 December 2023).

Faculty of Forensic & Legal Medicine (2023). Recommendations for the collection of forensic specimens from complaints and suspects – the evidence. https://fflm.ac.uk/wp-content/uploads/2023/01/Recommendations-Collection-of-Forensic-Specimens-the-evidence-FSSC-July-2023.pdf (accessed 12 November 2023).

Forensic Capability Network (2023). SARC glove process – briefing and FAQs. https://khub.net/group/fcn-sarc-accreditation-support/group-library/-/document_library/99SE3p242mAB/view_file/839900513?_com_liferay_document_library_web_portlet_DLPortlet_INSTANCE_99SE3p242mAB_redirect=https%3A%2F%2Fkhub.net%3A443%2Fgroup%2Fguest%2Fsearch%3Fp_p_id%3Dcom_placecube_digitalplace_communities_search_listings_web_SearchListingsPortlet (accessed 12 December 2023).

Forensic Science Regulator (2024). Guidance: DNA contamination controls – Forensic medical examinations (FSR-GUI-0017). https://assets.publishing.service.gov.uk/media/65a80392b2f3c6000de5d4c1/DNA_contamination_controls___Forensic_medical_examinations.pdf (accessed 24 January 2024).

Hedman, J., Jansson, L., Akel, Y. et al. (2020). The double-swab technique versus single swabs for human DNA recovery from various surfaces. *Forensic Science International: Genetics* 46: 102253.

Home Office (2016). Police and Criminal Evidence Act 1984 (PACE) - Code D Revised code of practice for the identification of persons by police officers. https://assets.publishing.service.gov.uk/media/5a7f9af2e5274a2e87db6dc2/57603_PACE_Code_D_2016_amended_221116.pdf (accessed 11 December 2023).

Hughes, V.K., Ellis, P.S., and Langlois, N.E. (2004). The perception of yellow in bruises. *Journal of Clinical Forensic Medicine* 11 (5): 257–259.

Kumar, V., Abbas, A., and Aster, J. (2021). *Robbins & Cotran Pathological Basis of Disease*, 10the. New York: Elsevier.

Langlois, N.E. and Gresham, G.A. (1991). The ageing of bruises: a review and study of the colour changes with time. *Forensic Science International* 50 (2): 227–238.

Maguire, S., Mann, M.K., Sibert, J., and Kemp, A. (2005). Can you age bruises accurately in children? A systematic review. *Archives of Disease in Childhood* 90 (2): 187–189.

Wilkinson, H. and Hardman, M. (2020) Wound healing: cellular mechanisms and pathological outcomes. *The Royal Society*. DOI:https://doi.org/10.1098/rsob.200223

FURTHER READING

FFLM | Standards of practice for forensic medical examination and collection of evidence | https://www.gov.uk/government/consultations/forensic-medical-exam-standard-for-sexual-assault-complainants/forensic-medical-examination-standard-document-fsr-c-116-accessible-version

Forensic Science Regulator | Code of Practice | https://www.gov.uk/government/publications/statutory-code-of-practice-for-forensic-science-activities/forensic-science-regulator-code-of-practice-accessible

Safeguarding

Amanda McDonough, Nicola Sheridan, and Mandy Smail

Mitie Care and Custody Health Ltd, London, UK

CHAPTER 14

AIM

This chapter will explore safeguarding children, adults at risk who have care and support needs and domestic violence and abuse. It will introduce the principles of safeguarding and protection from abuse, neglect and exploitation, providing the readers with an understanding of how to recognise and respond appropriately if they have concerns about a child or adult at risk, adhering to relevant legislation, local policies and referral pathways.

LEARNING OUTCOMES

Upon completion of this chapter, readers should be able to:

- Understand protection and safeguarding for children, young people and adults with care and support needs

- Recognise the signs and symptoms of abuse, neglect, exploitation and how to respond

- Understand the implications of the Domestic Abuse Act and its relevance in safeguarding, including the identification, assessment and appropriate response

---

SELF-ASSESSMENT

1. Define the different categories of abuse and provide examples of abuse. Outline how adults and children may be vulnerable to such types of abuse.

2. Outline the roles and responsibilities of healthcare professionals (HCP) working in custody concerning safeguarding adults and children, who may not be in custody.

3. Describe the boundaries of confidentiality and when to share information.

INTRODUCTION

This chapter will explore safeguarding children, adults at risk and domestic violence and abuse (DVA). It will introduce the principles of safeguarding and protection from abuse and neglect, providing readers with an understanding of how to recognise and respond appropriately, if they have concerns about a child or adult at risk, adhering to relevant legislation, local policies and referral pathways.

Every person has a right to feel safe; safeguarding all children under the age of 18 years and adults at risk is the responsibility of all agencies and individuals. HCPs have a statutory duty to safeguard and protect individuals from harm, abuse, neglect and exploitation. HCPs in a custody environment are working with some of the most vulnerable people in society and are in an ideal position to support the people they see. Practitioners must be alert to the potential indicators of

---

Police Custody Healthcare for Nurses and Paramedics, First Edition. Edited by Matthew Peel, Jennie Smith, Vanessa Webb, and Margaret Bannerman.
© 2025 John Wiley & Sons Ltd. Published 2025 by John Wiley & Sons Ltd.
Companion website: www.wiley.com/go/policecustodyhealthcare

abuse, neglect and exploitation, recognising risks and responding appropriately.

SAFEGUARDING CHILDREN

The United Nations Convention on the Rights of the Child (UNCRC) (1998) defines a child as anyone under the age of 18; this has been adopted in legislation by all four nations in the United Kingdom (UK). Therefore, in this chapter, the term child(ren) will refer to all those under the age of 18 years.

Safeguarding is supported by a legal framework, with many key pieces of legislation and statutory guidance outlined in both UK and international legislation.

The four nations in the United Kingdom – England, Northern Ireland (NI), Scotland and Wales have their own child protection systems and legislation. However, although different, they are all based on similar principles. HCPs need to be aware of and have a good understanding of both statutory and non-statutory guidance relevant to their area to safeguard children. Some of the main pieces of legislation and guidance are:

- The Children Act 1989 and 2004 (England and Wales)

- Working Together to Safeguarding Children 2018

- Children and Social Work Act 2017 (England)

- Social Services and Well-being (Wales) Act 2014

- The Children (Northern Ireland) Order 1995

- The Children (Scotland) Act 1995 and 2020

- Children and Young People (Scotland) Act 2014

- United Nations Convention on the Rights of the Child 1992

A key agency also in protecting children is the National Society for the Prevention of Cruelty to Children (NSPCC), founded in 1884 and dedicated to protecting children. They are the only UK charity with statutory child protection powers in England, Wales and NI to intervene to protect children from harm and abuse, having 'authorised person status', but excludes Scotland.

WHAT IS SAFEGUARDING?

Safeguarding is the broader term incorporating all aspects of promoting and protecting the health and well-being of children, from early help through to child protection. Child protection is part of the safeguarding continuum, which focuses on protecting children from significant harm or the likelihood, occurring inside and outside the family home and online.

The concept of significant harm and the paramount principle was first recognised in the Children Act 1989 (England and Wales) and is enshrined in The Children (Northern Ireland) Order 1995 and the Children (Scotland) Act 1995. This identifies the threshold which justifies compulsory intervention in family life, when it is in the best interest of the child.

BOX 14.1	DEFINITIONS

Harm	Ill-treatment or the impairment of health or development including, for example impairment suffered from seeing or hearing the ill-treatment of another (e.g. DVA)
Development	Physical, intellectual, emotional, social or behavioural development
Health	Physical or mental health
Ill treatment	Includes sexual abuse and forms of ill-treatment which are not physical'

Source: Adoption and Children Act 2002 / Crown / Public Domain.

There is no actual definition of what significant harm means; however, the Children Act 1989 indicates the health and development of the child should be compared to that which is reasonably expected of a similar child. For other definitions, see Box 14.1.

A single traumatic event may constitute significant harm, but more often, it is the accumulation of events, with consideration of the severity, duration and frequency, having a detrimental impact on the child.

If the HCP has a concern about a child, then a referral should be made to the local authority (LA) (or equivalent), where the child is living or is found. If there is reasonable cause to suspect a child has suffered, or is likely to suffer, the LA has a duty to make enquires to decide on what action is required, Section 47 Children Act 1989 (England and Wales), Article 50 The Children (Northern Ireland) Order 1995 and Children's Hearings (Scotland) Act 2011.

SIGNS AND INDICATORS OF ABUSE

It is vital that HCPs are aware of the signs and indicators of abuse, neglect and exploitation and know how to take appropriate action to safeguard and protect children.

Categories of Abuse

The main categories of abuse when a child is placed on a child protection plan/register are physical, sexual, emotional and neglect, although consideration must be given to other forms of abuse such as exploitation. Children can be subjected to more than one type of abuse. See Box 14.2 for examples of abuse categories.

There are threats to children in families (intra-familial harm), but harm, abuse and exploitation (see Box 14.3) can also occur outside of the family home, known as extra-familial harm. Extra-familial threats can occur in the community, at school, from peer and teenage relationship abuse, online abuse and from criminal and organised gangs in the forms of child criminal exploitation (CCE), including county lines and child sexual exploitation (CSE).

BOX 14.2	TYPES OF ABUSE
Physical	Involves causing any physical harm to the child; this can include hitting, biting, poisoning, burning, scalding, drowning or suffocating
Neglect	Is the failure to meet the child's basic needs: not providing adequate nutrition, shelter, hygiene, safety/supervision, warmth/affection or medical treatment, resulting in serious impairment of the child's health and development. This also includes the unborn baby due to maternal substance abuse
Emotional	The persistent emotional maltreatment of a child resulting in severe adverse effects on their emotional development. Can involve making the child feel worthless, unloved, ridiculing them, inappropriate expectations and can involve seeing or hearing the ill-treatment of another (DVA)
Sexual	Involves forcing/enticing a child to take part in sexual activities. This can be through physical sexual contact for example; inappropriate touching or rape, or non-contact activities such as, forcing children to watch/take part in pornography. Child sexual exploitation (CSE) is also sexual abuse; even if the relationship appears consenting, children cannot consent to their own abuse. Beckett et al. (2017) suggest these children have limited options and their choices are 'constrained choices', or 'survival strategies'. This could also be related to criminal exploitation. Sexual abuse is not solely perpetrated by adult males; females can commit acts of sexual abuse, as can other children
DVA	All children can experience and be adversely affected by DVA in their home life where DVA occurs between family members, including where those being abusive do not live with the child.

Source: Adapted from HM Government (2023).

BOX 14.3	EXPLOITATION

The abuse of power and control by perpetrators for their gain. It can include many forms of abuse such as child labour, slavery, domestic servitude, forcing them to take part in criminal activities: begging, financial fraud and cannabis cultivation. Additionally, child trafficking, CCE/CSE and county lines and the influences of extremism leading to radicalisation are included. Some indicators could be changes in behaviours, going missing, not attending school and unexplained gifts/money.

Source: Home Office (2023)/ Crown / Public domain.

All children can experience abuse, but there are factors that can make some more vulnerable, such as adverse childhood experiences (ACEs), drug and alcohol misuse, learning difficulties/disabilities, of both the child and parents, severe parental mental health issues and DVA. Children with care experience, known as looked-after children, are particularly vulnerable to exploitation due to the very nature that they have usually experienced trauma and abuse prior to going into care. Children with a disability are up to four times more likely to experience abuse than non-disabled children (Taylor et al. 2015). Also, consider children at risk of female genital mutilation (FGM).

Safeguarding children includes radicalisation and terrorism; it is crucial to recognise how extremists exploit their vulnerabilities. Often targeting those with social isolation or identity struggles, extremists use grooming tactics and manipulation similar to other forms of abuse. The internet plays a significant role, with children exposed to extremist content via social media and online forums. Isolating children from moderating influences, deepening their involvement in extremism. Concerned HCPs can also refer to prevent, part of the UK's counter-terrorism policy, aimed at stopping people supporting terrorism. It operates to safeguard individuals from radicalisation and challenge extremist ideology.

Beckett (2011) suggests there are three conditions required for abuse and exploitation to occur.

- **Source of harm**: Perpetrators who have access to children, motivation and mediums to cause harm.

- **Inadequate protective structures**: If not present to stop the sources of harm gaining access to children, then children cannot be safeguarded.

- **Children**: Children are vulnerable because they are children and abuse does not occur because of their vulnerability, but because of a perpetrator's choice and motivation to abuse, harm and exploit children.

WHAT TO DO IF YOU HAVE CONCERNS

Think Family

When the HCP sees an individual in custody, regardless of whether it is a child or an adult, always 'think family', if seeing a parent have professional curiosity and ask about any children they live with, or may have contact with, including the unborn baby.

The NSPCC (2018) identifies key principles for referring concerns known as the 4Rs:

Recognise: Signs of abuse, neglect or exploitation

Respond: Appropriately to any concerns

Record: All concerns and relevant information accurately and actions taken

Refer: Concerns to children's services

It is important for HCPs to recognise children can be both perpetrators of crime and also victims[1] and understand the need to protect and safeguard. All children must have an appropriate adult. See Chapter 4 – Appropriate Adults and Vulnerabilities.

Contextual Safeguarding

Contextual safeguarding is an approach to understanding and responding to young people's experiences of significant harm beyond their families. It recognises the different relationships young people form in their neighbourhoods, schools and online can feature violence and abuse. This approach extends traditional safeguarding models which focus on the family, to understand the impact of wider environmental factors on a young person's safety.

If the HCP has any concerns about a child (including the unborn), they have a duty to cooperate and refer to the LA, following their own organisational and regional policies and using the local threshold documents to assess the level of intervention. The quality of the referral is vital for the LA to assess the risk and impact on the child(ren); it needs to include all the significant information, clearly outline the concerns, risks and the impact on the child. Information should be clear and concise, with no jargon or abbreviations. Complete all sections of the referral form; if the individual is uncooperative or refuses to answer, then document this. Assessments should be child-centred and any decisions taken should always be made in the best interest of the child. To assess the level of risk, and if the threshold of significant harm has been met, the LA will convene a meeting to share information and agree an action plan. The welfare of the child is paramount and the HCP must not delay a referral because they do not have all of the information or do not have consent to share.

There is no agreed consensus on the threshold for safeguarding referral in police custody, with some areas identifying being in custody indicates a child is failing to thrive, whereas other areas consider a more targeted approach.

Information Sharing

Effective information sharing is crucial in safeguarding children and overrides all other considerations if the child is at risk of significant harm. The Data Protection Act 2018, the General Data Protection Regulation (GDPR) and human rights laws are not barriers to sharing information; they provide a framework to support and safeguard children (HM Government 2018). GDPR provides conditions for sharing personal information and although it is good practice to gain consent, it is not necessary for the purposes of safeguarding and promoting the welfare of a child, provided there is a lawful basis to share. The Data Protection Act 2018 contains 'safeguarding of children and individuals at risk', which allows practitioners to share information, without consent. The

information shared should be necessary, proportionate, relevant, accurate, timely and secure. If consent is not obtained, document it in the records and referral form (HM Government 2018).

HCPs should also familiarise themselves with the Caldicott principles; these apply within all health and social care organisations in relation to sharing of information. All four nations have Caldicott Guardians (UK Caldicott Guardian Council 2018).

Record Keeping

HM Government (2023) highlights the accountability and importance of good record keeping in safeguarding; it is crucial that HCPs practice good record keeping. Records must clearly identify the concerns and the impact on the child; they should be factual, accurate and contemporaneous. Including any discussions (what information was shared/not shared with and the reasoning and their designation), the decisions and actions taken.

SCENARIO 14.1   Child safeguarding

You are asked to see a 14-year-old child who has been arrested for theft of a motor vehicle, driving while over the legal limit for alcohol (Breath alcohol concentration 44 mcg/100 mg) and was found with cannabis. He was arrested at 03:04 and it is now 04:07 on a Saturday am. The police report he has not been reported missing and there is no one answering at his home address.

1. *Describe the various safeguarding concerns for this child.*

2. *What are the HCP's safeguarding responsibilities?*

3. *Outline the HCPs response and actions in response to their concerns.*

4. *How would the HCP's response change if the child was 17-year-old.*

SAFEGUARDING ADULTS

Safeguarding adults means protecting a person's right to live, free from abuse and neglect. The term vulnerable adult has now been replaced by the term 'adult at risk', ensuring the focus is on the situation causing the concerns rather than on the adult (Care Act 2014).

The Care Act 2014 identifies that safeguarding duties apply to any adult (18 years and over) who meets the following criteria:

- Has needs for care and support (regardless of whether the LA is meeting those needs)

- Is experiencing/at risk of, abuse or neglect

---

[1] We use the term 'victim' throughout but recognise individuals may not identify as such.

- As a result of those care and support needs, are unable to protect themselves from either the risk/or abuse or neglect

WHAT DOES SAFEGUARDING A VULNERABLE ADULT MEAN?

A vulnerable adult is anyone who may be either at risk or is mistreated, either physically, emotionally, mentally or financially. Adults who have been classified as vulnerable are more likely to experience mistreatment or being taken advantage of, whether it be a friend or family member.

PRINCIPLES OF SAFEGUARDING

There are six main principles that underpin all adult safeguarding work, as identified in the Care Act 2014. These include:

- **Empowerment**: To support vulnerable people to make their own informed decisions
- **Prevention**: To take action to stop abuse or neglect before it occurs
- **Proportionality**: Respond in the least intrusive manner appropriate to the risk identified
- **Protection**: Understand the best ways to protect and support vulnerable people
- **Partnership**: Work with organisations and local community to keep people safe
- **Accountability**: Noting safeguarding concerns if responsible for a vulnerable person

The main legislation governing safeguarding adults in England, Wales, Scotland and Northern Ireland include:

- The Care Act 2014
- The Adult Support and protection (Scotland) Act 2007
- The Social Services and well-being (Wales) Act 2014
- The Safeguarding Vulnerable Groups (Northern Ireland) Order 2007

The definition of safeguarding in Scotland somewhat differs from England, Wales and NI. A child is usually anyone under the age of 18 years. However, Scotland defines an adult as over the age of 16. The following definition for an adult comes from the Adult Support and Protection (Scotland) Act 2007, which defines a vulnerable adult over the age of 16 years old who is unable to safeguard their well-being, property rights and interests are at risk of harm because they are affected by a disability, mental disorder, or illness, physical or mental infirmity and are more vulnerable to be harmed. This is also known as the three-point criteria of which adults must meet all three.

SIGNS AND INDICATORS OF ABUSE

Signs of abuse and neglect can sometimes be difficult to identify when safeguarding adults, so it is important that HCPs recognise the signs and indicators of abuse, neglect and exploitation. And know how to take appropriate action to safeguard and protect an adult at risk.

CATEGORIES OF ABUSE

There are ten categories of abuse highlighted in the Care Act 2014. These can include but are not exclusive:

- **Physical abuse**: Any kind of physical harm, including inappropriate/unlawful restraints
- **Sexual abuse**: Making a person take part in sexual activity without their consent and can include contact or non-contact sexual activity or sexual exploitation
- **Financial/material abuse**: Fraud, stealing money, property or belongings
- **Neglect and acts of omission**: Failing to meet a person's needs can be deliberate, withholding care, medication or food
- **Self-neglect**: Unwilling or unable to care for themselves, including their health or an unsafe environment
- **Psychological or emotional abuse**: Controlling, intimidation, bullying or threats
- **Discriminatory**: Treating someone differently or unfairly because of the person's protected characteristics
- **Modern slavery**: Forced to work for no or little money, also includes trafficking, forced labour, exploitation both sexually and criminally
- **DVA**: Includes psychological, physical, financial, sexual, forced marriage, honour-based violence and FGM
- **Organisational abuse**: Poor care or lack of leadership or management structures, including insufficient staffing
- **Radicalisation**[2]: Influencing an individual to adopt extremist beliefs or ideologies, potentially leading to participation in terrorist activities

SAFEGUARDING REFERRAL PROCESS

HCPs will come across many vulnerable people daily due to the chaotic lives many individuals lead. The vulnerabilities the HCP will encounter include mental health, drug and alcohol issues, as well as learning disabilities and physical health issues.

When assessing individuals, it is important to ask vulnerability questions and observe their reactions.

- Do they understand what you are asking?

---

[2] Radicalisation is not included in the Care Act 2014.

- Are they under the influence of a substance?

- How is their mental health? Are they taking care of themselves or others?

If the HCP has concerns about the safety of an adult at risk, they have a duty to make a referral to the LA, under section 42 of the Care Act (2014) England, Adult Support and Protection (Scotland) Act 2007, Social Services and Well-being (Wales) Act 2014 and The Safeguarding Vulnerable Groups (Northern Ireland) Order 2007. If the individual has capacity, then consent should be gained before the referral unless they are in immediate danger. A safeguarding concern can be made without consent if someone else is at risk, a crime may have been committed, or the person does not have the capacity. For example, intoxication, substance abuse, fear or if consent is given under duress or coercion, such as those experiencing DVA or modern slavery. For those who lack capacity, the HCP should consider completing a best-interest decision on behalf of the adult.

SCENARIO 14.2   Adult safeguarding

You see a 76-year-old male who has been arrested for assault. It is alleged to pushed someone over at a bus stop. He normally lives with his wife, but she suffered a heart attack 2 weeks ago and is in a critical condition in hospital. He has been visiting her daily. He has no children or relatives, but a neighbour heard he was arrested and rang with concerns. He is normally always seen with his wife and does not go out alone. Since she has been in hospital, he has been seen wearing the same clothes for several days and leaving the front door open. They have also heard reports he is giving away money on the bus each day.

1. *Describe the safeguarding concerns for this gentleman*

2. *Assuming the police are not charging him and he does not need the emergency department, what are the safeguarding priorities?*

3. *The man does not want 'any fuss' and wants to go see his wife at hospital. He does not agree to a safeguarding referral being made – can he refuse?*

4. *Outline the HCP's actions and responsibilities.*

DOMESTIC VIOLENCE AND ABUSE

DEFINITION

The UK's definition of DVA is:

any incident or pattern of incidents of controlling, coercive, threatening behaviour, violence or abuse between those aged 16 or over who are, or have been, intimate partners or family members regardless of gender or sexuality. The abuse can encompass, but is not limited to psychological, physical, sexual, financial, emotional. (Home Office 2013)

FACTS AND STATISTICS

DVA is a crime and can impact all social and cultural groups. Generally committed in private behind closed doors, it is under-reported and recorded. It is however, far from being a private issue. DVA impacts the emotional, physical and psychological well-being of the individuals who are abused and the wider family and associated children who live with them.

In the year ending March 2020, an estimated 2.3 million adults aged 16–74 years experienced DVA in the last year (1.6 million women and 757,000 men) (Home Office 2022). The cost of DVA is estimated to be approximately £66bn for victims of DVA and more than one in ten of all offences recorded by the police are DVA related (Home Office 2022).

Official statistics show the number of incidents of DVA recorded by the authorities every year. But the problem is much bigger, as many do not tell anyone about their abuse, see Box 14.4.

BOX 14.4   DVA FIGURES

- Each year nearly 2 million people in England and Wales alone suffer some form of domestic abuse – 1.3 million female victims (7.9% of the population) and 695,000 male victims (4.2%).

- Each year, more than 100,000 people in the United Kingdom are at high and imminent risk of being murdered or seriously injured as a result of domestic abuse.

- Women are much more likely than men to be the victims of high-risk or severe domestic abuse: 94% of those going to Multi-Agency Risk Assessment Conference (MARAC) or accessing an independent domestic violence advisor (IDVA) service are women.

- In 2017–2018, the police recorded 599,549 domestic abuse incidents in England and Wales.

- 293 women were killed by a current or former partner in England and Wales between 2017 and 2018.

- 114,427 children live in homes where there is high-risk domestic abuse.

- 62% of children living with domestic abuse are directly harmed by the perpetrator of the abuse, in addition to the harm caused by witnessing the abuse of others

- On average, victims at high risk of serious harm or murder live with domestic abuse for 2.5 years before getting help.

Source: Adapted from CAADA_UK.

THE DOMESTIC ABUSE ACT 2021

The Domestic Abuse Act 2021 has created for the first time a statutory definition of DVA based on the existing cross-government definition to ensure DVA is properly understood, considered unacceptable and actively challenged across statutory agencies and the public's attitude.

The previous definition operated on a non-statutory basis. Putting the definition on a statutory footing, while also recognising the impact of DVA on children now ensures DVA is properly understood and victim support services are applying a common definition.

The Act provides several measures designed to address DVA, including:

- creation of Domestic Abuse Protection Notices (DAPN) and Domestic Abuse Protection Orders (DAPO)

- provides a statutory basis for the Domestic Violence Disclosure Scheme (Clare's law)

- creates a statutory presumption that victims of DVA are eligible for special measures in the criminal courts and prohibits offenders from cross-examining their victims in person in the family courts

- places a duty on local authorities to give support to victims of DVA and their children in refuges and safe accommodation

In addition, the Act also focuses on two central areas; the first being both parties must be aged 16 or over and 'personally connected' and the second defines what kinds of behaviour constitutes abuse. In defining the relationship between a perpetrator and victim, the criteria states that they must be '**personally connected**'. This definition now allows for different relationships to be captured and recognised as DVA, including, for the first time, ex-partners and family members.

The broad range of behaviours which may constituent DVA and may occur as a single incident, or a pattern of behaviour over time include:

- physical violence and abuse

- psychological and emotional abuse

- sexual abuse

- financial abuse

- coercive and controlling behaviours

- female genital mutilation (FGM)

- honour-based violence and forced marriage

Although it is acknowledged most victims are women, the definition is intentionally gender-neutral to ensure no victim is excluded from protection or access to services.

NON-FATAL STRANGULATION

Non-fatal strangulation is a dangerous, potentially fatal and pervasive form of DVA. Often compared with waterboarding, a form of torture that leaves victims feeling fearful they will die and helpless. Women being strangled as part of DVA are seven times more likely to be murdered than women experiencing DVA without strangulation. Recognising the destructive nature of strangulation, it is now a specific offence in England and Wales punishable by up to 5 years imprisonment, and in Northern Ireland, up to 14 years imprisonment

VIOLENCE AGAINST WOMEN AND GIRL'S STRATEGY

In July 2021, the government launched its cross-departmental Violence Against Women and Girls Strategy (VAWG), which sets out how the government intends to respond to, and prevent violence against women and girls, including the ambition to increase the levels of support available for survivors and their children and hold perpetrators to account.

The strategy has a broad remit and attempts to tackle the crimes, which disproportionately affect women and girls and the pervasive societal attitudes and prejudices which underpin these crimes. Its implementation is fundamental to how we respond to and prevent DVA as we know DVA is a highly gendered crime, with women overwhelmingly victims and perpetrators overwhelmingly men.

The 'Tackling violence against women and girls strategy' will complement the Domestic Abuse Act 2021 and the Government's Domestic Abuse Strategy, allowing for a 'once in a generation' opportunity to implement real change, reducing the prevalence of violence against women and girls (Home Office 2021). A large part of this will be to improve support and the response for victims and reduce domestic violence offences.

RECOGNISING DVA

Although we know DVA is a crime, it is also very much a health issue, as HPCs are often the first point, or the only point of contact for some victims experiencing DVA. Therefore, all HCPs should be aware of the recognised physical, emotional and behavioural indications of DVA, the forms it may take and impact it may have. More importantly, HCPs need to know how to respond appropriately.

ASKING ABOUT DVA

DVA is an isolating crime, so many victims feel unable to talk about their experiences. Evidence suggests victims find it very hard to raise the topic of DVA themselves and direct questioning gets positive results.

Therefore, HCPs are best placed and should always take a proactive approach to the identification of DVA using routine and selective enquiry. Even if a victim is not ready to disclose the abuse at the time of asking, it will send a clear message there is an understanding of this issue and there are professionals available to support them when they feel able to disclose. It may be necessary to ask the question several times before making a disclosure and never assume someone else will ask about it.

However, victims of DVA are at their most vulnerable and at the greatest risk of significant harm when they make a disclosure to someone and attempt to leave an abuser (or soon after leaving).

So, if any signs are apparent, or suspected DVA, it is vital all HCPs when asking, recognise this heightened period of risk. There may only be 'one chance' to manage the disclosure and associated risks, so knowing how to do the appropriate risk assessment and referrals is paramount.

Routine Enquiry

Never ask about DVA in front of anyone else; this includes partners, children and other members of the family if they are present. The individuals must be seen on their own. The following points are essential when asking routine enquiry questions:

- Ensure privacy – make sure you cannot be overheard.

- Avoid interruptions.

- Do not rush the person. Allow them to talk about their experience at their own pace.

- Never accept culture as an excuse for DVA.

- Consider whether an independent professional interpreter is needed.

- Ask the person if they would like to talk to someone else; they may prefer to talk to someone of the same sex.

- Provide every person with support services information regardless of their response.

- Ask direct questions sensitively such as:

  - Are you ever afraid at home?

  - Does your partner ever call you names or put you down?

  - Have you ever been forced to do anything sexually you did not want to do?

There are no set times when routine enquiry should be asked, but when there are concerns and when it is safe to do so, they should be asked about DVA. Research tells us that DVA starts or worsens during pregnancy. As such, routine enquiry is advocated at every contact with a pregnant woman.

Selective Enquiry

Outside of routinely asking, if health professionals see something that might indicate a person is experiencing DVA, HCPs have a responsibility to take the initiative and ask questions.

Responding to a Disclosure

Once disclosure of DVA has been made, HCPs should complete a risk assessment checklist, such as the CAADA-DASH (or regional variant). To identify the level of risk and whether the case should be referred to MARAC or alternative support.

High-risk If an individual scores 'high-risk', they should be informed a referral will be made to the MARAC to ensure a multi-agency safety plan can be put in place. Consent should be sought. However, if the victim refuses, a referral can still be made because of the level of risk. Those who have been victims of non-fatal strangulation should be considered high-risk.

Medium or low-risk Medium or low-risk should be offered a referral to other support agencies, with their consent. Where individuals are not high risk, but you have serious concerns, you can still share information without consent using 'professional judgement'.

Record Keeping and Information Sharing

Health records and effective information sharing between practitioners and agencies play an important role in responding to DVA. Ensuring records are contemporaneous, as they can be used in criminal proceedings against the perpetrator and information is only ever shared in accordance with the Data Protection Act 2018, GDPR and the Human Rights Act 1998.

Whilst it is good practice to gain consent, it is not always necessary to report DVA. The Data Protection Act 2018 outlines how to safeguard 'individuals at risk' and believes it is not always reasonable to expect an HCP to obtain consent, especially if doing so would enhance a person's risk.

GDPR permits the lawful sharing of personal information when necessary, proportionate, relevant, accurate, timely and secure. If consent is not obtained, this should always be documented in the records with the rationale for why you shared.

Using an Interpreter and Reasonable Adjustments

If interpreting services are required, you must always use a professional interpreter; this includes the use of sign-language interpreters for individuals who are profoundly deaf. Never use a family member, child or partner and try to get an interpreter of the same gender as the victim to prevent precluding discussion of certain subjects.

If a victim has a learning disability, consideration must be made as to whether a Learning Disability Advocate is needed to ensure the victim fully understands the question being asked. Reasonable adjustments should be made to ensure there is sufficient time to answer the questions. It may be relevant for the appropriate adult to be present if there is one.

If there is a reason to doubt a victim's capacity to consent to sharing information, a capacity assessment must be completed in line with the relevant mental capacity legislation. Consideration of using an Independent Mental Capacity Advocate (IMCA) should be made where necessary.

DVA AND CHILDREN

DVA is a significant safeguarding and child protection issue. Around 1:5 children have been exposed to DVA and it is a factor in over half of all Serious Case Reviews. Nearly three-quarters of children with a child protection plan nationally live in households where DVA occurs.

The Domestic Abuse Act (2021) recognises children living with DVA as a matter of concern and outlines children are impacted by DVA even when they have not been a direct witness of the abuse. Where it is known a child is living with DVA, it is important to assess the risk of harm to the mother and her children and to consider the need to make a referral to children's social care.

DVA AND THE LGBTQ+ COMMUNITY

Research into the prevalence of DVA within LGBTQ+ relationships shows that prevalence rates are equal, or at a higher rate, compared to non-LGBTQ+ couples. As such, the definition of DVA specifically includes reference to same-sex couples to recognise DVA does occur in LGBTQ+

| SCENARIO 14.3 | DVA |

You are asked to see a 37-year-old female who has been arrested for domestic assault against her partner. She reports she is the victim and that her partner is abusive and controls her. Today, because she reacted back, he 'got me arrested'. She lives with her partner and two children, aged 9 and 6 years old. She denies alcohol but reports smoking cannabis at night (when the children are asleep).

1. *Describe the safeguarding concerns outlined above.*
   a. *Why is DVA a child safeguarding issue even if the child has not been abused?*

2. *How do you approach the discussion around making a referral to the child safeguarding team?*

3. *How do you respond to someone refusing to provide detail, such as the children's date of birth, names and schools?*

relationships, so the use of routine and selective enquiry regardless of a person's sexuality is important.

CONCLUSION

Safeguarding is the responsibility of all those working with children and adults at risk, and the information and guidance provided in this chapter provide the knowledge and skills required to confidently identify concerns, assess the impact and act appropriately. Health professionals are in an ideal position to protect the most vulnerable in society and should always consider the risks and the impact on both children and adults. If HCPs have concerns, they must act immediately, following their organisational and regional procedures and not assume someone else will share the information.

| LEARNING ACTIVITIES |

1. Write a reflection on a safeguarding concern you had and how you dealt with it. Did you make a safeguarding referral? Consider how your experiences, attitudes, values and beliefs may have influenced your decision-making. Was it the outcome you had hoped for? If not, what could you possibly do in the future?

2. Research and create a list of relevant adult and children safeguarding resources and contact details. You could create two lists, one for colleagues and one for individuals.

3. Facilitate a group discussion on how HCPs can ensure they keep children and adults at risk at the centre of any decisions you make.

RESOURCES

Online

- Making every contact count (MECC) | https://www.mecclink.co.uk

- Royal College of Nursing | Safeguarding | https://www.rcn.org.uk/library/Subject-Guides/safeguarding

- SafeLives | Dash risk checklist | https://safelives.org.uk/sites/default/files/resources/Dash%20risk%20checklist%20quick%20start%20guidance%20FINAL.pdf

Organisations

- Barnardo's | https://www.barnardos.org.uk

- NSPCC | https://www.nspcc.org.uk

- SafeLives | https://safelives.org.uk

REFERENCES

Adoption and Children Act (2002). Adoption and Children Act 2002. https://www.legislation.gov.uk/ukpga/2002/38/contents (accessed 23 January 2024).

Adult Support and Protection (Scotland) Act (2007). Adult Support and Protection (Scotland) Act 2007. https://www.legislation.gov.uk/asp/2007/10/contents (accessed 23 January 2024).

Beckett, H. (2011). 'Not a world away'. The sexual exploitation of children and young people in Northern Ireland. https://www.barnardos.org.uk/sites/default/files/2020-12/13932_not_a_world_away_full_report.pdf (accessed 23 January 2024).

Beckett, H., Homes, D., and Walker, J. (2017). Child sexual exploitation: definition and guide for professionals – extended text. https://www.researchinpractice.org.uk/media/nvfotoo0/child_sexual_exploitation_practice_tool_2017_open_access.pdf (accessed 23 January 2024).

Care Act (2014). Care Act 2014. https://www.legislation.gov.uk/ukpga/2014/23/contents/enacted (accessed 23 January 2024).

Children Act (1989). Children Act 1989. https://www.legislation.gov.uk/ukpga/1989/41/contents (accessed 15 August 2024).

Children (Scotland) Act (1995). Children (Scotland) Act 1995. https://www.legislation.gov.uk/ukpga/1995/36/contents (accessed 23 January 2024).

Children's Hearings (Scotland) Act (2011). Children's Hearings (Scotland) Act 2011. https://www.legislation.gov.uk/asp/2011/1/contents (accessed 23 January 2024).

Data Protection Act (2018). Data Protection Act 2018. https://www.legislation.gov.uk/ukpga/2018/12/contents/enacted

Domestic Abuse Act (2021). Domestic Abuse Act 2021. https://www.legislation.gov.uk/ukpga/2021/17/contents/enacted (accessed 23 January 2024).

HM Government (2018). Information sharing; advice for practitioners providing safeguarding services to children, young people, parents and carers. https://assets.publishing.service.gov.uk/media/623c57d28fa8f540eea34c27/Information_sharing_advice_practitioners_safeguarding_services.pdf (accessed 23 January 2024).

HM Government (2023). Working together to safeguard children 2023. https://assets.publishing.service.gov.uk/media/65803fe31c0c2a000d18cf40/Working_together_to_safeguard_children_2023_-_statutory_guidance.pdf (accessed 23 January 2024).

Home Office (2013). Circular 003/2013: new government domestic violence and abuse definition. https://www.gov.uk/government/publications/new-government-domestic-violence-and-abuse-definition/circular-0032013-new-government-domestic-violence-and-abuse-definition (accessed 23 January 2024).

Home Office (2021). Tackling violence against women and girls strategy (accessible version). https://www.gov.uk/government/publications/tackling-violence-against-women-and-girls-strategy/tackling-violence-against-women-and-girls-strategy (accessed 23 January 2024).

Home Office (2022). Domestic abuse: statutory guidance. https://assets.publishing.service.gov.uk/media/62c6df068fa8f54e855dfe31/Domestic_Abuse_Act_2021_Statutory_Guidance.pdf (accessed 23 January 2024).

Home Office (2023). Criminal exploitation of children and vulnerable adults: county lines. https://www.gov.uk/government/publications/criminal-exploitation-of-children-and-vulnerable-adults-county-lines/criminal-exploitation-of-children-and-vulnerable-adults-county-lines (accessed 23 January 2024).

Human Rights Act (1998). Human Rights Act 1998. https://www.legislation.gov.uk/ukpga/1998/42/contents (accessed 23 January 2024).

NSPCC (2018). Procedures for what to do if you have a concern about a child. https://www.nspcc.org.uk/globalassets/documents/volunteering/essential-resources-for-volunteers/what-to-do-if-you-have-a-concern-about-a-child-for-those-who-do-work-directly-with-children-and-adults-at-risk-v1.pdf (accessed 23 January 2024).

Social Services and Well-being (Wales) Act (2014). Social Services and Well-being (Wales) Act 2014. https://www.legislation.gov.uk/anaw/2014/4/contents (accessed 23 January 2024).

Taylor, J., Stalker, K., and Stewart, A. (2015). Disabled children and the child protection system: a cause for concern. *Child Abuse Review* 25 (1): 60–73.

The Children (Northern Ireland) Order (1995). The children (Northern Ireland) order 1995. https://www.legislation.gov.uk/nisi/1995/755/contents/made (accessed 15 August 2024).

The Safeguarding Vulnerable Groups (Northern Ireland) Order (2007). The safeguarding vulnerable groups (Northern Ireland) order 2007. https://www.legislation.gov.uk/nisi/2007/1351/contents (accessed 23 January 2024).

The United Nations Convention on the Rights of the Child (1998). Convention on the rights of the child. https://www.unicef.org.uk/rights-respecting-schools/wp-content/uploads/sites/4/2017/01/UNCRC-in-full.pdf (accessed 23 January 2024).

UK Caldicott Guardian Council. (2018). A manual for Caldicott guardians. https://assets.publishing.service.gov.uk/government/uploads/system/uploads/attachment_data/file/581213/cgmanual.pdf (accessed 24 January 2024).

FURTHER READING

Barnardo's | Language matters | https://cms.barnardos.org.uk/sites/default/files/2023-04/Language_Mattters_2022_review.pdf

NSPCC | Definition and signs of child abuse | https://learning.nspcc.org.uk/media/1188/definitions-signs-child-abuse.pdf

Royal College of Nursing | Safeguarding children and young people – Every nurse's responsibility | https://www.rcn.org.uk/Professional-Development/publications/safeguarding-children-and-young-people-every-nurses-responsibility-uk-pub-009-507

CHAPTER 15

Writing Statements and Giving Evidence

Matthew Peel

Leeds Community Healthcare NHS Trust, Leeds, UK & UK Association of Forensic Nurses and Paramedics

---

AIM

This chapter explores the United Kingdom's (UK) criminal court system, emphasising the vital role of healthcare professionals in custody. By delving into the different witness types, the art of statement writing, and the importance of peer review, it aims to provide readers with the tools and knowledge to navigate the legal landscape confidently and precisely.

LEARNING OUTCOMES

After reading this chapter, you will be able to:

- Understanding the UK's criminal court system, differentiating between various courts and their functions and the roles of different types of witnesses

- Prepare clear and effective witness statements, recognising the importance of peer review in ensuring accuracy, credibility and professionalism

- Understand the duties, ethical considerations, and challenges faced by HCPs writing statements and giving evidence in court

SELF-ASSESSMENT

1. Describe the hierarchical structure of the UK's criminal court system and explain the significance of case law.

2. Define and differentiate between the three types of witnesses: Witness of Fact, Professional Witness, and Expert Witness. Provide examples of situations where each type of witness would be relevant.

3. Discuss the ethical considerations and challenges HCPs face when writing statements and giving evidence in court.

INTRODUCTION

This chapter outlines a comprehensive guide for HCPs in custody within the UK's complex criminal justice system. It aims to equip HCPs with the knowledge and skills to navigate legal procedures effectively. From understanding the hierarchical structure of the UK's courts to the roles and responsibilities of different types of witnesses, the chapter offers valuable insights. It also emphasises the critical role of well-prepared statements and the importance of peer review in ensuring the integrity and credibility of evidence presented in court. While this chapter does not specifically address the Coroner's Court (or Fatal Accident Inquiry in Scotland), the principles contained within apply.

Police Custody Healthcare for Nurses and Paramedics, First Edition. Edited by Matthew Peel, Jennie Smith, Vanessa Webb, and Margaret Bannerman.
© 2025 John Wiley & Sons Ltd. Published 2025 by John Wiley & Sons Ltd.
Companion website: www.wiley.com/go/policecustodyhealthcare

OVERVIEW OF THE CRIMINAL COURT SYSTEMS

The UK's criminal court system differs between the devolved nations, see Figure 15.1. Courts are hierarchical, meaning lower courts follow the decisions of higher courts, a system known as case law. The severity of the offence will determine where a case is heard, with less serious offences heard in the lower courts and more serious offences heard in the higher courts. The UK's Supreme Court is the highest court, which only hears appeals on points of law in cases of major public importance.

At court, individuals plead 'guilty' or 'not guilty'. Guilty pleas move to sentencing, with not-guilty pleas proceeding to trial. Cases heard before a court in England, Wales and Northern Ireland have two verdicts, 'guilty' and 'not guilty'. In Scotland, a third option currently exists, 'not proven'. Meaning there was not enough evidence to convict. In practical terms, both 'not proven' and 'not guilty', result in the accused being released without a conviction. However, 'not proven' can carry a social stigma.

The criminal courts are adversarial. This is a fundamental feature of the UK criminal justice system and is characterised by a two-sided structure in which legal representatives for the prosecution and the defence present their cases to an impartial judge and jury. Both sides present evidence and legal arguments. This includes questioning their own witnesses and cross-examining the opposition's witnesses.

This system is rooted in the belief that truth can best be discovered through the contest of opposing views.

TYPES OF COURT

England, Wales and Northern Ireland

Across England, Wales and Northern Ireland, there is a very similar court system, where a case will be heard depending on the offence type (see Box 15.1).

Magistrates' Court Almost all criminal court cases start and complete in the Magistrates' Court. However, more serious offences are passed up to the Crown Court for either sentencing (if guilty) or for trial.

There are no juries in Magistrates' Courts. Instead, cases are heard before several (typically three, but maybe two) Magistrates, or a District Judge. Magistrates are part-time volunteers trained to deal with the least serious cases, such as minor thefts, criminal damage, public disorder and motoring offences. District Judges are employed judiciary members who hear more serious and complex cases in Magistrates' Courts.

The Magistrates' Court has lesser sentencing powers than the higher courts. Depending on the offence, they can impose unlimited fines, bans, community orders and up to 12 months imprisonment (Sentencing Council 2023).

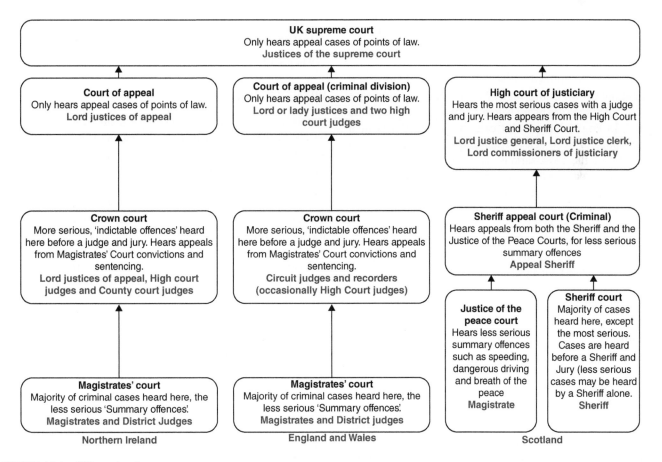

FIGURE 15.1 UK court system.

BOX 15.1	TYPES OF CRIMINAL CASES
Summary offences	Less serious offences, such as motoring offences and minor assaults, where the defendant is not usually entitled to trial by jury. These cases are completed in the Magistrates' Court.
Either-way offences	More serious offences such as theft and handling stolen goods, which can be heard by either Magistrates or a judge and jury at the Crown Court. Magistrates can decide to refer a case to the Crown Court for greater sentencing (if found guilty).
Indictable-only offences	Most serious offences such as murder, rape and robbery which must be heard at a Crown Court. Magistrates' Court will consider bail before referring the case to the Crown Court.

Youth Court Youth Courts are for children and young people aged 10–17 years old and work like a Magistrates' Court; cases are heard before several Magistrates or a District Judge without a jury. Unlike Magistrates' Court, hearings are not open to the public (except with permission) and individuals are referred to by name. Youth Courts have additional sentencing options such as referral orders, youth rehabilitation orders, along with detention and treatment orders.

Crown Court As outlined earlier, more serious offences are heard at the Crown Court (indictable or either-way offences). Crown Court cases are heard before 12 members of the public (a jury). In England and Wales, cases are presided over by a Circuit Judge or Recorder. A High Court Judge may preside over some of the most serious cases. In Northern Ireland, cases are presided over by a County Court Judge, or in some of the most serious cases, a High Court Judge. Crown Courts have greater sentencing powers, including a whole life order (Sentencing Council 2023).

In addition to the more serious offences and cases passed up from the Magistrates' Court, the Crown Court will hear appeals against a magistrates' conviction or sentencing.

Court of Appeal Hears appeals from the Crown Court.

Scotland

There are some distinct differences in the Scottish Court system.

Justice of the Peace Court Justice of the Peace Courts are unique to Scotland's criminal justice system. A Justice of the Peace is similar to a Magistrate and sits alone, or as a panel and hears the least serious cases, such as speeding, careless driving and breaches of the peace. The Court is limited to imposing a maximum fine of up to £2500 or 60 days imprisonment.

Sheriff Court The Sheriff's Court deals with more serious criminal cases, such as theft, assault and drug possession. Cases are heard before a Sheriff, similar to a Judge. Cases may be heard before a Sheriff alone. However, in these circumstances, the Sheriff's sentencing powers are limited to a £10,000 fine or 12-month imprisonment (Crown Office & Procurator Fiscal Service 2023). In cases heard before a jury, a Sheriff can impose an unlimited fine or up to five years imprisonment. Cases heard in the Sheriff's Court can be passed to the High Court for greater sentencing if necessary.

Sheriff Appeal Court The Court hears appeals against less serious criminal proceedings from both the Sheriff and the Justice of the Peace Courts. Appeals against conviction are heard by three appeal Sheriffs and appeals against sentencing are heard by two appeal Sheriffs.

High Court of Justiciary The High Court of Justiciary is both a trial court and a court of appeal. Criminal cases heard at the High Court of Justiciary include the most serious, such as murder, rape, armed robbery, drug trafficking and child sexual offences. The High Court of Justiciary has greater sentencing powers, up to life imprisonment.

WITNESSES

There are three types of witnesses.

WITNESS OF FACT

Witnesses of Fact, commonly referred to as an 'ordinary Witness' or 'Lay Witness', provide evidence based on their own personal knowledge or observations. They can only speak about what they have directly seen, heard or experienced. Unlike Expert Witnesses, they aren't permitted to give opinions, only facts.

The Witness of Fact role remains consistent throughout the United Kingdom. However, the specific procedures and legislative underpinnings vary, reflecting the unique legal traditions and systems in place in England and Wales, Scotland and Northern Ireland. Across all jurisdictions, the testimony of a Witness of Fact plays a crucial role in establishing the narrative of events.

PROFESSIONAL WITNESS

Custody HCPs attending court because of their professional duties will do so as a Professional Witness. While the term 'Professional Witness' is not defined in law, it refers to individuals who, due to their profession,[1] find themselves giving

---

[1] Medical professional (including nurse or paramedics), accountant, dentist or veterinary surgeon.

evidence in court. Professional Witnesses testify about their first-hand experiences and observations during their professional duties. The Professional Witness is a Witness of Fact, so they can only speak about what they have directly seen, heard, or experienced. Some limited opinion is allowed; for example HCPs can state it was their opinion an individual was fit to interview or there was a condition that might be due to drugs. HCPs, who understand the evidence base, may be able to provide an opinion of an injury type (i.e. bruise, abrasion or laceration). However, they should not give an opinion about what caused the injury, that is reserved for the Expert Witness. There is, however, no clear boundary where a Professional Witness becomes an Expert, leading to a lack of consistency in practice. Finally, the court can deem a Professional Witness an Expert to give an opinion based on their knowledge and experiences (Forensic Science Regulator 2020).

EXPERT WITNESS

Expert Witnesses play an important role in helping courts understand technical, scientific or specialised evidence that falls outside the scope of everyday knowledge. Unlike other witnesses, Expert Witnesses can provide an opinion based on their specialised knowledge, experience and training, usually after reviewing the full case bundle.

An Expert Witness's field of expertise must be relevant to the case and have a proven track record in their field, as their credentials, including education, publications and previous testimonies, might be examined.

Expert Witnesses may be instructed by either (or both) the prosecution or defence. However, their primary duty is to the court, not the party instructing them. Expert Witnesses provide unbiased, impartial and independent evidence to assist the court in the form of reports and oral evidence.

There is an increasing need for custody HCPs to develop themselves as Expert Witnesses. The UK Association of Forensic Nurses and Paramedics is developing an 'Expert Academy'. There are several key areas in custody HCPs can develop expertise:

- Interpretation of injuries
- Use of force, restraint and restraint-related deaths
- Road traffic legislation

SCENARIO 15.1 Witness type

You submitted a Statement after documenting some injuries several weeks ago. The prosecution team has come back asking for you to comment on what caused the bruise to the left arm.

1. *How do you respond to this request?*

STATEMENTS

Statements are usually requested by an Investigating Officer. Depending on the local agreement, officers may approach HCPs directly or via a single point of contact. Healthcare organisations and police forces should have a data-sharing agreement that includes the secure digital delivery of statements (i.e. secure email addresses). Completed statements should be retained by the HCP and submitted as a portable document file (PDF).

Witness Statements are factual reports, written in a particular format, relating to a specific event. Usually, they follow some forensic or medio-legal examination such as samples, body mapping or fitness to interview. Across England and Wales, the Criminal Justice Act 1967 (section 9) allows courts to accept statements without oral evidence, where it is accepted by both the prosecution and defence. Similar rules apply in Northern Ireland[2] and Scotland.[3]

Statements should be typed and well presented on a specific template provided by the police, see Box 15.2. Statements reflect the HCP's quality, attention to detail and thoroughness. Poorly written, grammatical errors or illogical format may give the impression of poor quality, which may introduce doubt into the integrity of their evidence. The need for well-prepared and presented statements is obvious beyond the need to maintain a professional impression. They aid investigations and assist courts in reaching a verdict. It has often been said a good statement avoids the need to attend court. While it is true a poor statement is more likely to require the HCP to attend court, a good statement, well detailed and presented, giving the impression of a high-quality assessment, may also be called to court, as the high-quality evidence may boost the case.

Peer Review

There are several benefits to peer reviewing statements before submission for the HCP, justice and the forensic healthcare organisations (see Box 15.3). Peer review may involve simple grammar and spelling checks, or a more detailed review of the contemporaneous notes to ensure accuracy and objectivity. A peer, typically another experienced forensic HCP, is chosen to review the statement (they should not have had any direct or indirect involvement in the case to maintain impartiality). During the review, the peer assesses the statement for clarity, accuracy and completeness. They ensure the statement remains unbiased and is rooted solely in objective findings and observations. The reviewer also checks for potential omissions or inconsistencies. Although this is considered best practice, coaching a witness is not allowed in the legal system and each area has mechanisms to consider how this is applied.

---

[2] The Criminal Evidence (Northern Ireland) Order 1988.
[3] Criminal Justice and Licensing (Scotland) Act 2010.

BOX 15.2	WRITING A WITNESS STATEMENT

Style

- Typed using a clear font, size 12
- Signed and dated by the HCP on all pages
- Appropriate use headings
- One topic per paragraph
- Chronological order
- Avoid abbreviations (or state in full at first use)
- Avoid medical terminology (or explain in brackets)

Contents

- HCP's name
- HCP's up-to-date qualifications and professional registration details
- HCP's broader clinical experience
- HCP's experience in forensic healthcare
- Date, start and end time of examination
- Who requested the examination and the full name and pin number of the police officer/staff member requesting the examination
- Any information given to the clinician by the police officer/police staff member
- State there are healthcare notes from which the Statement is made.
- Provide availability to act as a witness for at least the following 6 months (separate form).

BOX 15.3	BENEFITS OF PEER-REVIEW

Benefits for the HCP:

1. **Professional development**: Peer review provides an opportunity for learning and professional growth, as HCPs can gain insights into best practices and potential areas for improvement

2. **Increased confidence**: Knowing that their work has been scrutinised by peers can boost the confidence of HCPs when writing future statements or providing oral testimony in court

Benefits for the justice system:

3. **Quality assurance**: The review process acts as a quality control mechanism, ensuring that the statements meet certain standards before being submitted

4. **Reduced risk of errors**: The likelihood of factual errors or omissions that could affect the outcome of a case is minimised

5. **Streamlined proceedings**: Courts can proceed more efficiently when they can rely on the quality and accuracy of the statements, potentially speeding up the judicial process

Benefits for the organisation:

6. **Reputation management**: Organisations that implement rigorous peer-review processes are likely to be viewed as more credible and reliable, which can enhance their reputation

7. **Standardisation**: Peer review helps maintain a consistent standard of reporting across the organisation, making it easier to manage quality

Following review, the peer provides feedback, including suggestions, revisions, corrections, clarifications or additional information the HCP should consider incorporating. Once any necessary revisions are made, the statement is ready for submission. Documenting the entire peer-review process, including feedback and revisions, is important and would form part of the undisclosed materials, although this does not necessarily need to be submitted with the Statement (Faculty of Forensic & Legal Medicine 2021).

STATEMENT STRUCTURE AND CONTENT

Statements should be structured using headings, following a logical sequence, being concise and relevant, see Box 15.4. Avoid including unnecessary extraneous details. Headings should be changed depending on the individual circumstances.

The author should be identified by name and repeated on each page. Each page is numbered sequentially, with footer space for the author's and a witness's signature. The date of birth need only be stated if not 18 years old; otherwise, 'over 18 years' is sufficient. Finally, the witness's occupation is included.

Before the main body of the statement, the perjury clause must be signed and dated. Declaring what is stated is truthful. A signed statement knowingly dishonest amounts to perjury and can lead to imprisonment.

Introduction

Outline the basis for the statement, who requested it and what it relates to. Where applicable, include a statement indicating the statement is based on your contemporaneous notes.

| BOX 15.4 | EXAMPLE OF A STATEMENT (ENGLAND AND WALES HEADER) |

WITNESS STATEMENT
Criminal Procedure Rules, r 16.2; Criminal Justice Act 1967, s. 9

Statement of: Nora Tracewell

                 RN (Adult), BSc (Hons)

Age: Over 18 years

Occupation: Custody Healthcare Professional (Nurse)

This Statement (consisting of one page, each signed by me) is true to the best of my knowledge and belief and I make it knowing that if it is tendered in evidence, I shall be liable to prosecution if I have wilfully stated in it anything that I know to be false or do not believe to be true.

Date: 25/11/2024

Signature:

1. Introduction

1.1 This is a Professional Witness Statement requested by Detective Constable Ethan FOREN (DC5590F) of Westshire Constabulary. Regarding my examination of Rigor HEALMAN on 28 August 2024.

1.2 This Statement is made using the contemporaneous notes made at the time.

2. Author

2.1 My name is Nora TRACEWELL. I am a Registered Nurse (Adult), Registration Number: 12A3456B. I qualified in 2012 with a BSc (Hons) Nursing Studies (Adult) and have undertaken further academic study and work-based training. I have 6 years of experience as a nurse in acute and emergency settings. I am currently employed by Forentech Health Solutions as a Custody Healthcare Practitioner. Forentech Health Solutions provides custody healthcare to Westshire Constabulary. I have worked continuously in custody healthcare since May 2018.

2.2 As a Custody Healthcare Practitioner, I am required to assess fitness to detain and interview. Conduct mental health assessments and suicide risk. I also undertake detailed examinations and documentation of injuries. Finally, I am sometimes required to take forensic samples.

3. Background

3.1 HEALMAN was referred to me by DC FOREN (DC5590F) for a fitness-to-interview assessment. DC FOREN (DC5590F) advised me HEALMAN was arrested for an allegation of assault.

3.2 On 21 August 2024 at 10:50, while on duty at Holmesville Custody suite, I attended Rigor HEALMAN, aged 46 years (DOB: 13/12/1977), custody reference: X123Y456Z, in the medical room. HEALMAN was unaccompanied.

3.3 I concluded the assessment at 11:45.

4. Consent

4.1 I introduced myself to HEALMAN and explained my role. I ensured he understood what was explained to him and he provided written consent for a clinical assessment and if subsequently requested, a Statement.

5. History

5.1 HEALMAN stated he had no significant past medical history or current medication.

6. Examination

6.1 HEALMAN was alert (awake) and orientated (an awareness of self, place, time and situation). HEALMAN walked to the medical room independently with a steady gait. HEALMAN remained seated throughout and was cooperative. His speech was normal and conversations were logical and coherent. He was appropriately dressed. He made eye contact and did not appear distracted. There was no evidence of any intoxication or withdrawal syndrome.

7. Treatment and advice

7.1 No treatment or advice was given.

8. Recommendations

8.1 I advised the custody officer HEALMAN was fit to detain and interview and recommended 30-minute checks at Level 1.

9. Conclusion

9.1 I was asked to assess HEALMAN's fitness for interview. I found HEALMAN fit to interview. I had no further contact with HEALMAN.

_____END OF STATEMENT_____

Correspondence address;

c/o Forentech Health Solutions,

123 Helix Drive, Geneton

Author

HCPs should outline their name, professional background (i.e. nurse or paramedic), registration details and current role (including a brief summary). Include any relevant experience and qualifications. However, do not provide a full curriculum vitae. Remain concise and relevant.

Background

Introduce the individual's full name, date of birth and unique identifiers such as custody reference number. Indicate the date, time, and specific location of the examination and the reason for examination or contact. Indicate the details of others present, such as an appropriate adult, police officer or colleague. If background information or history was provided and relevant to the assessment or decision-making, including who provided the information or history, it may be appropriate to include the details.

Consent

Demonstrate consent was sought for treatment, examination, sample and statement. There is no need to routinely provide evidence (e.g. signed consent forms).

History

Note any relevant past medical history, mental health history, drug history, allergies and social history (including drugs and alcohol history). As always, only relevant information should be shared. This will depend on the individual circumstances of the case. For example, it would not be relevant to routinely note evidence of immunisations or blood tests. However, if someone claims needle phobia, these may be useful to the court. Where extraneous, irrelevant details are not included, close the paragraph stating, 'Further irrelevant information is available'.

Examination

Provide a concise summary of any relevant positive and negative assessment findings. Start with a general overview of their presentation, followed by any relevant specific areas examined. Any injuries should be documented as outlined in Chapter 13 – Evidence Collection (Documenting injuries and samples). If submitting body maps with the statement, these must be referred to within the statement's body.

If an individual made a significant comment during the assessment, these could be included in a statement. For example, 'I didn't mean to kill her'. Such comments should be noted verbatim using speech marks.

Forensic Samples (If Appropriate)

Any forensic samples taken should be listed with their unique exhibit number and description. Note if samples were taken per the recommendations or indicate any deviations and a rationale. Finally, demonstrate the continuity of the chain of evidence by indicating when and to whom samples were handed.

BOX 15.5	EXAMPLE STATEMENT EXCERPT FOR A BLOOD SAMPLE

7. Road traffic procedure.

   7.1 Using the 'RTA Blood Sampling Kit' (BN:AB34, Exp: 01/2026) I demonstrated to HEALMAN the seal was intact. I opened the kit, breaking seal no.: J123456789, in the presence of HEALMAN.

   7.2 At 10:15, on the 21 September 2024, I took 9 ml of blood from HEALMAN. The sample was obtained on the first attempt and there were no complications.

   7.3 The sample was divided into two vials, which were agitated by myself for thirty seconds. The samples were labelled (WAP01234567) and sealed in containers at 10:19. Both samples were handed to PC Miles SPEEDON (RTP6574) at 10:20. HEALMAN was offered a sample by the officer.

   7.4 PC SPEEDON explained to HEALMAN the option of having their sample tested independently of the police.

   7.5 A HO/RT5 was completed and handed to the officer.

Road Traffic Procedures (If Appropriate)

If the statement pertains to a road traffic procedure and sample taking, it is important to include all the relevant details, including times. Box 15.5 outlines an approach to documenting the taking of road traffic samples (in addition to the detail in Box 15.4).

Treatment and Advice (If Appropriate)

If appropriate, outline the details of any treatment and advice provided.

Recommendations

Outline any recommendations provided to the police, such as fitness to detain and interview and the need for an appropriate adult.

Conclusion

Provide a summary of the statement and conclude by indicating any further contact or interaction with the named patient.

ATTENDING COURT

HCPs may receive notice to attend court informally, such as by an officer or more formally by summons. A summons compels attendance with failure, liable for a fine, imprisonment or both.

BEFORE COURT

Providing evidence in court is stressful. Preparation is key, review any notes, statements or reports concerning the case

BOX 15.6	PROHIBITED ITEMS

- Blades (including scissors, knives and razors)
- Other sharp articles (i.e. knitting needles and darts)
- Glass
- Metal cutlery
- Syringes (unless accompanied with a prescription)
- Toy or imitation guns
- Tools (i.e. screwdrivers, hammers and nails)
- Ropes and chains
- Alcohol liquids (including oils, perfumes, lighter refills and cleaning products)
- Full-length umbrellas
- Crash helmets

Source: UK Government (2021)/with permission of Crown.

and identify any apparent strengths or weaknesses. Bring all necessary documentation to the court, such as your statement and other relevant material. Witnesses are usually permitted to review their notes. However, try to avoid bulky or unnecessary items.

DRESS

Dress comfortably but professionally, demonstrating your respect to the court and the seriousness of the matters being considered.

ARRIVING AT COURT

Punctuality is essential. Usually, a specific time is given when attendance is required. Arrive early, as the airport-style security measures may cause delays, see Box 15.6 for a list of prohibited items. Attention should be paid to the location of the court, as not all cases are tried locally. If unfamiliar with the court, it is wise to rehearse the journey. Where parking requires upfront payment, pay sufficient in case of delays. Finally, ensure phones or similar devices are turned off or set to silent.

Witnesses cannot observe proceedings before giving evidence. On arrival, HCPs should make themselves known to the Witness Care service to register attendance, who can also help with any queries and provide a waiting area. If unfamiliar with court layout, you may request to visit an empty court to familiarise yourself (if available).

ORAL EVIDENCE

Providing oral evidence in court can cause anxiety, especially if unfamiliar. When in the witness box, adopt a somewhat detached, dignified and professional appearance. Remaining composed despite what may feel like provoking, or even aggressive questioning. Reassuringly, it is rare for counsel to use intimidating tactics as often seen on TV, with such behaviour quickly curtailed by the court.

While in the witness box, HCPs should pay particular attention to their speech. Speak at a measured pace; conscious anxiety may cause accelerated speech. Often, the Judge or Magistrate will take notes whilst speaking, this can be a good indicator of the speed of your speech is appropriate. Do not shout, but speak clearly to be heard throughout the court. See Box 15.7 for tips to do and avoid and Box 15.8 for addressing the court.

Courts are unlike any normal interaction. While HCPs are asked questions by a legal advocate, their answers are addressed to the judge (or sheriff), jury or magistrate. Defying the normal rule of conversation. To overcome the instinct to respond to the individual asking the question, HCPs should stand with their feet facing the judge, jury or magistrate.

Always allow questions to be asked in full before replying, never assume a question and interrupt. Once asked, take a second to consider the question and frame a response. Respond only to the question asked. Responses will vary; some will simply rely on a 'Yes' or 'No'. Others may require a more in-depth discussion and explanation. Avoid jargon or technical words.

HCPs may have omitted confidential material from a statement because the individual did not consent or they felt it was unnecessary. However, they may be asked about

BOX 15.7	DO'S AND DON'TS

Do	Don't
• Act professional	• Be afraid to say 'I do not know'
• Try to appear confident	• Get angry
• Take a deep breath before answering	• Take questions personally
• Speak slowly and clearly, directing answers towards the Judge, Jury or Magistrate	• Be tempted to appear 'all-knowing'
	• Use sarcasm
• Consider all questions before answering	• Use humour
• Ask for any unclear or poorly worded question to be repeated	• Provide emotional responses

BOX 15.8 ADDRESSING THE COURT

Magistrates' Court

- Magistrate* – 'Sir' or 'Madame'
- District Judge – 'Sir' or 'Madame'

Crown Court

- High Court Judge – 'My Lord' or 'My Lady'
- Circuit Judge - 'Your Honour'
- Recorders – 'Your Honor', 'His Honor' or 'Her Honour'

Sheriff Court (Scotland)

- Sheriff – 'My Lord' or 'My Lady'

Justice of the Peace Court (Scotland)

- Justice of the peace – 'Your Honour'

High Court

- High Court Judges – 'My Lord' or 'My Lady'

*In Northern Ireland, address Magistrates as 'Your Worship'.

this confidential material while giving evidence. In such cases, the HCP should advise the judge or similar, they do not have permission to share this information. The judge or similar, will direct the HCP on whether to answer or not (Medical Defence Union 2021). Sharing confidential material after being directed by the court if permitted. Indeed, HCPs refusing to follow the court's direction may find themselves in contempt of court, punishable with a fine, imprisonment or both (UK Government 2022).

Declaration of Truth

Before entering the witness box, HCPs will be asked how they wish to declare truth by oath or affirmation. Once in the witness box, the HCP will read aloud their declaration. When making the declaration, nurses should speak clearly and look towards the magistrate, judge (or sheriff) or jury.

Evidence in Chief

Following the declaration, HCPs will be taken through their evidence. First, being led to state their name, qualifications, experience and role. This helps demonstrate the significance and relevance of the evidence and provides a gentle introduction to speaking in court. Evidence in chief is relatively straightforward; HCPs are typically taken through their written statement and asked if it is correct. HCPs may be asked to provide additional comments or explain how

decisions or conclusions were reached. Evidence in chief, indeed all oral evidence, is not a memory test. If necessary, ask the court to refer to any notes.

It is good practice to prepare yourself by writing down and rehearsing, saying who you are, your professional qualifications, affiliations, pre- and post-nominal titles, how long you have been in practice and broadly how many cases you have seen.

Cross-examination

Following the evidence in chief, the opposing council (typically the defence) can cross-examine. Cross-examination allows the opposing council to test the evidence for weaknesses and highlight these to the court, including trying to discredit their testimony or highlight inconsistencies. Cross-examination is likely to be the most challenging aspect of giving evidence. As outlined earlier, prepare by reviewing the statement for weaknesses and likely opportunities for cross-examination.

Re-examination

After the cross-examination, the initial council can re-examine the HCP. However, this re-examination should only focus on addressing specific points raised during the cross-examination.

SCENARIO 15.2 Giving evidence

You are giving evidence at the Magistrate's Court in relation to a drug driving offence. You have given your evidence in chief and are being cross-examined. The defence is suggesting you, along with the police, bullied and intimidated the defendant into providing a blood sample and that he did not freely consent.

1. *How do you react to this line of questioning?*
2. *How do you respond to this line of questioning?*

CONCLUSION

The chapter provides a thorough understanding of the legal landscape that HCPs in police custody settings must navigate. It underscores the importance of being well-prepared, not just in the clinical aspects of the role but also in the legal responsibilities that come with it. The guidance on writing statements and the benefits of peer review serves as practical tools for HCPs to enhance their professional development and contribute effectively to the justice system.

LEARNING ACTIVITIES

1. Engage in role-playing activities where you take on the role of Professional Witness. Present evidence or a statement in a mock Court setting. Afterwards, reflect on the challenges and importance of clarity, accuracy and impartiality. Ask peers for feedback on your performance.

2. Review your witness statements. Identify strengths, weaknesses, and areas of potential cross-examination. Reflect on the importance of peer review in ensuring the integrity and credibility of evidence presented in court.

3. Visit a local court and observe a trial or hearing, ideally where a colleague gives evidence. Take notes on the roles of different witnesses, the presentation of evidence and the overall court proceedings. Reflect on the experience and the importance of HCPs understanding the legal landscape.

RESOURCES

Online

- Faculty of Forensic and Legal Medicine | Forensic clinicians as witness in criminal proceedings | https://fflm.ac.uk/wp-content/uploads/2020/12/Forensic-clinicians-as-witnesses-in-criminal-proceedings-Prof-K-Rix-Oct-2020.pdf

- Medical Defence Union | Acting as a Professional Witness | https://www.themdu.com/guidance-and-advice/guides/acting-as-a-professional-witness

- Royal College of Nursing | Statements: how to write them | https://www.rcn.org.uk/Get-Help/RCN-advice/statements

Organisations

- Bond Solon | https://www.bondsolon.com

- Courts and Tribunals Judiciary (England and Wales) | https://www.judiciary.uk

- Department of Justice (Northern Ireland) | Courts and Tribunals - https://www.justice-ni.gov.uk/topics/courts-and-tribunals

- Scottish Courts and Tribunals | https://www.scotcourts.gov.uk

REFERENCES

Criminal Justice Act (1967). Criminal Justice Act 1967. https://www.legislation.gov.uk/ukpga/1967/80/section/9 (accessed 06 October 2023).

Crown Office & Procurator Fiscal Service (2023). The justice process. https://www.copfs.gov.uk/the-justice-process/scotland-s-criminal-justice-system/#:~:text=Sheriff%20courts&text=In%20a%20solemn%20case%2C%20the,maximum%20fine%20of%20£10%2C000 (accessed 06 October 2023).

Faculty of Forensic & Legal Medicine (2021). Peer review in sexual offences. https://fflm.ac.uk/wp-content/uploads/2021/05/Peer-review-in-sexual-offences-Dr-C-White-April-2021.pdf (accessed 05 December 2023).

Forensic Science Regulator (2020). DNA anti-contamination: forensic medical examination in sexual assault referral centres and custodial facilities. https://www.gov.uk/government/publications/sexual-assault-referral-centres-and-custodial-facilities-dna-anti-contamination (accessed 11 December 2023).

Medical Defence Union (2021). Disclosure without consent. https://www.themdu.com/guidance-and-advice/guides/disclosure-without-consent (accessed 21 April 2022).

Sentencing Council (2023). Going to court. https://www.sentencingcouncil.org.uk/going-to-court/#step1 (accessed 16 August 2024).

UK Government (2021). Going through security at a court or tribunal building. https://www.gov.uk/entering-court-or-tribunal-building (accessed 26 November 2021).

UK Government (2022). Contempt of court. https://www.gov.uk/contempt-of-court (accessed 21 April 2022).

FURTHER READING

Peel, M. (2023). Understanding the nurse's role as a professional witness. *Nursing Standard* 38: 29–34.

Special Circumstances

CHAPTER 16

Matthew Peel[1] and Thomas Bird[2]

[1] Leeds Community Healthcare NHS Trust, Leeds, UK & UK Association of Forensic Nurses and Paramedics

[2] Mitie Care and Custody Health Ltd, London, UK & UK Association of Forensic Nurses and Paramedics

AIM

This chapter will explore several special circumstances within police custody; this includes those detained for terror-related offences, pregnancy, children and those suspected of concealing drugs internally. Allowing healthcare professionals to provide appropriate care.

LEARNING OUTCOMES

Upon completion of this chapter, readers should be able to:

- Understand the terrorism legislation and the legal and procedural differences between this and Police and Criminal Evidence Act 1984 (PACE), or equivalent. Finally, HCPs should understand their responsibilities

- Understand the typical progression of pregnancy from conception to birth, along with the complications associated with pregnancies and their signs. Finally, HCPs should understand the increased risk to maternal and unborn child from substance misuse

- Understand the need to recognise all children in custody as special circumstances, with their own unique vulnerabilities and risk, such as child sexual exploitation. HCPs should have a firm understanding of the issues of consent in children

- Understand the immediate and longer-term assessment and management of individuals suspected of concealing drugs internally. Finally, HCPs should understand the associated risks and provide appropriate advice to the individual and officers

SELF-ASSESSMENT

1. List the relevant differences between the terror legislation and PACE (or equivalent).

2. What are the potential risks associated with pregnancy and substance misuse?

3. What role do HCPs have in advocating for the rights of children in custody?

4. List the different methods individuals can conceal drugs internally, and their short- and longer-term risk and complications.

INTRODUCTION

In the complex and sensitive environment of police custody, healthcare professionals (HCPs) are often confronted with special circumstances that require tailored approaches. This chapter delves into four distinct scenarios: terrorism-related detentions, pregnancies, juvenile detention and individuals suspected of concealing drugs. Each of these scenarios presents unique challenges, risks and healthcare needs, demanding a nuanced and informed response.

Terrorism-related detentions often involve heightened security measures and stress, influencing both their psychological and physical health. Pregnancies in custody require a delicate balance of care, considering both maternal and foetal health, while navigating the constraints of the custody environment. Children, due to their age and developmental stage, present distinct psychological and physical health needs that differ significantly from adults. Lastly, individuals suspected of concealing drugs pose unique medical emergencies, where timely and accurate healthcare intervention can be lifesaving. Understanding the specific healthcare requirements, legal considerations and ethical dilemmas inherent in each situation is crucial for providing appropriate and empathetic care to this vulnerable population.

TERRORISM ACT 2000

The Terrorism Act 2000 (TACT) legislation applies throughout the United Kingdom (UK), providing a unified legal framework for dealing with terrorism-related offences. Those arrested under TACT are not subject to the Police and Criminal Evidence Act 1984, Police and Criminal Evidence (Northern Ireland) Order 1989 or Criminal Justice (Scotland) Act 2016, while similar, there are some important differences (see Box 16.1). It is important to note there may be variations in how the act is implemented and enforced across the devolved nations.

The United Kingdom is a member of the Optional Protocol to the Convention against Torture (OPCAT) and the European Convention on Human Rights (ECHR) (see Box 16.2); two significant international instruments designed to protect human rights and prevent miscarriages of justice. Given the heightened security, prolonged detention and often severe nature of terrorism charges, there is a risk of harsh treatment. The OPCAT, an additional protocol to the United Nations Convention against Torture, aims to prevent torture and other cruel, inhuman or degrading treatment or punishment through the National Protective Mechanism (NPM). The NPM conduct regular, independent, unannounced and unrestricted visits to all places where persons are deprived of their liberty. This includes TACT suites. HCPs must be cognisant and attentive to any signs or reports of breaches to both OPCAT and the ECHR.

Section 41 of TACT grants police the power to arrest a person without a warrant if they reasonably suspect the individual is a terrorist, defined as a person who is or has been involved in the commission, preparation or instigation of acts of terrorism.

BOX 16.1	IMPORTANT DIFFERENCES IN TACT

Police procedures

- It is the inspectors' responsibility to review the necessity of detention.

- Detention should be reviewed every 12 hours. After the first 24 hours, reviews must be carried out by an officer of at least Superintendent rank.

- Can be detained for up to 14 days.

- A Superintendent must authorise any intimate samples.

Healthcare differences

- Individuals are subject to a medical examination in detention.

- Individuals are offered a medical examination on release.

- Visited by an HCP daily (after 96 hours but usually done routinely).

- The detention clock does <u>not</u> stop if transferred to the hospital.

- Intimate samples (except for urine) can only be taken by a registered medical practitioner (doctor).

BOX 16.2	RELEVANT ECHR ARTICLES

Article 3 – Prohibition of torture	This is particularly relevant for terrorism change for suspects, as it ensures protection against torture and inhuman or degrading treatment, regardless of the gravity of the charges against them.
Article 5 – Right to liberty and security	The ECHR safeguards the rights of individuals to fair treatment regarding arrest and detention. Under terrorism charges, where detentions can be extended, this article's provisions ensure that such detention is lawful and not arbitrary.
Article 6 – Right to a fair trial	This is crucial in the context of terrorism charges. It ensures detainees have access to a fair legal process, which is essential in cases that often involve complex legal and ethical considerations.

Terrorism is defined as the use or threat of action designed to influence the government or an international governmental organisation, or to intimidate the public to advance a political, religious, racial or ideological cause. The United Kingdom faces several terrorism threats, with a recent rise in extreme right-wing terrorism, see Box 16.3 for the current landscape in Great Britain.

BOX 16.3 TERRORIST LANDSCAPE IN GREAT BRITAIN

Categorisation of terrorism events	
• Domestic	12%
• International	77%
• Northern Ireland	5%
• Not classified	6%
Sex	
• Male	91%
Age	
• Under 18 years	5%
• 18–20 years	9%
• 21–24 years	16%
• 25–29 years	22%
• 30 years or over	49%
Nationality	
• British	60%
• African	10%
• Asian	9%
• Middle East	9%
Length of detention	
• Less than one day	37%
• 1 to less than 7 days	50%
• 7 to less than 14 days	13%
Outcome	
• Released	56%
• Charged	37%
• Other	7%

Source: Adapted from Allen et al. (2022).

TERRORISM SUITES

TACT suites are specially equipped to house suspected terrorists. The Secretary of State is responsible for designating places where terrorism suspects can be detained. Across England and Wales, there are five TACT suites that are hosted by the local police force. Scotland and Northern Ireland each have a single TACT suite. For this reason, not all HCPs will be exposed to individuals detained under TACT.

Security

As expected, the security is higher and may include a search on entry. Items such as phones and laptops may be prohibited. HCPs should be vetted to an appropriate level.

Finally, because of the heightened security risks, HCPs should maintain a degree of anonymity. This includes removing any identification (name or identity badges) and signing documents (electronically or physically) using police identifying number rather than their name.

Cells

Cells within TACT suites are designed to a different standard. They are typically larger and include moulded furniture such as desks and beds. Individuals may have access to a limited selection of movies.

INITIAL ASSESSMENT

Individuals are subject to an initial clinical assessment when detained. While the Faculty of Forensic & Legal Medicine (2023b) recommends a forensic physician with membership or fellowship undertake the initial assessment, legislation does not require this.

Fitness to Detain

The fitness to detain follows the process laid out in Chapter 3 – Fitness Assessments. However, because of the prolonged nature of detention, consideration should be given to securing and continuing all normal medication. Consider the individual's access to hygiene, exercise, privacy, sleep and diet. Because of the prolonged detention, individuals may be allowed a family or friend to visit on welfare grounds. Additionally, because of the risk of hunger strikes, take an initial weight and height. Finally, any referral to a hospital will present a security risk. If necessary, consideration should be given to remote consultations or arranging consultations within the TACT. However, this will depend on the acuity and severity of the condition.

Children detained under TACT present a special challenge, especially if detained for an extended period. HCPs should therefore apply safeguarding considerations, including considering the risk of radicalisation.

Fitness to Interview

The fitness-to-interview assessment and safeguards remain the same as in Chapter 3 – Fitness Assessments. Most terrorists involved in group activities do not have a mental illness (Ho et al. 2018). However, 43% of lone-actor terrorists have a history of mental illness, including schizophrenia, delusional disorder, antisocial personality disorders and autism spectrum disorders (Ho et al. 2018). Personality traits can influence interviews, terrorists are associated with paranoid and antisocial traits and suicide bombers are linked to dependent and avoidant or impulsive and emotionally unstable personality traits (Ho et al. 2018).

DAILY REVIEW

Daily HCP reviews following the initial assessment are mandatory after 96 hours, but typically commence immediately. Ideally, reviews should occur in the morning, assessing their ongoing fitness to detain and interview. HCPs should consider and document the individual's access to hygiene, exercise, privacy, sleep and diet. Note the presence or absence of any injuries or complaints.

SCENARIO 16.1	Terrorism detention – initial assessment

You are asked to complete an initial assessment for a 55-year-old male with type 2 diabetes and a metallic heart valve who has been arrested for engaging in the preparation of acts of terrorism. He is currently prescribed warfarin 7 mg daily and metformin 500 mg twice daily. He is currently well; the examination is unremarkable and his blood glucose is 10.9 mmol/l.

1. *Describe your approach to the fitness to detain and interview assessment.*

2. *Are they fit to be detained and interviewed?*
   a. *What are the foreseeable risks?*
   b. *Provide a care plan for the police, including a recommended level and frequency of observations with a rationale.*

3. *Outline the healthcare plan for medication, blood glucose checks and the rationale.*

4. *They are due an INR blood test in three days; outline your approach to this.*

PREGNANCY

Pregnancy is generally considered a natural, physiological process rather than an illness, see Box 16.4. However, it should be considered a special circumstance in custody, with HCPs conscious about the health and well-being of both mother and unborn child. Pregnant women in custody can often suffer a mix of mental illness, substance misuse and domestic violence and may have not sought any antenatal care.

ASSESSMENT

Pregnant women should be assessed for their fitness to detain as outlined in Chapter 3 – Fitness Assessments. HCPs should take a detailed social history and enquire about any domestic violence, child safeguarding procedures (current or past) and substance misuse. Note any previous pregnancies and births, along with any complications. Check they are registered with a midwife and receiving antinatal care, see Box 16.5.

If a woman suspects she is pregnant, she should be offered a pregnancy test. Modern pregnancy tests are very sensitive and can detect very early pregnancies. If gestational

BOX 16.4	CONCEPTION TO BIRTH

0–4 weeks	Conception and first trimester
	• Placenta begins to form
5–8 weeks	Embryonic stage
	• Heart starts beating and major organs begin to develop
	• About the size of a kidney bean
9–12 weeks	Foetus stage
	• Fingers and toes are fully formed
	• Can make a fist and open and close mouth
13–16 weeks	Second trimester
	• May start to suck its thumb
	• Mum may feel movements
17–20 weeks	• Growing rapidly
	• Movements more noticeable
	• Can hear external noises
21–24 weeks	• Viable outside of the womb (with intensive medical support)
	• Lungs not yet fully mature
25–28 weeks	Third trimester (28 weeks)
	• Brain rapidly developing
	• Eyes opening and close
	• Now sleeps and wakes regularly
29–32 weeks	• Gains weight and body fat
	• Able to regulate own temperature
33–36 weeks	• The lungs are nearly fully mature
	• The foetus moves into a head-down position (in preparation for birth)
37–40 weeks	Full-term
	• Considered full-term at 37 weeks
	• Continues to gain weight
Around 40 weeks	Birth

BOX 16.5	ROUTINE ANTENATAL CARE

Weeks	
0	Conception
10	'Booking appoint' where the pregnant woman meets the midwife for the first time. The appointment is important to screen for complications.
11–14	Ultrasound scan (dating, twins and complications)
20	Ultrasound scan (to check for anomalies)
28	Full blood count and antibody assessment
40	Birth
42	Induction of labour by this time

BOX 16.6	CALCULATING GESTATIONAL AGE

1. Identify the **first** day of the LMP (the date when the last menstrual bleeding started).

2. Count the number of weeks and days from the LMP to the current date.

For example: If the LMP began on 16 October 2024, and today's date is 9 December 2024, the estimated gestational age is 7 weeks and 5 days.

age is unknown, estimate based on the last menstrual period (LMP), see Box 16.6.

Be sure to check the blood pressure and urine for protein if the woman is over 20 weeks pregnant. If agreeable, consider screening urine for drugs of abuse if available.

SUBSTANCE MISUSE

The misuse of substances can lead to significant risks and complications for both the foetus and the mother, see Box 16.7. As such, the management of such cases requires senior input and oversight. The Royal College of Psychiatrists (2020) advocates a low threshold for referral to hospital, see Box 16.8.

SAFEGUARDING

Safeguarding referrals for pregnant women are made to ensure the safety and well-being of both the expectant mother and her unborn child due to various concerns, including domestic abuse, substance misuse, mental health issues or situations where the pregnant woman's behaviour or circumstances, put her or her unborn child at risk.

No specific gestational age dictates when a safeguarding referral must be made. Referrals are based on the presence of risk factors or concerns, regardless of the stage of pregnancy. However, the greater the gestational age, the greater the relative risk. While safeguarding is a priority, it is also essential to handle such referrals with respect for confidentiality and where possible, with the pregnant woman's consent.

COMPLICATIONS

Ectopic Pregnancy

An ectopic pregnancy occurs when the embryo implants outside of the uterus, usually in a fallopian tube. Ectopic pregnancies can easily be missed and should be considered with any women of child-bearing age with abdominal pain and a pregnancy test performed, see Box 16.9.

BOX 16.7	RISKS AND COMPLICATIONS

Alcohol

Intoxication
- Risk of maternal aspiration and hypoxia
- Reduced foetal movement

Withdrawal
- Foetal distress
- Miscarriage and preterm labour

Overall risk
- Foetal alcohol spectrum disorder
- Low birth weight
- Neurodevelopment complications

Heroin (and other opioids)

Intoxication
- Risk of maternal aspiration and hypoxia
- Hypoxia or hypotension in overdose
- Reduced foetal movements

Withdrawal
- Foetal distress
- Miscarriage and preterm labour

Overall risk
- Neonatal abstinence syndrome
- Premature birth
- Low birth weight
- Birth defects

Cocaine (including crack cocaine)

Intoxication
- Fluctuations in blood pressure

Overall risk
- Placental abruption
- Premature birth
- Low birth weight

Amphetamines

Intoxication
- Foetal distress due to reduced uterine blood flow

Overall risk
- Premature birth
- Low birth weight
- Birth defects

Benzodiazepines

Intoxication
- Risk of maternal aspiration and hypoxia
- Hypoxia or hypotension in overdose
- Reduced foetal movements

Withdrawal
- Foetal distress
- Miscarriage and preterm labour

Overall risk
- Neonatal withdrawal syndrome
- Cleft lip and palate
- Floppy infant syndrome

BOX 16.8	RED FLAGS – SUBSTANCE MISUSE AND PREGNANCY

- Acute intoxication and drowsiness
- Reduced or active foetal movements
- Uterine tightening
- Alcohol or drug withdrawal
- Drug-dependent and not already on treatment (i.e. opioid substitution therapy)
- Cocaine or crack cocaine misuse
- Benzodiazepine misuse
- Multiple or high-risk injection sites, ulcers or abscesses
- Homeless
- Detained over night or at the weekend

Source: Adapted from Royal College of Psychiatrists (2020).

BOX 16.9	SIGNS OF ECTOPIC PREGNANCY

- Vaginal bleeding
- Abdominal pain
- Shock (tachycardia and/or hypotension)

BOX 16.10	SIGNS OF SPONTANEOUS MISCARRIAGE

- Vaginal bleeding
- Abdominal cramps
- Fluid or tissue discharge from the vagina

Spontaneous Miscarriage

Any pregnancy where the foetus dies before 24 weeks is a spontaneous miscarriage, see Box 16.10. The majority occur within the first 12 weeks and it is estimated 15% of known pregnancies end in miscarriage.

Anyone suspected of suffering a spontaneous miscarriage should ideally be referred directly to an early pregnancy unit (EPU) and avoid the Emergency Department. EPUs care for women experiencing complications or concerns in early pregnancy (up to 16–18 weeks). Services differ nationally and may not offer a 24/7 service.

After 16–18 weeks, women suspected of spontaneous miscarriage should be referred to the Maternity Assessment Centre (MAC). MACs provide urgent and emergency care during pregnancy and sometimes in the weeks following birth. This service is distinct from regular antenatal appointments and addresses immediate and unexpected concerns during pregnancy.

Pre-eclampsia

Pre-eclampsia is a complication that occurs in 6% of pregnancies, characterised by high blood pressure and protein in the urine after 20 weeks, see Box 16.11. It is a serious condition because it can lead to complications for both the mother and the foetus.

Suspected pre-eclampsia can be referred directly to the MAC.

Eclampsia

Pre-eclampsia can lead to the development of eclampsia, a severe and potentially life-threatening complication of pregnancy characterised by the onset of seizures. Treatment requires the immediate delivery of the child. Because of the severity of the illness, individuals should be referred to the Emergency Department via ambulance.

SCENARIO 16.2	Pregnancy in custody

A young woman, in her early twenties, is arrested and denies being pregnant initially. However, physical examination and her history suggest she is in her late second trimester. She has a history of alcohol and cocaine use and is currently exhibiting signs of alcohol intoxication. She previously gave birth to a baby, which was taken into care and has therefore not sought any antenatal care.

1. *Describe your approach to the fitness to detain and wider pregnancy assessment.*

2. *Are they fit to be detained in custody?*
   a. *What are the foreseeable risks?*

3. *What are the pregnancy complications associated with intoxication, withdrawal or long-term use of:*
   a. *Alcohol?*
   b. *Cocaine?*

4. *Describe your approach and responsibilities in safeguarding the mother and unborn child.*

CHILDREN IN CUSTODY

A child is defined by the United Nations as anyone under the age of 18 years (UNICEF 1989). In England, Wales and Northern Ireland, the age of criminal responsibility is 10 years old. In Scotland, the age was raised from 8 to 12 years old in

---

BOX 16.11 · SIGNS OF PRE-ECLAMPSIA

- Usually asymptomatic
- BP ≥ 140/90
- Proteinuria (≥ +1 protein on a urine dipstick test)
- Headache (mild – severe)
- Oedema (peripheral or pulmonary)
- Visual disturbances

BOX 16.12 · SUMMARY OF CONCORDANT ON CHILDREN IN CUSTODY

- Whenever possible, charged children will be released on bail.
- Children denied bail will be transferred whenever practicable.
- Secure accommodation will be requested only when necessary.
- Local Authorities will always accept requests for non-secure accommodation.
- The power to detain will be transferred to the Local Authority.

Source: Adapted from Home Office (2017).

2019. Children below these ages cannot be arrested or charged with an offence and will, therefore, not be seen in custody. There are other procedures to deal with behaviours or concerns in children below the age of criminal responsibility. However, the focus of this chapter is children in custody.

Children account for about 6–8% of all detentions. The number of children detained has fallen over the last 10 years by 58%, which is higher than adults, who have only seen a reduction of 36% during the same time. This reflects the National Police Chiefs' Council (2022) strategy to only use custody as a last resort. Officers must avoid keeping children and young people in custody any longer than necessary, pre- and post-charge. On average, children are detained for just under 11 hours and adults almost 13.5 hours. Finally, In England, officers must comply with the 'Concordant on children in custody', see Box 16.12.

Children in custody represent a unique and vulnerable group, facing a higher likelihood of complex health and social challenges. These young individuals often present with mental health issues, such as ADHD, conduct disorder or depression and may require regular medication. Many have histories of self-harm, suicide attempts or substance misuse. Their educational levels, particularly literacy and numeracy, frequently fall below national expectations for their age and they may struggle with communication, decision-making and low self-esteem.

Additionally, these children might be navigating difficult living situations, such as inadequate housing or being asylum seekers without guardians. They often carry the weight of past emotional, physical or sexual abuse and may be involved with child protection services, in care or transitioning out of care. Their backgrounds may include experiences of neglect, trauma or bullying, which can manifest in both their behaviour and their interactions with others and are often referred to as adverse childhood experiences.

Given these multifaceted risks, it is crucial HCPs recognise and address the heightened needs of detained children. A thorough understanding of these risk factors is essential for providing appropriate support, ensuring their safety and well-being while in custody and determining the need for specialised referrals.

Consent

Consent in custody varies depending on the reason for referral.

Clinical If the nature of the contact is clinical, such as responding to a clinical complaint, medication or fitness to detain, then children aged 16–17 can consent and the Mental Capacity Act applies. Consent must be valid (i.e. voluntary, informed and with capacity).

Children below 16 may have the capacity to give valid if they demonstrate sufficient maturity, intelligence and understanding of what the treatment entails. This ability to consent, based on their cognitive and emotional maturity, is referred to as Gillick competence.

Forensic examinations and samples This includes medico-legal examinations such as fitness to interview or charge, documentation of injuries and forensic samples (except road traffic). While children aged 16–17 year can consent to forensic examination, the HCP must be satisfied they understand the purpose and nature of the examination, including any samples. It is good practice to also seek consent from someone

---

BOX 16.13 · PARENTAL RESPONSIBILITY

- A mother
- A father if he is either:
  - married to the child's mother
  - listed on the birth certificate (after a certain date, depending on which part of the United Kingdom the child was born in)
- Adoptive parent
- Guardian
- Local authority (usually shared with parents and cannot consent to non-urgent procedures alone)
- Foster parents **do not** have parental responsibility

with parental responsibility, see Box 16.13 (Faculty of Forensic & Legal Medicine 2023a). The police have their own rules around requesting samples of children under 18 years old.

Where the child is under 16 years old, then HCPs must seek consent from someone with parental responsibility. HCPs must also have the consent and cooperation of the child. Forensic examinations or samples should not be taken without consent and cooperation. Consider the safeguarding needs of children who are being examined for sexual offences as the perpetrator (see *Resources* at the end of the chapter).

Child Sexual Exploitation

Child sexual exploitation (CSE) is a form of child sexual abuse. It occurs when an individual or group takes advantage of an imbalance of power to coerce, manipulate or deceive a child into sexual activity in exchange for something the child needs or wants. The exchange can be for tangible items like money, drugs, alcohol or less-tangible things like affection or status.

When a child is brought into custody, it may be because they have been arrested for activities related to their exploitation, such as theft, drugs or violence. It is crucial to recognise they may be victims of CSE (see Box 16.14). HCPs can be a critical intervention point to identify and safeguard children at risk of or experiencing CSE. Children who display disruptive or challenging behaviour are sometimes at risk of being overlooked as victims of CSE. It is essential for HCPs to challenge these misconceptions and advocate for the child's welfare and access to appropriate support services.

Child Criminal Exploitation and County-lines

Child criminal exploitation (CCE) is a form of abuse where children are manipulated and coerced into committing crimes. The model of 'county lines' is a prevalent form of CCE, where urban gangs extend their drug networks to provincial areas, often using children and vulnerable adults to carry and sell drugs across county boundaries.

BOX 16.14	SIGNS OF CHILD SEXUAL EXPLOITATION

- Unexplained gifts or new possessions
- Changes in behaviour, such as becoming secretive or withdrawn
- Unexplained absences from home or school
- Physical signs of abuse and/or sexual activity
- Relationships with older individuals or groups
- Evidence of drug, alcohol or substance misuse
- Fearful, anxious or submissive behaviour
- Signs of psychological trauma including self-harm or suicidal thoughts

BOX 16.15	SIGNS OF CHILD CRIMINAL EXPLOITATION AND COUNTY LINES

- Unexplained absences from school or home
- Large amounts of drugs, money or multiple phones
- Relationships with controlling, older individuals or group
- Evidence of physical injury or assault
- Use of drug-related language or acronyms
- Unexplained acquisition of money or expensive gifts
- Acts that appear out of character, such as shoplifting or theft
- Fearful or anxious behaviour, particularly around certain individuals

Children involved in CCE may come into custody having been arrested for crimes such as drug trafficking, theft, carrying weapons or violence. It is important to recognise these children may be victims as it can trigger safeguarding interventions and help to divert from further exploitation and to appropriate support services (see Box 16.15). Children involved in county lines may also be at risk of 'going country', which refers to travelling to rural areas to sell drugs. They may be reported missing or found in areas away from their home region.

SCENARIO 16.3	Children in custody

A 14-year-old girl in custody is identified as a potential victim of child sexual exploitation. She is withdrawn, reports multiple older boyfriends and presents with signs suggestive of child sexual exploitation. She's reluctant to discuss her situation and police want the HCP to perform a pregnancy test.

1. *Outline your approach to trying to get the young girl to engage.*

2. *Describe your safeguarding responsibilities and actions.*

3. *Outline your approach to consent for performing a pregnancy test.*

4. *Describe your rationale for performing a pregnancy test (or not).*

DRUG CONCEALMENT (PACKER, STUFFER AND PUSHER)

Concealing drugs within body orifices presents a high risk in custody, necessitating careful management to detect deterioration and prevent fatality in the event of complications.

BOX 16.16	CONCEALMENT TERMINOLOGY
Packers or 'mules'	Individuals ingest drugs, often cocaine, in tightly wrapped, usually machine-manufactured packages, which are later expelled and sold. Although machine manufacturing has reduced the risk of rupture, any leakage could lead to severe or fatal poisoning. Border Force authorities, particularly air, sea or land ports, typically discover this sophisticated method, which is frequently employed by international organised crime syndicates.
Stuffers	Individuals who hide or swallow drugs wrapped in cling film (or similar packaging) to avoid detection. However, due to inadequate protection within the digestive system, there is a higher likelihood of poisoning. More typically seen in police custody.
Pushers	Individuals concealing drugs in their rectum or vagina to evade detection. These items are usually well wrapped, often using condoms or in plastic receptacles like 'Kinder eggs', resulting in lower risks compared to other methods. More typically seen in police custody.

BOX 16.17	RISK OF DRUG CONCEALMENT
Toxicity	If a package ruptures or leaks, individuals may be exposed to a fatal dose of a drug. Toxicity refers to the harmful effects that can occur when drugs are ingested in quantities that exceed the body's capacity to metabolise or eliminate. Toxicity will be dependent on the type of drug, purity, quantity, individual tolerance and metabolism.
Infection	The process of packaging drugs may not be sterile, leading to potential infections.
Injury	The act of concealing drugs, such as swallowing or inserting them, can lead to physical injury or damage to internal organs. This could include a bowel obstruction or ileus.

There are three common methods employed by individuals involved in drug concealment: packers or 'mules', stuffers and pushers (see Box 16.16).

COMPLICATIONS

Individuals should be informed of the complications associated with drug concealment (see Box 16.17), which should be documented in the clinical record. There are several factors that increase the risk of complications, see Box 16.18.

BOX 16.18	RISK FACTORS

- Improvised/home-made packaging
- Large quantity of drugs (especially for body stuffers)
- High number of packets (>50)
- Large size of packets
- Delayed passage (>48 h)
- Poisoning in a co-transporter
- Previous abdominal surgery (greater risk of obstructing secondary to adhesions)
- Concomitant drug usage, especially constipating agents

Source: Adapted from Royal College of Emergency Medicine (2020).

INITIAL ASSESSMENT (PRE-HOSPITAL REFERRAL)

Individuals suspected of concealing drugs should be treated as needing urgent medical attention and transferred directly to the hospital before arriving in custody (College of Policing 2021). However, suspicion may arise after arrival in custody. In such cases, the priority should be the assessment and management of A-B-C-D-E as outlined in Chapter 19 – Emergencies, followed by a referral to the hospital.

At Hospital

The Royal College of Emergency Medicine (2020) provides guidelines for managing suspected drug concealment. In summary, they recommend a low-dose CT scan of the abdomen and pelvis, after which asymptomatic packers can be discharged back to custody. However, stuffers and pushers should be observed for eight hours post-ingestion. Further management will depend on their presentation and results.

Hospitals should report any CT scan results as either positive, negative or indeterminate. However, it should be stressed a negative result does rule out drug concealment.

Intimate Searches

In England, Wales and Northern Ireland, police Inspectors can authorise[1] an intimate search by HCPs (nurses and doctors) for someone suspected of concealing Class A drugs.[2] In Scotland, they may be carried out under the authority of a sheriff's warrant. An intimate search is an examination of any bodily orifices other than mouth, such as ears, nose, rectum or vagina. Any such examinations must only be performed with the individual's informed consent and in a hospital with full

---

[1] Section 55 PACE and PACENI.
[2] Cocaine, heroin, ecstasy, heroin, LSD, magic mushrooms, methadone and methamphetamine.

resuscitation facilities. However, the Royal College of Emergency Medicine (2020) does not recommend intimate searches due to the risk to the individual and the HCP. Police cannot compel HCPs to undertake such searches.

SUBSEQUENT ASSESSMENT AND MANAGEMENT (POST-HOSPITAL DISCHARGE)

Assessment

Those suspected of drug concealment may face extended periods of detention[3] and require a comprehensive and well-documented fitness to detain assessment as outlined in Chapter 3 – Fitness Assessments. Using the opportunity to establish a rapport, explain ongoing management and encourage compliance. The assessment is a chance to identify any physical or mental health needs impacted by prolonged detention. It is important to consider medication requirements and ensure adequate resources are available.

All clinical assessments should take place in the medical room for twofold reasons. Firstly, privacy and dignity, allowing individuals to speak with the HCP in private outside the presence of an officer. Secondly, movement and exercise are encouraged to promote normal bowel movements. If feasible, this private conversation should aim to gather critical details such as the time of concealment, the specific drug, the quantity and any information regarding the packaging. This approach enhances transparency and assists in ensuring their safety and well-being.

As a minimum record vital signs (including NEWS2), blood glucose and pupils or clearly document any refusal. Organisations may wish to use a 'Refusal to Accept Treatment/Referral to Hospital' waiver, signed in the presence of a witness. Capacity assessment and decisions should be appropriately documented.

Enquire about any recent diet and intentions to eat and drink while in custody.

Management

Any signs or symptoms of drug toxicity (see Box 16.19) at any point should be recognised as requiring emergency admission to hospital and emergency equipment should be made immediately available.

Police should document all food and drinks provided and the amount consumed on the custody record and make it available to the HCP. Recommend a normal diet and regular exercise. Both will encourage normal bowel movements. Acknowledging the constraints of food available in custody, advise may include police sourcing alternative options. However, this should be coordinated by the police rather than HCP. Recommended alternative options include:

- Wholewheat biscuits such as Weetabix or plain shredded whole grain options such as Shredded wheat or porridge oats

---

[3] In 2018, a 24-year-old man was held in police custody for 47 days. He was eventually released without charge following medical advice after not opening his bowels during this time, despite eating and drinking.

BOX 16.19	TOXICITY SIGNS OR SYMPTOMS
Tachycardia or arrythmia	Bradycardia
Hypertension	Hypotension
Pyrexia	Hypothermia
Dilated pupils	Pinpoint pupils
Tachypnoea	Reduced respiratory rate
Agitation	Reduced consciousness
Nausea	Vomiting
Seizures	
Chest pain	
Abdominal pain	

- Wholemeal or granary bread, wholemeal pasta or brown rice
- Nutrient-rich sources like beans, lentils and chickpeas
- A variety of vegetables
- Fresh, dried or canned fruit and fruit juices
- Nutrient-dense seeds or nuts

Individuals may avoid passing stools to prevent the detection of concealed drugs, which often lead to constipation. The use of laxatives is not recommended; a rapid increase in peristalsis can potentially damage concealed packages.

Level of observations Because of the level of risk, as a minimum recommend Level 3 – Constant Observations. However, consideration should be given to Level 4 – Close Proximity to spot any deterioration early and prevent the individual from expelling and swallowing a package. At a minimum, individuals should be roused every 30 minutes for the first eight hours post-concealment. Technology, such as camera-based vital sign alarms, should not be used to replace Level 3 or 4 observations.

Officers should be advised to challenge any daytime sleeping. Overnight, individuals sleeping should be roused at four hourly intervals.

Healthcare reviews Considering the inherent unpredictability of concealed packages and their potential to leak or rupture, it is strongly advised that all individuals undergo regular reviews (see Box 16.20). There is currently no consensus on how often individuals should be reviewed. However, for the first 24–48 hours, four hourly reviews are reasonable, followed by 8-hourly reviews.

Furthermore, it is essential to review following any bowel movements, as there is a possibility bowel movements could cause damage to a concealed package. There is no consensus on how many clear stools are necessary.

| BOX 16.20 | HEALTHCARE REVIEWS |

- Wake if sleeping

- Review recent diet and fluid intake

- Check for signs or symptoms of toxicity

- Check for any signs of bowel obstruction

- Check consciousness level, pulse, respiratory rate, SpO_2 and pupils

FOOD OR FLUID REFUSAL

Those suspected of drug concealment may refuse food or fluid. Food or fluid refusal is defined as someone refusing food for 48 hours, or food and fluids for 24 hours (Home Office 2022). Anyone refusing food or fluids should be weighed and have a blood glucose checked daily. HCPs should engage with individuals to identify reasons for food or fluid refusal and warn about the risks, including death. Where individuals persistently refuse both food and fluid referral to liaison and diversion, or local mental health teams for further assessment.

Prolonged (over five days) refusal of food or fluid may risk refeeding syndrome, a potentially severe condition characterised by significant electrolyte and fluid imbalances resulting from the reintroduction of nutrition after inadequate intake (see Box 16.21).

In cases of food and fluid refusal, it is important to carefully consider the potential impact of administering medications. These decisions should be made in consultation with senior clinicians to ensure the individual's safety and well-being.

| SCENARIO 16.4 | Drug concealment |

A 30-year-old man, suspected of 'stuffing' drugs (heroin and crack cocaine) when arrested is brought into custody. He denies concealing drugs but shows signs of discomfort and anxiety.

1. Outline your approach to the fitness to detain assessment.

2. Are they fit to be detained?
   a. What are the foreseeable risks?
   b. Provide a care plan for the police including a recommended level and frequency of observations with a rationale.

Eighteen hours later, he returned from hospital and complained of opioid withdrawal. At the hospital, he was monitored for several hours and had a low-dose CT, which did not demonstrate any packages. On examination, there are clinically objective signs of opioid withdrawal, including diarrhoea.

3. Outline your approach to opioid withdrawal assessment.

4. What are the risks and benefits of:
   a. Offering no treatment (i.e. dihydrocodeine or symptomatic relief)?
   b. Offer symptomatic relief only?
   c. Offering dihydrocodeine (or equivalent) and symptomatic relief)?

5. Outline your ongoing care plan.

6. Outline your advice to the police.

| BOX 16.21 | RISK OF REFEEDING SYNDROME |

| At risk | Little or no food for >5 days |
| High risk | Any **ONE** of the following: |

- BMI <16 kg/m²
- Little to no food for >10 days
- Unintentional weight loss >15% in the last 3–6 months

Any **TWO** of the following:

- BMI <18.5 kg/m²
- Little to no food for >5 days
- Unintentional weight loss >10% in the last 3–6 months
- History of alcohol abuse or the use of some drugs, including insulin, chemotherapy, antacids or diuretics

| Severe risk | Any **ONE** of the following: |

- BMI <14 kg/m²
- Very little or no nutrition for >15 days

Source: Adapted from Brighton and Sussex University Hospital (2017).

CONCLUSION

This chapter has illuminated the unique and complex challenges faced by HCPs in managing special circumstances within custody. From the heightened security and stress in terrorism-related detentions to the delicate care required for pregnant women, each situation demands a specialised approach. Children and individuals suspected of concealing drugs further underscore the diverse range of scenarios encountered. This exploration not only enhances understanding of these distinct needs but also emphasises the importance of a tailored, empathetic approach in these sensitive environments. It is our hope this chapter empowers HCPs with the knowledge and skills necessary to navigate these challenges effectively, ensuring the provision of high-quality, ethical and compassionate healthcare to all detained individuals, regardless of their circumstances.

LEARNING ACTIVITIES

1. Write a reflection for each of the special circumstances outlined earlier. Consider how your attitudes, values and beliefs may have impacted your approach to the assessment, advice and ability to communicate with officers and the individual.

2. Liaise with local antenatal services (e.g. EPU or MAC) to establish referral criteria and route. Produce a handy poster (or similar) for colleagues.

3. With colleagues, run a tabletop exercise where you manage the care of an individual with a prolonged detention due to suspected drug concealment. Use various scenarios to explore the various complications.

RESOURCES

Online

Terrorism

- Terrorism Act (2000) – https://www.legislation.gov.uk/ukpga/2000/11/contents
- College of Policing | Terrorism Act 2000 – https://www.college.police.uk/app/detention-and-custody/terrorism-act-2000-tact
- Police and Criminal Evidence Act 1984 (PACE) Code H | Code of practice for the detention, treatment and questioning by Police Officers of persons in police detention under section 41 of, and Schedule 8 to, the Terrorism Act 2000 (https://assets.publishing.service.gov.uk/government/uploads/system/uploads/attachment_data/file/1135849/Revised_PACE_Code_H_-_2023_revisions.pdf)
- Police and Criminal Evidence (Northern Ireland) Order 1989 (PACENI) Code H | Code of Practice for the Detention, Treatment and Questioning of Persons under Section 41 of, and Schedule 8 to, the Terrorism Act 2000 (https://www.justice-ni.gov.uk/sites/default/files/publications/doj/pace-code-h-2015.pdf)
- Police Scotland | Care and Welfare of Persons in Police Custody (https://www.scotland.police.uk/spa-media/0mfjn3pa/care-and-welfare-of-persons-in-police-custody-sop.pdf)

Pregnancy

- NHS | Pregnancy | https://www.nhs.uk/pregnancy/
- North Yorkshire Safeguarding Children Partnership | Safeguarding unborn babies | https://www.safeguardingchildren.co.uk/professionals/procedures-practice-guidance-and-one-minute-guides/safeguarding-unborn-babies/

Children in Custody

- Centre of expertise on child sexual abuse | Sibling sexual abuse and behaviour | https://www.csacentre.org.uk/research-resources/practice-resources/sibling-sexual-abuse/
- Brook and British Association for Sexual Health and HIV | Spotting the signs tool | https://www.brook.org.uk/wp-content/uploads/2023/09/Spotting-the-signs-tool_FINAL-FILLABLE-2.pdf

Drug Concealment

- Faculty of Forensic & Legal Medicine | Recommendations for healthcare professionals asked to perform intimate body searches | https://fflm.ac.uk/wp-content/uploads/2021/03/Recommendations-for-healthcare-professionals-asked-to-perform-intimate-body-searches-FFLM-and-BMA-March-2021.pdf
- Royal College of Emergency Medicine | Management of suspected internal drug trafficker | https://rcem.ac.uk/wp-content/uploads/2021/10/Management_of_Suspected_Internal_Drug_Trafficker_December_2020.pdf

Organisations

- Counter Terrorism Policing | www.counterterrorism.police.uk
- Toxbase | https://www.toxbase.org/

REFERENCES

Allen, G., Burton, M. and Pratt, A. (2022). *Terrorism in Great Britain: The Statistics*. London: House of Commons Library. https://researchbriefings.files.parliament.uk/documents/CBP-7613/CBP-7613.pdf (accessed 04 April 2023).

Brighton and Sussex University Hospital (2017). Refeeding syndrome guideline for adults. https://www.bsuh.nhs.uk/library/wp-content/uploads/sites/8/2019/06/RefeedingJuly2017.pdf?UNLID=47313861202381352335 (accessed 08 November 2023).

College of Policing (2021). Alcohol and drugs. https://www.college. police.uk/app/detention-and-custody/detainee-care/alcohol-and-drugs (accessed 20 October 2023).

Faculty of Forensic & Legal Medicine (2023a). Consent from children and young people in police custody in England and Wales for medical examinations. https://fflm.ac.uk/wp-content/uploads/2019/03/ Consent-from-CYP-in-Police-Custody-in-England-and-Wales-for-Medical-Examinations-Oct-2023.pdf (accessed 08 November 2023).

Faculty of Forensic & Legal Medicine (2023b). Medical Care of Persons Detained Under the Terrorism Act 2000. https://fflm.ac.uk/ wp-content/uploads/2019/05/Medical-Care-of-Persons-Detained-Under-the-Terrorism-Act-2000-Dr-A-Gorton-July-2023.pdf (accessed 21 July 2023).

Ho, C.S.H., Quek, T.C., Ho, R.C.M., and Choo, C.C. (2018). Terrorism and mental illness: a pragmatic approach for the clinician. *BJPsych Advances* 25 (2): 101–109.

Home Office (2017). Concordant on children in custody: preventing the detention of children in police stations following charge. https:// assets.publishing.service.gov.uk/media/5a82211140f0b6230269afee/ Concordat_on_Children_in_Custody_ISBN_Accessible.pdf (accessed 08 November 2023).

Home Office (2022). Care and management of detained individuals refusing food and/or fluids. https://assets.publishing.service. gov.uk/government/uploads/system/uploads/attachment_data/ file/1107746/DSO_-_03-2017_Care_and_management_of_detainees_ refusing_food_and_or_fluid.pdf (accessed 08 November 2023).

National Police Chiefs' Council (2022). National strategy for police custody. https://www.npcc.police.uk/SysSiteAssets/media/downloads/ publications/publications-log/criminal-justice/2023/national-strategy-for-police-custody.pdf (accessed 08 November 2023).

Royal College of Emergency Medicine (2020). Management of suspected internal drug trafficker. https://rcem.ac.uk/wp-content/ uploads/2021/10/Management_of_Suspected_Internal_Drug_ Trafficker_December_2020.pdf (accessed 20 October 2023).

Royal College of Psychiatrists (2020). *Detainees with Substance Use Disorders in Police Custody: Guidelines for Clinical Management*, 5the. https://fflm.ac.uk/wp-content/uploads/2020/12/college-report-cr227. pdf (accessed 27 December 2023).

UNICEF (1989). The United Nations convention on the rights of the child. https://www.unicef.org.uk/wp-content/uploads/2016/08/unicef-convention-rights-child-uncrc.pdf (accessed 08 November 2023).

FURTHER READING

Royal College of Psychiatrists and Faculty of Forensic & Legal Medicine| Detainees with substance use disorders in police custody: Guidelines for clinical management. https://fflm.ac.uk/wp-content/ uploads/2020/12/college-report-cr227.pdf (accessed 16 August 2024).

Governance

Vanessa Webb

Nurture Health and Care Ltd, Norwich, UK

CHAPTER 17

AIM

The chapter will address key areas such as clinical effectiveness, risk management, leadership and quality improvement, ensuring that healthcare provision in police custody aligns with national healthcare standards while recognising the specific needs and constraints of the custodial setting. This approach ensures a dual focus: upholding the rights and well-being of individuals in custody and maintaining the highest standards of professional healthcare practice as outlined in NHS clinical governance principles and our professional organisations.

LEARNING OUTCOMES

Upon completion of this chapter, readers should be able to:

- Identify the legislative and regulatory frameworks that impact our practice

- Can identify the key principles of the NHS Patient Safety Strategy

- Can identify your role in clinical governance

SELF-ASSESSMENT

1. Can you describe a time you raised a clinical concern and discuss how this aligns to national strategy in the NHS?

2. Can you identify a quality improvement project in your organisation and discuss how the front-line staff contribute to this?

3. Can you describe how you demonstrate leadership skills as a healthcare professional (HCP)?

INTRODUCTION

Clinical governance is a framework for ensuring high-quality, safe and effective healthcare services.

Clinical governance ensures HCPs are trained and competent, including visible leadership. HCPs should adhere to evidence-based practices and be accountable for their performance but be aware that the complexity of our environments requires professional judgement and person-centred approaches. Clinical governance involves identifying standards for best practice, monitoring and evaluating these systems, ensuring a patient focus, identifying areas for improvement and implementing changes to improve the quality of care.

It encompasses a range of activities, including quality assurance, risk management, clinical audit, education and training, research and continuous improvement.

THE LEGISLATIVE STANDARDS

The legislation that governs the delivery of forensic clinical practice includes aligning services with the Health and Social Care Act, complying with the Police and Criminal Evidence

---

Police Custody Healthcare for Nurses and Paramedics, First Edition. Edited by Matthew Peel, Jennie Smith, Vanessa Webb, and Margaret Bannerman.
© 2025 John Wiley & Sons Ltd. Published 2025 by John Wiley & Sons Ltd.
Companion website: www.wiley.com/go/policecustodyhealthcare

Act, The Road Traffic Act and ensures The Human Rights Act, The Children's Act, Health and Safety at Work Act, Mental Health Act, Data Protection Act, Care Act, Mental Capacity Act, Equality Act and their equivalence across the four nations are applied.

REGULATORY ENVIRONMENT

The landscape of regulatory oversight in forensic clinical practice is intricately structured and overseen by distinct yet interconnected bodies across the United Kingdom. At its core, the HM Inspectorate of Constabulary and Fire & Rescue Services (HMICFRS), alongside the Forensic Science Regulator (FSR), set the foundational guidelines for practice within England and Wales. In Scotland, oversight is specifically managed by the HM Inspectorate of Constabulary in Scotland, which focuses on the inspection of custody services, while Northern Ireland is overseen by Criminal Justice Inspection Northern Ireland.

Parallel to these, the regulatory framework is complemented by healthcare-specific bodies: the Care Quality Commission (CQC) in England, the Care Inspectorate in Scotland, the Regulation and Quality Improvement Authority in Northern Ireland, and the Care Inspectorate Wales. This creates a complex tapestry of standards that, while grounded in common principles, leads to nuanced approaches across the United Kingdom.

Healthcare services within police custody are expected to adhere to the same high standards prevalent in other healthcare environments. However, the application of these standards within the criminal justice system often sparks tension, reflecting varied interpretations and implementations across the four nations. This variance underscores the challenge of ensuring uniform quality and safety in forensic clinical practice, amidst differing regulatory landscapes.

As an example, the HMICFRS has developed a framework for inspection of custody arrangements for all police forces in England and Wales. This framework is focused on the treatment and conditions of those detained and has expectations grouped under five inspection areas:

- Leadership, accountability and working with partners

- Pre-custody: first point of contact

- In the custody suite: booking in, individual needs and legal rights

- In the custody cell, safeguarding and healthcare

- Release and transfer from custody.

Whereas the CQC supports the HMICFRS across five domains: safe, effective, caring, responsive and well-led, and measure evidence in relation to these domains. Benchmarking across different standards creates tensions for healthcare providers in identifying best practice.

HEALTHCARE EXPECTATIONS IN POLICE CUSTODY

Healthcare provision within police custody settings is premised on the fundamental right of individuals to have 'equivalency of care' to their services to that in the community (Royal College of General Practitioners 2018), underpinned by robust governance standards. In England, the national commissioning specification outlines the framework for healthcare in police custody and liaison and diversion services (NHS England 2024). However, local adaptations ensure that healthcare delivery is tailored to the specific needs of each police force and provider, resulting in varied practices across the United Kingdom, including Scotland and Northern Ireland. It is imperative that systems are in place for seamless information sharing, ensuring continuity of care that matches community standards, and addressing the health needs of those detained during custody, upon transfer and following release.

HCPs must be readily available round-the-clock to meet the emergent health needs of those detained. Each police force area has its own model of delivery, with a comprehensive induction for HCPs, coupled with ongoing training and regular, documented supervision to maintain professional competencies. Moreover, clinical facilities within custody suites are required to adhere to rigorous medicines management and infection control standards, equipped with suitable, well-maintained and calibrated instruments to ensure they are fit for purpose.

Navigating the intricate balance between the duty of care owed by HCPs and the public protection mandate of the police presents a unique challenge. Healthcare providers in these settings must adeptly manage their dual responsibilities: delivering therapeutic care while also contributing to the evidence-gathering process as an objective professional.

QUALITY AND SAFETY FOR HEALTHCARE IN POLICE CUSTODY

Quality and safety in healthcare require that the provision of healthcare services should be efficient, effective and patient-centred, while minimising risks and harm to patients. Every organisation should then be able to capture these in their systems and be able to demonstrate these when required.

CLINICAL EFFECTIVENESS

Providers should deliver evidence-based care, ensuring patients receive the right treatment at the right time based on the best available evidence. In police custody settings, research, evaluation and the evidence base related to this unique environment are limited.

Resources to consider are:

- National Institute for Health and Care Excellence, which is built on principles of evidence-based medicine and reviews the robustness of research outcomes. This may have limited transferability to police custody due to the lack of representation of our population to the research participants and our unique role; however, this should be considered as part of our approach.

- Faculty of Forensic & Legal Medicine, Royal Colleges and United Kingdom Association Forensic Nurses & Paramedics, provide guidelines that usually are based on expert opinions and consensus statements. The expert opinions are based on the clinical experience of HCPs or expert panels, while consensus statements are developed through a formal process involving multiple experts. They provide the lowest level of evidence, as they are not based on rigorous research methods and therefore should be taken in conjunction with wider evidence sources but often form the foundation of forensic practice due to the limited research with our population and in our environment.

- Forensic Science Regulator is built on principles of systems management, evidence and continuous improvement. Currently, it is not implemented in custody, although the Sexual Assault Referral Centres (SARCs) are currently undertaking accreditation to ISO 15189 (Forensic Science Regulator 2024). Research papers inform the collection and interpretation of evidence and are captured in *'Recommendations for the Collection of Forensic Specimens from Complainants and Suspects'* updated 6 monthly.

PATIENT EXPERIENCE

Patient experience refers to the sum of all interactions and perceptions patients have while receiving healthcare services. It encompasses every aspect of care, from the clinical encounter itself to the physical environment, communication and emotional support. A positive patient experience is an essential component of high-quality healthcare, as it can directly impact patient satisfaction, treatment adherence and health outcomes.

In mainstream health services, including secure environments, ensuring that equivalency of care is crucial, especially in a system where those detained may experience negative attitudes, stereotypes and unequal treatment. These barriers can have significant consequences for the health and well-being of those detained; however, patient feedback is currently not routinely sought in police custody as part of quality improvement.

In police custody, our principal role is to provide objective forensic practice. Confidentiality is not guaranteed in relation to disclosure and medical records can be requested as part of court evidence and therefore consent includes the lack of confidentiality in this environment. We still retain our professional duty of care to demonstrate dignity and respect disclosing only information relevant to their detention but we share information in relation to their safe detention and where it is relevant to the criminal justice system.

To address stigma and discrimination in custody healthcare, providing ethical care is critical (see Chapter 18 – Professional Ethics), so education and training content should include the unique needs of those detained, cultural competency and considerations of concepts such as bias in reducing stigma and improving care.

Peer support, which involves individuals with lived experience in the development and delivery of police healthcare services, is still in its infancy; however, this is increasing and can help counteract stigma and foster understanding and is utilised within mainstream healthcare as an important element to include in high-quality healthcare systems.

HCPs understand the provision of comprehensive and integrated care that addresses physical, mental and substance use disorders in a holistic assessment, which creates an opportunity to access the wider health systems to address multiple needs.

As part of our role as HCPs, we should advocate for policies that promote equitable access to healthcare services and address underlying social determinants alongside traditional healthcare services and our experience of collaboration between healthcare providers, community organisations and the criminal justice system places us at the forefront of understanding the complexity of need of our client group.

We do have the possibility of empowering patients with knowledge about their conditions, acknowledging patient concerns, respecting their choices and creating access to wider services.

Our unique environment means individuals may present differently to mainstream healthcare than in a custody environment. Exaggerating symptoms, for example may enable the avoidance of an interview or detention; playing on emotion to attempt to create tension may present as a feature of their history or reflect their state of arousal considering the impact of arrest. The HCP's role includes not only a holistic assessment to ensure their safe detention, undertaking forensic samples and documenting injuries but also in understanding how different behaviours might need to be considered in our care plans.

The HCP should maintain professional boundaries, communicate effectively to share information and discuss concerns and choices where possible. This should be documented accurately and thoroughly, including time stamps of medical encounters and observations, documentation of incidental injuries and verbatim quotes of significant statements.

Our interventions should retain a patient-centred approach with safety and provision of evidence-based care informing our practices and documenting the rationale for our decision-making.

PATIENT SAFETY

Providers must actively identify and mitigate risks, continuously monitoring and learning from incidents to prevent harm to patients. Nationally, healthcare providers share little safety data in relation to incidents related to police custody.

Although not implemented in police custody, in 2019, NHS England and NHS Improvement published the 'NHS Patient Safety Strategy' (NHS England 2019), which aims to create a comprehensive approach to improve patient safety. Key components could be utilised to build a safer custody environment across the four nations as good practice.

Dame Elish Angiolini QC, led an independent review of deaths and serious incidents in police custody in England and Wales, which was published in 2017 (Angiolini 2017). The review made 110 recommendations aimed at improving the way police custody is managed and reducing the number of deaths and serious incidents that occur. This included improving the quality and consistency of healthcare provision in custody, including mental health support.

As HCPs, we should encourage a culture of safety where staff feel comfortable reporting errors, near misses and unsafe practices without fear of blame or punishment. This helps to identify potential risks and implement corrective actions and is embodied within the 'just culture' from the NHS, see Figure 17.1.

Through incident reporting and analysis, including adverse events, near misses and concerns, this data can be used to identify trends, prioritise improvement efforts and track progress over time and local systems should be able to understand and act on their own incidents and complaints.

This resulting improvement often through standardisation of processes and procedures whenever possible to reduce variability and minimise the potential for errors, should also be supplemented due to the complexity of our environments using critical thinking, judgement and aids such as decision-making tools and these should be considered as part of our education and competency frameworks.

By incorporating these components into a patient safety strategy, healthcare organisations can work towards reducing harm, improving the overall quality of care and ensuring a safer environment. We would welcome a national incident collection system and analysis of emerging themes to create insight into our unique environment.

Although patient safety is often considered in the remit of a governance department, all staff should understand the principles of the complaints process, the investigation in relation to patient safety and human resources (not to be confused with the police investigation into crime) and how to participate as an HCP and to consider your role in a systems approach to change. Reflective practice should also include recognition of how systems, culture, values and beliefs all impact our practice.

Deaths in police custody have a statutory investigation process and must be referred to the Independent Office for Police Conduct in England and Wales, the Scottish Fatalities Investigation Unit in Scotland and the Police Ombudsman in Northern Ireland. When faced with this situation as an HCP, this is often overwhelming as whole custody may be 'locked down' and will be managed in accordance with your own organisational policies and that of the local police force.

Undertaking an investigation within healthcare governance has multiple steps that require careful planning, execution and analysis. We are moving away from Root Cause Analysis and Five Whys, due to the simplicity of this approach, which led to a single point of failure and rarely to successful improvement and incorporating the principles of the NHS Patient Safety Strategy, the approach of the Health Services Safety Investigations Body (HSSIB) and Systems Engineering Initiative for Patient Safety (SEIPS) as an analysis framework that can ensure a comprehensive, systematic and robust process (HSSIB 2024).

Identification of Incident or Issue

Whether it is an unexpected patient outcome, a near miss, or a pattern of errors, the first step is to report the incident. Increasingly, we are looking at how positive outcomes should also be seen as a learning opportunity. This should be completed through your own organisational reporting structures.

If as an HCP, you are asked to investigate, clearly define the incident or issue to be investigated. This can be defined in a 'Terms of Reference' (ToR) that outlines the purpose, scope (and what are the boundaries of the activity), and structure of the investigation as a project plan. It serves as a guide or blueprint, detailing what is to be achieved, how it will be achieved, and the roles and responsibilities of those involved, along with the key milestones.

Data Collection

It is important to gather detailed data about the incident. As an HCP, you might be interviewed if involved in an adverse event or may be asked to be part of the evidence-gathering process. This usually includes a timeline, with decision-making points identified and could include reviewing medical records, staff interviews, equipment logs, audits and rota analysis. The HSSIB suggests investigations should be thorough and impartial, using a variety of sources to understand all aspects of an incident.

Systems Analysis

As an HCP, it is unlikely that you will be a lead investigator but appreciating how a critical analysis using a framework such as the SEIPS model enables understanding of the complex interplay of various factors that contribute to safety outcomes. It emphasises patient safety is influenced by the characteristics of people, human factors, tasks, tools and technologies, the physical environment and the organisation. Analysing the incident using this model can help identify how these elements interacted to contribute to the incident. Other models may be used by your organisations.

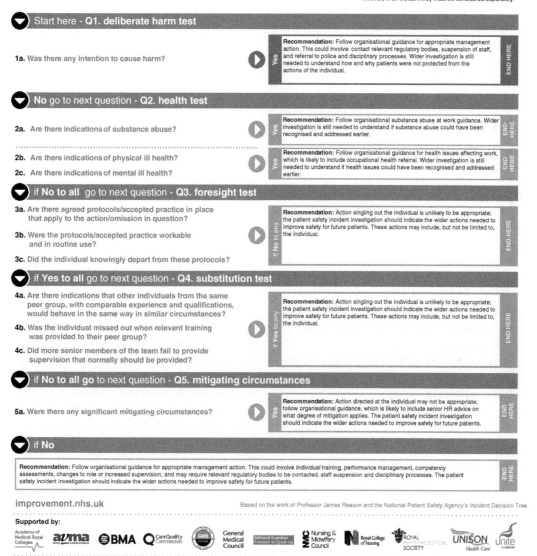

FIGURE 17.1 A just culture guide. *Source:* NHS Improvement / CROWN COPYRIGHT / Public Domain.

Identify Factors and Themes

Using the data collected and your analysis tool, the factors that contribute to the incident are identified. This should include not just the immediate causes of the incident but also the underlying system factors, such as lack of staffing or delayed 999 responses. Insight can be created by using our experience as an HCP to contribute to the analysis of data.

Develop Recommendations or Safety Action Plans

Based on the findings of the investigation, action plans that could prevent similar incidents in the future will be implemented. As an HCP, you will be involved in the implementation of these action plans. These will address the contributing factors identified and may include changes to procedures, training, equipment or organisational culture, but should move away from blame and as an HCP, you will be required to respond to the change process.

Implementation and Monitoring, Sharing Findings and Learning

As an HCP, you may monitor the effectiveness of changes over time. Adjustments may need to be made as they are put into practice and their impact is evaluated. The NHS Patient Safety Strategy promotes the use of Patient Safety Incident Response Framework (PSIRF) to manage and learn from patient safety incidents.

IMPROVING OUTCOMES IN POLICE CUSTODY

Measurement of outcomes and quality will be identified as part of the service delivery for each provider and reported as part of contract management.

Currently, the priority is often access to healthcare monitoring the timelines, such as initial health assessments upon request and any follow-up care or referrals.

High-quality services should also consider the following:

- **Continuity of care**: Assess the effectiveness of coordination between police custody healthcare services and community healthcare providers. This may include the transfer of relevant medical information and follow-up care after their release.
- **Clinical outcomes**: Track specific health-related outcomes.
- **Patient experience**: Measure satisfaction with the healthcare services provided in police custody settings.
- **Safety incidents**: Monitor the occurrence of patient safety incidents within police custody healthcare settings, such as medication errors, adverse events, or near misses.

- **Staff experience**: Assess staff satisfaction and well-being within the police custody healthcare setting. This may include measuring staff retention, job satisfaction and perceptions of workplace safety and support.
- **Compliance with guidelines and protocols**: Evaluate the extent to which healthcare services in police custody settings adhere to established guidelines, protocols and best practices. This may include assessing the use of evidence-based practices, completion of mandatory training and audit of documentation of care.
- **Resource utilisation**: Analyse the efficiency and effectiveness of resource utilisation within police custody healthcare settings. This may involve monitoring staffing levels, use of medical supplies or other resources.
- **Mental health and alcohol/substance misuse**: Evaluate the provision and effectiveness of risk assessments within police custody, including timely identification of needs, access to appropriate care and coordination with community services upon release.

By measuring these outcomes, healthcare providers and policymakers can gain valuable insights into the quality and effectiveness of healthcare services within police custody settings. This information can then be used to guide improvements, enhance accountability and ensure the delivery of safe and effective care.

AUDIT AND CONTINUOUS IMPROVEMENT

In the UK, national clinical audits are a critical component of quality improvement across the healthcare systems. They involve the systematic collection and analysis of clinical data to assess the quality of care against established benchmarks and identify areas for improvement. The results of these audits are used to inform evidence-based practice, guide policy decisions and drive service improvement.

Several organisations are involved in coordinating and conducting national clinical audits in the UK, including the Healthcare Quality Improvement Partnership (HQIP), the Royal Colleges and other professional healthcare bodies.

National clinical audits typically focus on specific aspects of healthcare delivery, such as a particular condition (e.g. diabetes and stroke), patient population (e.g. children and older adults), or clinical intervention (e.g. surgery and medication management). They often involve the collection of data from healthcare providers across the country, allowing for the comparison of performance on a national scale. Forensic practice has lacked national clinical audit, although the work of the Forensic Science Regulator is increasingly implementing a quality management process.

Clinical audit is still in its infancy in forensic healthcare, and therefore, supporting local clinical audit is a key component of your care. Each provider will undertake local audits, and traditionally, these will include health and safety audits, medicines management audits and notes audits, but we would encourage clinical audit to become part of your own opportunity to make a difference.

The clinical audit process can be broken down into the following steps:

- **Identify a topic or issue**: Choose a specific aspect of healthcare service delivery you want to evaluate, such as a particular clinical intervention, a diagnostic test, or a care process. The topic should be relevant to your organisation and have the potential for significant improvement.

- **Define the audit criteria and standards**: Develop a clear set of criteria and standards based on evidence-based guidelines, best practices or expert consensus. These criteria will serve as the benchmark against which current practices will be compared.

- **Collect data**: Gather data on current practices related to the selected topic. This may involve reviewing medical records, observing clinical procedures, conducting interviews or administering surveys. Ensure that the data collection methods are consistent and reliable.

- **Analyse the data**: Compare the collected data against the predefined criteria and standards. Identify any gaps or discrepancies between current practices and the desired level of performance.

- **Develop an action plan**: Based on the findings of the data analysis, create a detailed action plan outlining the steps needed to improve clinical practices and close the gaps identified during the audit. The plan should include specific, measurable objectives, as well as a timeline and assigned responsibilities for each action item.

- **Implement the action plan**: Execute the action plan and make the necessary changes to clinical practices. This may involve revising policies and procedures, providing additional training, or modifying workflows.

- **Monitor and evaluate the changes**: Continuously monitor the impact of the implemented changes on clinical practices and patient outcomes. Evaluate the effectiveness of the changes by conducting follow-up audits and comparing the new data against the original criteria and standards. Adjust the action plan as needed based on the findings of the follow-up audits.

- **Share the results and lessons learned**: Communicate the results of the clinical audit and the lessons learned to relevant stakeholders. Sharing the findings can promote organisational learning and encourage the adoption of best practices across the organisation and due to the lack of

published work, we would encourage consideration of publishing your own audits.

This process promotes continuous learning, fosters a culture of improvement, and supports the delivery of safe, effective and patient-centred care, often using methodology such as PDSA cycles (Plan, Do, Study, Act).

The force, commissioners and providers should work together to ensure clinical governance arrangements enable continual improvements in the quality of patient care through effective partnership working and the auditing and monitoring of standards.

INTRODUCTION TO LEADERSHIP

Clinical leadership is essential for the effective functioning of healthcare systems. It is now recognised in our professional roles that we all play a role in leadership and that as clinical leaders, we ensure patients receive high-quality care and treatment. As an HCP, we all have leadership responsibilities ensuring we help develop and implement clinical policies and practices that improve patient outcomes, participating in quality improvement, collecting data and supporting the development of evidence-based practices, to monitor and improve the quality of care and mentoring and support others to become competent practitioners. There are three common leadership styles, see Box 17.1.

As leaders, HCPs work across police, healthcare teams and wider organisations to ensure everyone is working together effectively and as part of our role, we create a culture of collaboration and communication that enables teams to work together and enable continuity of care.

In a police forensic healthcare environment, where patients are in custody, leadership that prioritises patient safety and security is essential, but due to the need to represent human rights and consider ethical dilemmas and communication across organisations, some types of leadership may be good to explore.

HCPs all need to be self-aware to consider their own communication style and how they can influence others even in roles that sit outside management and leadership. Reflective practice is critical and this should be included in our portfolio of evidence to demonstrate ongoing professional development and to support revalidation, where applicable.

The NHS Leadership Academy has resources to build your skills in leadership, which can be available to roles outside the NHS and as a model considers nine dimensions:

- Inspiring shared purpose

- Leading with care

- Evaluating information

- Connecting our service

BOX 17.1	COMMON LEADERSHIP STYLES
Authoritarian	This style is characterised by individual control over all decisions with little input from group members. Leaders dictate policies and procedures, decide what goals are to be achieved and direct all activities to achieve these goals without any meaningful participation by the subordinates.
Democratic	Democratic leaders involve group members in the decision-making process. They encourage collaboration and ensure that each member's voice is heard before making a final decision. This style is associated with respect for team members' opinions and is used to build consensus and commitment among the team.
Laissez-faire	A hands-off approach where leaders provide little or no direction and give team members as much freedom as possible. All authority or power is given to the employees, and they must determine goals, make decisions and resolve problems on their own.
Transformational leadership	Transformational leaders inspire and motivate their teams to achieve shared goals. They encourage creativity, innovation and collaboration and foster a positive work environment.
Servant leadership	Servant leaders prioritise the needs of their team and work to serve them. They listen actively, provide support and empower their team members to achieve their full potential seeking to serve others.
Situational leadership	Situational leaders adapt their leadership style by assessing the situation and adjusting their leadership style to ensure their team can achieve its goals. In a police forensic healthcare environment, situational leaders could adapt their style to meet the unique challenges of working with patients in custody.
Distributed leadership	Distributed leadership is a style that distributes leadership roles and responsibilities across organisations. It encourages collaboration, shared decision-making and empowerment and is good to consider in relation to our close working across organisations with different professional regulatory frameworks.
Values-based leadership	Values-based leadership is a style that emphasises ethical and moral values as the foundation for decision-making. It promotes a culture of trust, respect and accountability and forms the foundation of trauma-informed care.
Place-based leadership	Place-based leadership is a style that focuses on the unique needs and characteristics of a specific location or community. It prioritises collaboration and engagement with local stakeholders, to identify and address local challenges.

- Sharing the vision
- Engaging the team
- Holding to account
- Developing capability
- Influencing for results

By developing leadership skills, we will be confident in managing differences of professional opinion, be a positive role model for those around and create a safe environment for person centred care.

CONCLUSION

In conclusion, the integration of robust NHS clinical governance principles within police custody settings, and the unique challenges and responsibilities of HCPs in such settings demand adherence to professional codes of practice with a commitment to continuous learning and skills development. This includes engaging in mandatory and statutory training, actively participating in supervisory and appraisal processes and embracing various learning, including those that support the competency of the HCP.

Central to our role as HCPs is the upholding of organisational policies and procedures and the ability to escalate concerns appropriately. This ensures that our practice not only meets the high standards set by bodies like the National Police Chiefs' Council, the Care Quality Commission and Her Majesty's Inspectorate of Constabulary or their equivalent in the four nations but also aligns with our professional responsibilities. Accurate record-keeping and documentation are critical in the criminal justice system and require meticulous attention to detail, including recording times, verbatim disclosures and examination findings.

Furthermore, demonstrating curiosity and a willingness to delve beyond surface presentations in our practice enhances our risk assessments and ongoing professional development. This approach requires us to acknowledge and mitigate biases, consider wider perspectives managing differences in professional opinion and participating in quality improvement initiatives, being receptive to new ideas and change, which are crucial components of effective clinical governance. Raising concerns and following serious incident processes are not only part of our governance obligations but also our commitment to high standards of care and patient safety.

In essence, the role of HCPs in governance within police custody settings is multifaceted and integral to delivering healthcare that is not only effective and safe but respectful of the rights and needs of those in custody. By aligning our practice with these governance standards and principles, we contribute significantly to the overarching goal of ensuring excellence in healthcare, regardless of the challenging contexts in which we operate.

LEARNING ACTIVITIES

1. Review a clinical incident that you have raised and undertake an analysis to review and identify recommendations for change.

2. Undertake a clinical audit and share the findings with your team.

3. Review a national policy or guideline that is relevant to custody to see how current practice aligns with the approach.

RESOURCES

Online

- British Medical Association | Forensic and secure environments ethics toolkit | https://www.bma.org.uk/advice-and-support/ethics/working-in-detention-settings/forensic-and-secure-environments-ethics-toolkit

- Royal College of General Practitioners | Resources for Secure Environments | https://elearning.rcgp.org.uk/mod/book/view.php?id=13151&chapterid=618#:~:text=The%20RCGP%20Secure%20Environments%20Group,the%20health%20and%20justice%20system

- Each of the regulators and police forces has its own website and can be a source of information.

Organisations

- Faculty of Forensic and Legal Medicine | www.fflm.ac.uk

- Forensic Science Regulator | https://www.gov.uk/government/organisations/forensic-science-regulator

- National Institute for Health and Care Excellence | www.nice.org.uk

- NHS Leadership Academy | https://www.leadershipacademy.nhs.uk

- UK Association of Forensic Nurses and Paramedics | www.ukafnp.org

- Royal College of Nursing | www.rcn.org.uk

REFERENCES

Angiolini, E. (2017). Reports of the independent review of deaths and serious incidents in police custody. https://assets.publishing.service.gov.uk/media/5a821d1040f0b6230269ae98/Report_of_Angiolini_Review_ISBN_Accessible.pdf (accessed 19 February 2024).

Forensic Science Regulator (2024). Guidance DNA contamination controls: forensic medical examination. https://www.gov.uk/government/publications/dna-contamination-controls-forensic-medical-examinations/dna-contamination-controls-forensic-medical-examinations-accessible#introduction (accessed 19 February 2024).

Health Services Safety Investigation Body (2024). The investigator's toolkit: SEIPS. https://www.hssib.org.uk/news-events-blog/the-investigators-toolkit-seips/ (accessed 19 April 2024).

NHS England (2019). The NHS patient safety strategy. https://www.england.nhs.uk/patient-safety/the-nhs-patient-safety-strategy/ (accessed 19 February 2024).

NHS England (2024). Health and justice. https://www.england.nhs.uk/commissioning/health-just/ (accessed 19 February 2024).

Royal College of General Practitioners (2018). Equivalence of care in secure environments. https://www.rcgp.org.uk/representing-you/policy-areas/care-in-secure-environments#:~:text=%27Equivalence%27%20is%20the%20principle%20by,environments%20are%20afforded%20provision%20of (accessed 19 February 2024).

FURTHER READING

Healthcare Quality Improvement Partnership | Best Practice in Clinical Audit | https://www.hqip.org.uk/resource/best-practice-in-clinical-audit/

NHS England | Patient Safety Incident Response Framework | https://www.england.nhs.uk/patient-safety/patient-safety-insight/incident-response-framework/

CHAPTER 18

Professional Ethics

Vanessa Webb

Nurture Health and Care Ltd, Norwich, UK

AIM

This chapter explores how the legal and ethical frameworks impact assessments in police custody. It will introduce the approach that considers how to manage risk and uncertainty in decision-making and how to record decision-making in line with their professional regulator standards and explore how Human Rights Legislation and dual obligations should form part of our critical thinking.

LEARNING OUTCOMES

Upon completion of this chapter, readers should be able to:

- Understand how ethical frameworks and legislation impact decision-making in police custody

- Explore bias and how this impacts decision-making

- Appreciate that the police work within a different professional framework to a healthcare professional (HCP)

SELF-ASSESSMENT

1. Why is decision-making in relation to healthcare different in police custody to traditional health environments?

2. List the four ethical principles in Beauchamp and Childress model.

3. Describe how confirmation bias has been reflected in your own professional practice.

INTRODUCTION

The safety and well-being of those detained in police custody are paramount and extend beyond determining the fitness to be detained and interviewed, obtaining evidential samples or documenting injuries. It includes assessment, diagnosis, treatment and referral, ensuring continuity of care, safeguarding and professional practice.

The history of forensic medicine in police custody captured in Chapter 2 – History of Forensic Science, revealed the changing landscape of professionals, which has now expanded to include forensic medical examiners and forensic HCPs. These are supported by wider multidisciplinary teams and work within a complex system of healthcare, criminal justice and social care.

Increasing human rights has been considered in the application of justice to those detained in police custody. Examples of injustice and failure to observe basic human rights or rights enshrined in statute can be read about at Inquest, a campaigning third-sector organisation campaigning for 'No More Deaths' in public sector organisations. The input of healthcare is critical, acting as advocates for those who are vulnerable and reinforces the need for HCPs to be aware of those human rights issues.

Our role requires the ability to be an agent for the court and gather medical evidence to assist in the prosecution or defence, which should be impartial and objective, whilst providing a therapeutic role and organise medical care to ensure safety and well-being of individuals, meeting professional standards and obligations.

Police Custody Healthcare for Nurses and Paramedics, First Edition. Edited by Matthew Peel, Jennie Smith, Vanessa Webb, and Margaret Bannerman.
© 2025 John Wiley & Sons Ltd. Published 2025 by John Wiley & Sons Ltd.
Companion website: www.wiley.com/go/policecustodyhealthcare

A 32-year-old male, who is a known personality disorder, was arrested due to a Public Order offence with intoxication. He is no longer intoxicated and is not withdrawing from substances, but your assessment, which included questions regarding his mental health revealed him to be suicidal, stating he has had enough of being on this Merry-go-round. He states when released, he is going to a bridge and ending things.

It is out of hours, and there are no on-site services such as Liaison and Diversion. You contact the crisis team, who state he is known to the services, and is under the community team. They believe this is a pattern of behaviour and that he would not be 'sectionable' and that he should be released as he has capacity, is aware of his behaviours and knows where to seek help if needed.

1. *The police are not accepting of this approach. What does the HCP consider?*

INTRODUCTION TO ETHICS

Ethics in healthcare plays a crucial role in guiding HCPs in making moral decisions and providing quality care to patients. It involves a set of principles and values that help navigate the complex and often challenging situations, which arise in the practice of medicine.

It encompasses the procedures, policies and principles designed to guide HCPs in their practice and helps address a wide range of moral dilemmas, including issues related to patient care, research, consent and confidentiality and provides a framework for HCPs to make decisions that are respectful, equitable and effective. It ensures patients' rights and autonomy are respected, and healthcare providers act in the best interest of their patients but also consider resource allocation and conflict of interest.

Several ethical principles guide HCPs in their decision-making process. In The Principles of Biomedical Ethics, Beauchamp and Childress (1979) listed four ethical principles: autonomy (respecting patients' right to make decisions about their care), beneficence (acting in the best interest of the patient), non-maleficence (doing no harm) and justice (fair distribution of healthcare resources).

INTRODUCTION TO LAW

Law in healthcare is a complex and multifaceted field that encompasses the legal issues related to healthcare, including medical malpractice, patient rights and healthcare legislation.

Legislation establishes the boundaries of acceptable practice, offers protection to patients and practitioners and ensures a framework for decision-making that is both ethical and just.

Criminal court deals with criminal offences, such as assault, robbery, murder, arson, rape, road traffic offences and other crimes which can result in punishment, such as imprisonment. The burden of proof in criminal cases is 'beyond a reasonable doubt', meaning the evidence must prove the defendant's guilt to a high degree of certainty.

Criminal cases start in the Magistrates' Court, with more serious cases referred to the Crown Court.

Civil Court handles disputes or problems between individuals or entities, such as contractual disputes, personal injury claims, property disputes and family law matters. The burden of proof in civil cases is usually 'preponderance of the evidence', meaning the evidence must show it is more likely than not the defendant is liable.

The Coroner's court is a specialised court that investigates the causes of unexpected, unnatural, violent, or accidental deaths. Scotland has a Fatal Accident Inquiry. It is neither criminal nor civil and does not determine guilt or liability. Coroners conduct inquiries, not trials, to determine the cause and circumstances of a person's death and may make recommendations to prevent similar deaths or accidents in the future.

Key legislation varies across the four countries but includes parallel law:

- The Health and Social Care Act governs healthcare services, embodying principles that should be reflected in police custody, including the concept of equivalency.

- The Human Rights Act incorporates European Convention rights into UK law, including the right to life and a ban on inhumane treatment, relevant to healthcare.

- The Data Protection Act aligns with the EU's GDPR and is crucial for HCPs, managing how personal data is handled and stored to maintain patient confidentiality.

- The Mental Health Act outlines the detention and treatment protocols for those with severe mental disorders, including without consent.

- The Mental Capacity Act governs decision-making for individuals who may lack capacity, focusing on best-interest decisions.

- The Children's Act emphasises child welfare and sets the foundation for child protection and care.

- The Care Act consolidates adult social care legislation, outlines local authorities' responsibilities in care provision and funding.

- The Medicines Act controls the manufacture, supply and licensing of medicines.

- The Health and Safety at Work Act mandates compliance with workplace health and safety regulations.

- The Equality Act prevents discrimination based on protected characteristics like race, gender and religion.

Across the four nations, the legislation differs, although the key principles are mirrored.

HCPs must adhere to legal frameworks but, in addition, adhere to their professional guidelines from their respective regulatory bodies, such as the General Medical Council (GMC), Nursing and Midwifery Council (NMC) and Health and Care Professionals Council (HCPC).

The police must understand numerous laws defining their roles, responsibilities and limits, which again vary across the four countries; key to these are the following:

- Police and Criminal Evidence Act (PACE) or equivalent in the four nations to outline police powers like stop and search, arrest and evidence collection.

- The Terrorism Act provides special police powers for terrorism-related situations, including suspicion-less stop and search under specific conditions.

- The Misuse of Drugs Act establishes the legal framework for controlled drugs, granting police search, seizure and arrest powers for drug-related crimes.

- The Road Traffic Act covering vehicle and driving offences, including driving under the influence, speeding and dangerous driving.

Across the four nations, the legislation differs, although the key principles are mirrored.

HEALTHCARE, LAW AND ETHICS AND THEIR INTERFACE

Forensic healthcare, especially when providing care within police custody settings, occupies a unique interface between the realms of law and healthcare. The overlap between the two domains in this context is intricate and multidimensional and can lead to differences in professional opinion.

DUTY OF CARE FOR HCPs

HCPs owe a duty of care to ensure the patients they serve receive effective, safe and high-quality care that meets the standards of our professional regulators.

Rights of the Individual are the primary focus of the healthcare duty of care with the well-being of the individual patient at the centre. This includes both their physical and mental well-being and are required to ensure valid consent, confidentiality with specific limitations and management of patients that is evidence based.

Although there are specific requirements about statutory reporting and risk to the public, these are associated with specific circumstances and do not usually inform daily practice.

DUTY OF CARE FOR POLICE OFFICERS

Police officers owe a duty of care to protect individuals and the public from harm. This can encompass a wide range of activities, from preventing crime to responding to emergencies.

The primary duty of a police officer is to protect the public, even if this sometimes means overriding the rights of an individual. For instance, detaining a suspect to prevent them from committing a crime. A significant part of their duty of care is ensuring laws are enforced and justice is served.

In conclusion, while both HCPs and police officers have a duty of care, the primary focus and how this duty manifests in practice can differ significantly based on the inherent goals and principles of each profession.

CONSENT AND THE MENTAL CAPACITY ACT

VALID CONSENT

It is a general legal and ethical principle that informed and valid consent, should be freely given by a person with the capacity to make that decision independently and must be obtained before commencing an examination, starting treatment or physical investigation, or providing care.

MENTAL CAPACITY ACT

The Mental Capacity Act (2005) and the equivalent in the four nations, has two main purposes: to protect the autonomy of individuals who have the capacity to make their own decisions and to protect those who lack capacity by ensuring their involvement in decisions relating to them and acting in their best interests.

It is underpinned by five principles:

- **Presumption of capacity**: Everyone over the age of 16 is presumed to have the capacity to make their own decisions, unless it is proven otherwise

- **Support to make a decision**: People should be given all appropriate help and support to make their own decisions

- **Ability to make unwise decisions**: People have the right to make decisions others might regard as unwise or eccentric

- **Best interest**: Anything done for, or on behalf of a person who lacks capacity must be done in their best interests

- **Least restrictive**: Anything done for, or on behalf of a person who lacks capacity should be the least restrictive of their basic rights and freedoms

See Chapter 16 – Special Circumstances for consent in children.

These principles are of such importance that they are set out at the start of the Act, before the legal test, to determine if a person lacks mental capacity. The principles aim to protect and empower individuals who may lack the mental capacity to make their own decisions about their care and treatment.

The Mental Capacity Act is guided by four key questions, which are used to determine whether a person lacks the capacity to make a **specific decision**. These questions are:

1. Can the person understand the information relevant to the decision? This question assesses whether the person can comprehend the information provided to them.

2. Can the person retain the information long enough to make the decision? This question assesses whether the person can remember the information provided to them long enough to make a decision.

3. Can the person weigh up the information to make the decision? This question assesses whether the person can use the information provided to them to weigh up the pros and cons of different options.

4. Can the person communicate their decision? This question assesses whether the person can communicate their decision in any way, such as through speech, sign language or other means.

These questions are used to determine whether a person lacks the capacity to make a specific decision. If it is determined the person lacks capacity, decisions must be made in their best interests, considering their past and present wishes, beliefs, values and any other relevant factors.

Individuals with limited decision-making ability can often be supported to make as many decisions as possible for themselves. It encourages the provision of appropriate support and assistance to help individuals understand and participate in the decision-making process.

The Mental Capacity Act and the principle of valid consent overlap. Valid Consent requires that the patient has the capacity to make decisions about their care, while the Mental Capacity Act provides a framework for assessing capacity and making decisions on behalf of individuals who lack capacity.

CONSENT AND PROFESSIONAL REGULATORS

Nursing and Midwifery Council

'It is a general legal and ethical principle that informed and valid consent, freely given by a person with the capacity to make that decision independently, must be obtained before commencing an examination, starting treatment or physical investigation, or providing care.' (NMC 2018)

General Medical Council

The GMC (2020) has seven principles in relation to consent:

Principle one: All patients have the right to be involved in decisions about their treatment and care and be supported to make informed decisions if they are able.

Principle two: Decision-making is an ongoing process focused on meaningful dialogue, the exchange of relevant information specific to the individual patient.

Principle three: All patients have the right to be listened to, and to be given the information they need to make a decision and the time and support they need to understand it.

Principle four: Doctors must try to find out what matters to patients, so they can share relevant information about the benefits and harms of proposed options and reasonable alternatives, including the option to take no action.

Principle five: Doctors must start from the presumption that all adult patients have the capacity to make decisions about their treatment and care. A patient can only be judged to lack the capacity to make a specific decision at a specific time and only after assessment in line with legal requirements.

Principle six: The choice of treatment or care for patients who lack capacity must be of overall benefit to them and decisions should be made in consultation with those who are close to them or advocating for them.

Principle seven: Patients whose right to consent is affected by law should be supported to be involved in the decision-making process and to exercise choice if possible.

This requires that relevant and accurate information be provided. This includes disclosing the nature, risks, benefits and alternatives, as well as any potential consequences of refusing.

Health and Care Professions Council

The HCPC (2021) mirror the guidance from the NMC and GMC.

'For consent to be valid, it must be voluntary and informed, and the person giving consent must have the capacity to make the decision'.

The GMC (2020), states that 'making decisions about treatment and care when a patient's right to consent is affected by law' states that a patient's right to make a healthcare decision for themselves can be affected by mental health or other legislation and by common law powers of the courts. Patients may be required by law to comply with assessment or treatment because they present a risk to themselves, to their health or to others. There are strict safeguards around using these legal powers to restrict or restrain individuals, and these determine what is permitted without consent. You should be aware of what treatment is, and is not, legally permissible.

If you consider it necessary to use these legal powers to treat or assess a patient without consent, you must follow the procedures set out in the relevant legislation, statutory guidance and paragraph 96 of the GMC (2020) guidance, see Box 18.1. If you need advice or support, you should contact your defence body, professional association or seek independent legal advice.

BOX 18.1	TAKING A PATIENT-CENTRED APPROACH

You must take a patient-centred approach even if the law allows you to assess or treat a patient without their consent. For example, you must:

a. Be polite and considerate and respect your patient's dignity and privacy.

b. Protect your patient's rights and freedoms and, if restriction or restraint is necessary, use it for the minimum time and in the least restrictive way possible.

c. Support your patient to be involved in decisions about their care, let them know if they can exercise choice about any aspect of their treatment, and respect their choices if possible.

d. Keep your patient informed about the progress of their treatment and regularly review decisions.

Source: Adapted from General Medical Council (2020).

This is an area with **no consensus in practice** in how we manage consent in a forensic environment, although the most robust document is the British Medical Association's 'Forensic Ethics Toolkit', see Resources.

The Mental Capacity Act is decision-specific, so day-to-day decisions that are low risk, and low harm usually meet the threshold that individuals have the capacity to make their own choices, whereas complex decisions may meet the threshold for a documented Mental Capacity Act assessment, which records the decisions made.

SCENARIO 18.2 Mental capacity

A 22-year-old female, with learning disabilities (known to attend a school for special educational needs) and you consider at risk of exploitation, has been found with substances which she stated she has swallowed.

The ambulance has been called to transfer her to hospital in line with your local policy for those who have swallowed substances. She refuses to go stating that she wants her interview and to go home. The ambulance staff state she has the capacity to refuse conveyance. The police are happy to hold her if you deem her fit for detention and interview.

1. *What does the HCP consider?*

CONFIDENTIALITY

Confidentiality in police custody for healthcare is subject to legal and ethical considerations. The duty of confidentiality is not absolute and disclosure of patient information may be justified in certain circumstances. Any disclosure of confidential patient information to the police must be supported by either the explicit consent of the individual concerned or be sufficiently in the public interest to warrant the disclosure.

The GMC provides guidance for doctors on confidentiality in relation to handling patient information, which can be seen on their website, and provides decision-making toolkits.

Confidentiality is an important legal and ethical duty, but it is not absolute.

- Doctors must respect patients' privacy and confidentiality and only use patient information for the purposes for which it was given.

- Doctors must disclose information if they are required to do so by law or if there is a public interest in doing so.

- Doctors must balance the duty of confidentiality with the wider duty to protect the health of the public and prevent harm.

- Doctors must ensure patients are aware of the circumstances in which their information may be disclosed.

- Doctors must ensure patient information is kept secure and not disclosed to unauthorised individuals.

- Doctors must be aware of their obligations under data protection legislation.

The GMC guidance provides a framework for considering when to disclose a patient's personal information and applies that framework to disclosures to patients, other HCPs, employers, insurers and the police.

According to the NMC (2018), confidentiality is defined as a duty owed by nurses, midwives and nursing associates, to all those who are receiving care. This includes ensuring patients' personal information is kept private and secure and only used for the purposes for which it was given. The NMC Code emphasises the importance of respecting patient's privacy and confidentiality, ensuring patients are aware of the circumstances in which their information may be disclosed.

According to the HCPC (2021), confidentiality means protecting personal information, which includes details of a service user's lifestyle, family, health and treatment. Health and care professionals have a legal obligation to handle patient's information privately and securely and to ensure patients are aware of the circumstances in which their information may be disclosed. The HCPC provides guidance on confidentiality, which includes advice on how to handle confidential information, when to disclose information and how to obtain consent. The HCPC emphasises the importance of respecting patient's privacy and confidentiality, ensuring patients' personal information is kept secure and not disclosed to unauthorised individuals.

The three professional regulating bodies all recommend the management of patient data, confidentiality similarly.

The Caldicott Principles act as a useful framework (Department of Health and Social Care 2020):

- Justify the purpose(s) for using confidential information.

- Use confidential information only when it is necessary.

- Use the minimum information that is required.

- Access to confidential information should be on a strict need-to-know basis.

- Everyone with access to confidential information must be aware of their responsibilities.

- Understand and comply with the law.

- The duty to share information can be as important as the duty to protect patient confidentiality.

- Inform patients about how their confidential information is used.

If a matter related to sharing information or confidentiality arises, ask for advice from colleagues or use your escalation processes; however, remember to consider consulting with the Caldicott Guardian.

The Faculty of Forensic and Legal Medicine (FFLM), Royal College of Nursing, United Kingdom Association of Nurses and Paramedics (UKAFNP) and Royal College of General Practitioners: Secure Environments give no additional guidance in addition to the above. The British Medical Association summarises this well in their document 'Confidentiality toolkit', see Resources.

Each police force should have an information-sharing agreement with healthcare providers embedded within the tender documentation or a policy for those employed by the police, which should clarify how and when information is provided and documented in the police custody record, with clear and unambiguous instructions given. All other information should be recorded in healthcare notes.

The Criminal Procedure and Investigations Act has Codes of Practice that require medical records to be disclosed under certain circumstances to the Crown Prosecution Service (CPS). However, in normal circumstances, health records must not be shown, or given to the police without the written consent of the patient, unless one of the exceptions applies. The Police and Criminal Evidence Act – PACE – Code H states information about a person's health must be kept confidential. The four nations have their own policies and processes. Consent is sought to ensure information can be shared in relation to their well-being in custody, but also includes if they have revealed anything relevant to the crime and the records would form part of the undisclosed material for court. The four countries will vary in their application of information governance.

Where information needs to be passed to the police concerning the individual's health and their need to be given medication, or kept under observation while in custody, only the information necessary to safely fulfil this requirement should be disclosed.

Custody officers should be provided with clear and detailed instructions about any medications needed, any additional needs and any medical reviews required, including the frequency of observations needed. In providing this information, they should bear in mind police officers are not medically qualified and cannot be expected to interpret complicated medical terminology.

Where there is a forensic or evidential potential, the purpose and use of this should be made clear to the individual being examined, with appropriate consent obtained early and any duty to disclose made clear.

The joint Police Scotland and NHS Scotland (2015) guideline considers this area of practice.

If the patient refuses to consent, an examination should not be undertaken, although observation should occur where there are any acute concerns, with advice given based on observation only.

SCENARIO 18.3   Limited assessment

You have been asked to assess a 45-year-old male for fitness to detain as he is complaining of ankle pain. You are aware that the nature of his arrest is for an attempted murder that involves knives and that the male escaped from an upstairs window and was caught in the back garden. He is not intoxicated and is able to consent to his examination.

You examine him and his Ottawa assessment indicates he requires an X-ray, which he agrees to; however, whilst assessing his leg, you notice an open wound (incision) to his calf, which he declined to give information on but is actively bleeding. You notice injuries to his knuckles on his right hand and also see there is blood on his trousers at a thigh height, but he will not let you assess his upper leg and says he will not allow documentation of injuries and refused further assessment.

1. *What does the HCP consider?*

USING A DECISION-MAKING FRAMEWORK TO SUPPORT CRITICAL THINKING

When considering complexity, professional differences of opinion, or management of risk and uncertainty, consideration should be given to the legal, regulatory or evidence-based guidance or organisational policies.

However, these may not fit the specific nature of case; therefore, an ethical framework can be considered to identify additional actions that can be considered.

Using an ethical framework like Beauchamp and Childress (1979) can support complex decision-making in healthcare in police custody.

- **Autonomy:** The principle of autonomy means the patient has the right to make their own decisions about their healthcare. In police custody, HCPs must respect the autonomy of the patient, despite the system where police detention allows little autonomy for those detained.

- **Beneficence:** The principle of beneficence means HCPs must act in the best interest of the patient. In police custody, HCPs must balance the actions requested as part of police custody and any possible harm that might result.

- **Non-maleficence:** The principle of non-maleficence means HCPs must not harm the patient. In police custody, HCPs must ensure any interventions cause minimal harm, although often the act of being in custody has a psychological impact.

- **Justice:** The principle of justice means healthcare resources should be distributed fairly, but in a police custody setting, HCPs must ensure that individuals have access to the same level of healthcare, regardless of their background, or circumstances, but also consider Human Rights, Right to Justice or Public Protection.

By applying the Beauchamp and Childress framework, HCPs can ensure they are making ethical decisions that respect the patient's rights. It can also help to provide a rational way to defend a particular course of action and assist in the analysis of the issues involved in complex decision-making, in healthcare in police custody.

Appreciating the different professional perspectives is a critical component of decision-making, enabling different viewpoints to be considered and included in decision-making.

| **SCENARIO 18.4** | Unconscious blood sample (not road traffic related) |

You have been asked to go to hospital and take bloods for toxicology from an individual who has been found in the road and is now unconscious and ventilated in intensive care due to a significant head injury.

The police feel it is important to have toxicology as this is a possible incident that has involved alcohol in both parties. There is no indication of a sexual assault and the police have stated we are the only people that can take the sample.

1. *What does the HCP consider?*

ACTING IN AN OBJECTIVE AND IMPARTIAL MANNER

As forensic HCPs, our dual obligations include those of our professional identity but also to act objectively and impartially so we can be an agent for the court.

Human brains are designed to recognise patterns, take shortcuts and use past experiences to support decision-making, which means they are liable to bias (Klocko 2016). They are risk-averse and respond to threats by creating a protective mechanism to escape danger. These, however, all impact on decision-making if humans are unaware of their presence.

More attention is paid to information easily available, as it is familiar and then we overweight memories which are more easily retrievable. This makes us likely to misdiagnose serious illness for alcohol and substance intoxication, or withdrawal and mental health issues. If we then only seek information that confirms our assessment, rather than a holistic assessment (confirmation bias), this will lead to misdiagnosis, which is a key finding in many incidents.

Once we make an initial decision or judgement, this provides a mental anchor which acts as a source of resistance to reaching a significantly different conclusion as new information becomes available. It is what happens when one has made a snap judgement and then disregards feedback that is inconsistent with this position.

Therefore, HCPs should **always undertake a full assessment** and try to exclude wider diagnosis other than the obvious, to ensure all differential diagnosis is considered and that we document our findings with neutrality (Skellern 2015).

Another important internal behaviour is to maintain a sense of control over events and the environment and we will often give greater weight to information that shows us in a favourable light (self-serving bias), or through trying to be part of the team and belong, which is a safety strategy, where we are safer in a herd; however, this means it is harder to challenge the status quo, often copying others, especially when dealing with complexity. Which can lead to copying poor practices or being compliant with police requests rather than make a decision which is unpopular (Forensic Science Regulator 2020).

The psychology of risk is an interesting bias, as we tend to avoid risks, especially if the outcome is severe and we lack control over the outcome. This means HCPs may choose not to act or choose the most risk-averse options, which can lead to the overuse of other services or delegation of decision-making to the next shift.

Get in the habit of reframing problems: Think about the information relied on for the decision – to what extent have you been biased towards information that is easily retrievable or available? How may this have affected your thinking? What other possibilities are there?

Diagnostic momentum, once labels are attached to patients, they tend to become stickier and stickier. What started as a possibility, gathers increasing momentum until it becomes permanent and other possibilities are excluded. In a repeat attendee to custody, do you assume their diagnosis is the same as last time?

Your thinking is shaped by prior assumptions and preconceptions, for example ageism, stigmatism and stereotyping:

- If this was a person who is not in custody, would you look at this the same way?

- If this person was older or younger, would you look at this the same way?

- If they were a member of your family, would you look at this the same way?

This forms the basis of reflective and reflexivity as part of HCP practice and should be recorded as part of your own learning journey and create opportunities for supervision to discuss how complexity in decision-making can challenge.

CONCLUSION

In this chapter, we have delved into the multifaceted realms of legal, ethical and professional frameworks that guide decision-making in police custody, especially from the perspective of HCPs. The intricate balance between upholding the law, adhering to ethical principles and fulfilling professional duties has been explored in detail, highlighting the unique challenges faced in the custody environment.

As HCPs, we safeguard the rights and well-being of individuals, ensuring their access to equitable healthcare services and the necessity of a multidisciplinary approach in managing their care. Through real-world scenarios, we have seen how HCPs navigate complex dilemmas, balancing the need for safety, legal obligations and the ethical imperative to do no harm.

As we conclude, it is clear that decision-making in police custody is not just about clinical assessments; it is deeply intertwined with ethical considerations, legal requirements and the professional standards set by regulatory bodies. HCPs working in this environment must be adept at critical thinking, applying ethical frameworks like Beauchamp and Childress's principles, and understanding the legal context of their work. This includes recognising the impacts of bias and striving for objectivity and impartiality in their assessments and care provision.

LEARNING ACTIVITIES

1. Use a risk template for calculating risk for a clinical dilemma and consider whether the risk is acceptable, or what actions can be put in place to mitigate risk. Alternatively, you can escalate the risk to others or halt the action by placing them as unfit to detain.

2. Reflect on a challenging case in which you felt the need for senior advice. What was the dilemma that presented and what were the legal frameworks, professional frameworks, ethical frameworks and your own critical thinking to manage this case?

RESOURCES

Online

- British Medical Association | Core ethics guidance | https://www.bma.org.uk/media/rsfly3zd/core-ethics-guidance.pdf

- British Medical Association | Forensic and secure environments ethics toolkit | https://www.bma.org.uk/advice-and-support/ethics/working-in-detention-settings/forensic-and-secure-environments-ethics-toolkit

- Royal College of Nursing | Confidentiality | https://www.rcn.org.uk/Get-Help/RCN-advice/confidentiality

Organisations

- General Medical Council |https://www.gmc-uk.org/

- Health and Care Professions Council | | https://www.hcpc-uk.org/

- INQUEST | https://www.inquest.org.uk

- Nursing and Midwifery Council https://www.nmc.org.uk/

REFERENCES

Beauchamp, T. and Childress, J. (1979). *The Principles of Biomedical Ethics*. New York: Oxford University Press.

Department of Health and Social Care (2020). The eight Caldicott principles. https://assets.publishing.service.gov.uk/media/5fcf9b92d3bf7f5d0bb8bb13/Eight_Caldicott_Principles_08.12.20.pdf (accessed 19 February 2024).

Forensic Science Regulator (2020). Cognitive bias effects. https://assets.publishing.service.gov.uk/media/5f4fc26ce90e074695f80977/217_FSR-G-217_Cognitive_bias_appendix_Issue_2.pdf (accessed 19 February 2024).

General Medical Council (2020). Decision making and consent. https://www.gmc-uk.org/professional-standards/professional-standards-for-doctors/decision-making-and-consent (accessed 19 February 2024).

Health and Care Professions Council (2021). Consent and confidentiality. https://www.hcpc-uk.org/standards/meeting-our-standards/confidentiality/guidance-on-confidentiality/ (accessed 19 February 2024).

Klocko, D.J. (2016). Are cognitive biases influencing your clinical decisions? *Clinical Reviews* 26 (3): 32–39.

Nursing and Midwifery Council (2018). The code. https://www.nmc.org.uk/globalassets/sitedocuments/nmc-publications/nmc-code.pdf (accessed 19 February 2024).

Police Scotland and NHS Scotland (2015). National guidance on the delivery of police custody healthcare and forensic medical services. http://www.knowledge.scot.nhs.uk/media/10840614/national%20guidance%20on%20the%20deliveryof%20police%20care%20healthcare%20and%20forensic%20medical%20services%20v2.0.pdf (accessed 19 February 2024).

Skellern, C. (2015). Minimising bias in the forensic evaluation of suspicious paediatric injury. *Journal of Forensic and Legal Medicine* 34 (2015): 11–16. https://doi.org/10.1016/j.jflm.2015.05.002.

FURTHER READING

Bowen, R.T. (2010). *Ethics and the Practice of Forensic Science (International Forensic Science and Investigation)*. Boca Raton, FL: CRC Press.

British Medical Association | Confidentiality toolkit | https://www.bma.org.uk/advice-and-support/ethics/confidentiality-and-health-records/confidentiality-and-health-records-toolkit

Jonsen, A.R. (2000). *A Short History of Medical Ethics*. Oxford: Oxford University Press.

Emergencies

Matthew Peel[1], Nick Hart[2], and Nick Skinner[2]

[1] Leeds Community Healthcare NHS Trust, Leeds, UK & UK Association of Forensic Nurses and Paramedics
[2] Leeds Community Healthcare NHS Trust, Leeds, UK

CHAPTER 19

AIM

This chapter aims to provide an in-depth understanding of the approach to managing a wide range of emergencies in custody, with a focus on the A-B-C-D-E approach. Readers will gain knowledge about various specific emergencies relevant to the setting and learn how to manage these situations effectively.

LEARNING OUTCOMES

Upon completion of this chapter, readers should be able to:

- Describe the A-B-C-D-E approach in emergencies and its importance in prioritising patient care

- Identify common emergencies in custody, including medical, psychiatric and substance-related conditions

- Recognise the key signs and symptoms of specific emergencies and develop strategies for effective assessment, management and escalation when necessary

SELF-ASSESSMENT

1. List three types of common emergencies you face and outline the assessment and management.

2. Outline the dose, indication, frequency and contraindications for three emergency drugs commonly available in your area. Explain how you would decide which drug to use in an emergency.

3. What are the major toxidromes (a group of signs and symptoms that collectively indicate a specific drug overdose) and their signs and symptoms. Outline the management of each toxidrome in police custody.

INTRODUCTION

There are some emergencies like acute behavioural disturbance, alcohol ketoacidosis, delirium tremens, overdose and Wernicke's encephalopathy, more likely to present in custody than in other settings due to the demographics. Some emergencies will arise from a long-term condition, such as asthma exacerbation, hypoglycaemia, hyperglycaemia and seizures. Finally, some emergencies occur suddenly and without warning, just as they do among the general population.

HCPs must have the necessary knowledge, skills and equipment to respond to emergencies. HCPs may have only some of the equipment listed in Box 19.1 and therefore, may be unable to complete all steps laid out in managing emergencies. However, this information is included to cover the varying levels of equipment available. All HCPs must be trained at Resuscitation Council UK's Immediate Life Support level for adults and basic life support for children. Training should include their local automated external defibrillator (AED) and available equipment with relevant clinical scenarios.

BOX 19.1   **EMERGENCY EQUIPMENT (VARIES LOCALLY)**

Bag	• Durable, tear-resistant, and wipeable
	• Easily identifiable and removable compartments
Protective equipment	• Personal protective equipment; gloves, aprons, gowns, eye protection, face masks
	• Sharps bin
	• Tuff-cut scissors
Airway	• Battery-operated portable suction with yankauer and catheters
	• Oropharyngeal airways ISO 5.5-10.0 (previously size: 0–4)
	• Nasopharyngeal airways (size: 5.5–7)
	• i-gel® O$_2$ Resus Pack (size: 3–5)
	• Laryngoscope
	• Magill forceps
Breathing	• Pocket mask with oxygen port
	• Bag-mask with reservoir (adult and child)
	• Catheter mount
	• Oxygen cylinder
	• Simple oxygen mask (adult and child)
	• High-concentration oxygen mask (adult and child)
	• Nebuliser mask (adult and child)
	• Large spacer for inhalers
Circulation	• AED and pads
	• Razors
	• Extremity tourniquet
	• Various dressings and bandages
	Dependent on skill mix
	• *Intravenous (IV) cannulas (size: 16–20 gauge), tourniquet and dressings*
	• *IV fluid-giving sets*
Disability	• Capillary blood glucose meter
	• Capillary blood ketone meter
Exposure	• Emergency foil blanket
	• Cling film for burns
Drugs	<u>Non-injectables</u>
	• Aspirin 300 mg tablets
	• Diazepam 10 mg/2.5 ml rectal solution or midazolam 10 mg/2 ml oromucosal solution
	• Glyceryl trinitrate 400 mcg spray
	• Salbutamol 5 mg/2.5 ml nebuliser
	• Salbutamol 100 mcg inhaler
	<u>Injectables</u>
	• Adrenaline 1 mg/1 ml (1:1000) for anaphylaxis
	• *Adrenaline 1 mg/10 ml (10,000) for cardiac arrest (if IV cannula stocked)*
	• Glucagon 1 mg
	• Naloxone 400 mcg/1 ml (or 1.8 mg nasal spray)
	• *Glucose 10% 500 ml (if IV cannula stocked)*
	• *Normal saline 0.9% 1 l (if IV cannula stocked)*

Because emergencies will involve police staff, regular cardiac arrest drills may improve teamwork.

AMBULANCE TRANSPORT

Most of the emergencies described in this chapter warrant an ambulance. Ambulance services sometimes operate a limited service, prioritising Category 1 calls such as cardiac arrest, anaphylaxis, life-threatening asthma, obstetric emergencies, airway compromise and cardiovascular collapse (including septic shock). Meaning other calls are delayed or not responded to. HCPs facing such delays should first discuss their concerns with the ambulance service. In the event of an unsatisfactory response, the HCP needs to consider the risks and benefits of a clinically unsupervised transport by police to hospital or remaining in custody. These are complex decisions; Box 19.2 outlines an approach to documenting such decisions.

SCENARIO 19.1	Ambulance transport

You were summoned to an unconscious 53-year-old male in a cell with a blood glucose of 1.5 mmol/L. He was initially unresponsive and very sweaty. You requested an ambulance and administered 1 mg of glucagon. His blood glucose is now 5.4 mmol/l; they have a history of type 1 diabetes but are otherwise well. They are still sweaty and a little confused about time and place. They are a little tachycardic and hypertensive, but otherwise, observations are normal. The ambulance was called 37 minutes ago and they cannot give you any idea when they might arrive; it could be several hours.

1. *Outline your approach to this assessment.*

2. *Outline the risk and benefits of police transferring him to hospital.*

3. *Outline the risk and benefits of waiting for the ambulance.*

CARDIAC ARREST

Nationally, most adult out-of-hospital cardiac arrests are due to a cardiac issue. However, in custody, they are a mix of natural, substance misuse and self-harm. Among children,

BOX 19.2	DOCUMENTING DECISIONS

I have requested an ambulance, but they are unable to provide an ambulance in a satisfactory timeframe due to excessive demand. They are currently prioritising Category 1 calls only. I have discussed with the custody officer the risks and benefits of police transporting to hospital or keeping the patient here. We both agreed the least risky option is for police to make the 10-minute journey to the hospital, rather than risking the patient deteriorating and running out of oxygen.

the primary cause is hypoxia from a secondary illness (i.e. asthma or choking).

MANAGEMENT

Management differs between adults and children (see Figures 19.1 and 19.2). However, the primary focus is recognition, getting help, high-quality, minimally interrupted chest compressions and early defibrillation. HCPs may be the only HCP present and must lead and direct others, see Figure 19.3.

Airway and Ventilation

Take a stepwise approach to the airway. If an i-gel is inserted, deliver uninterrupted chest compressions and ventilate 10 breaths per minute (or 10–15 breaths per minute for children). In the event of a significant air leak, revert to minimally interrupted chest compressions.

Chest compressions Perform high-quality, minimally interrupted chest compressions at a rate of 100–120 per minute to a depth of 5 cm (or one-third of the chest depth for children). For children, depending on their size, use one or two hands. Allocate two chest compression operators, rotated every two minutes. If resuscitation is prolonged, operators may need to be changed.

Defibrillation AEDs are designed to be used without specialist training. Attach pads as directed and follow commands. When delivering a shock, the bag-mask should be kept at least one metre away from the chest unless attached to an i-gel.

Adult pads can be used on children over 8 years old. Pads should be placed as directed unless there is little separation, where one pad should be placed in the centre of the chest and one on the back.

Identify and Treat Any Reversible Causes

While resuscitation efforts are ongoing, assess and treat any reversible causes.

SCENARIO 19.2	Cardiac arrest

You are summoned to a cell with a 27-year-old male who was found not breathing and without a pulse on a routine cell check. He has been in custody 6 hours and according to his risk assessment, he has a history of drug use and epilepsy. CPR is already being performed and you note vomit in the mouth.

1. *Outline your immediate priorities.*

2. *Consider the reversible causes and comment on their likelihood and management.*

3. *Outline your responsibilities post-incident (i.e. transported to hospital).*

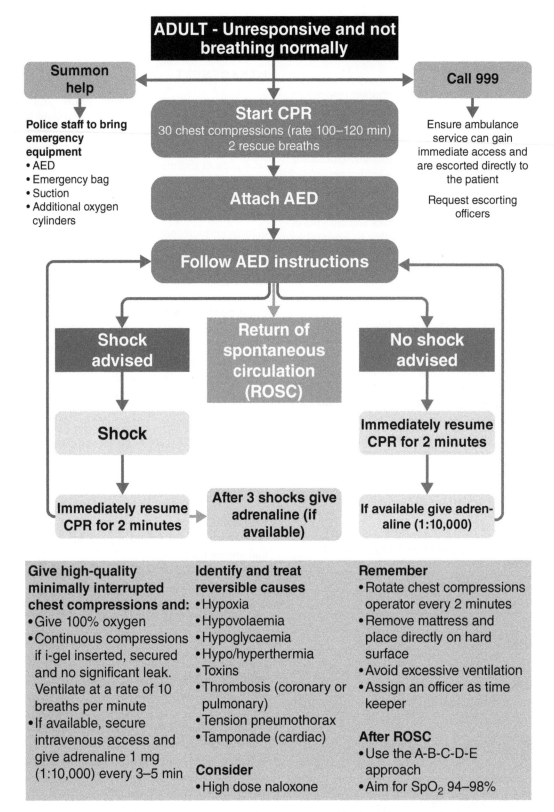

ADULT - Unresponsive and not breathing normally

Summon help

Police staff to bring emergency equipment
• AED
• Emergency bag
• Suction
• Additional oxygen cylinders

Call 999

Ensure ambulance service can gain immediate access and are escorted directly to the patient

Request escorting officers

Start CPR
30 chest compressions (rate 100–120 min)
2 rescue breaths

Attach AED

Follow AED instructions

Shock advised

Return of spontaneous circulation (ROSC)

No shock advised

Shock

Immediately resume CPR for 2 minutes

Immediately resume CPR for 2 minutes

After 3 shocks give adrenaline (if available)

If available give adrenaline (1:10,000)

Give high-quality minimally interrupted chest compressions and:
• Give 100% oxygen
• Continuous compressions if i-gel inserted, secured and no significant leak. Ventilate at a rate of 10 breaths per minute
• If available, secure intravenous access and give adrenaline 1 mg (1:10,000) every 3–5 min

Identify and treat reversible causes
• Hypoxia
• Hypovolaemia
• Hypoglycaemia
• Hypo/hyperthermia
• Toxins
• Thrombosis (coronary or pulmonary)
• Tension pneumothorax
• Tamponade (cardiac)

Consider
• High dose naloxone

Remember
• Rotate chest compressions operator every 2 minutes
• Remove mattress and place directly on hard surface
• Avoid excessive ventilation
• Assign an officer as time keeper

After ROSC
• Use the A-B-C-D-E approach
• Aim for SpO_2 94–98%

FIGURE 19.1 Adult life support algorithm. *Source:* Based on Resuscitation Council (UK) Adult Advanced Life Support Algorithm.

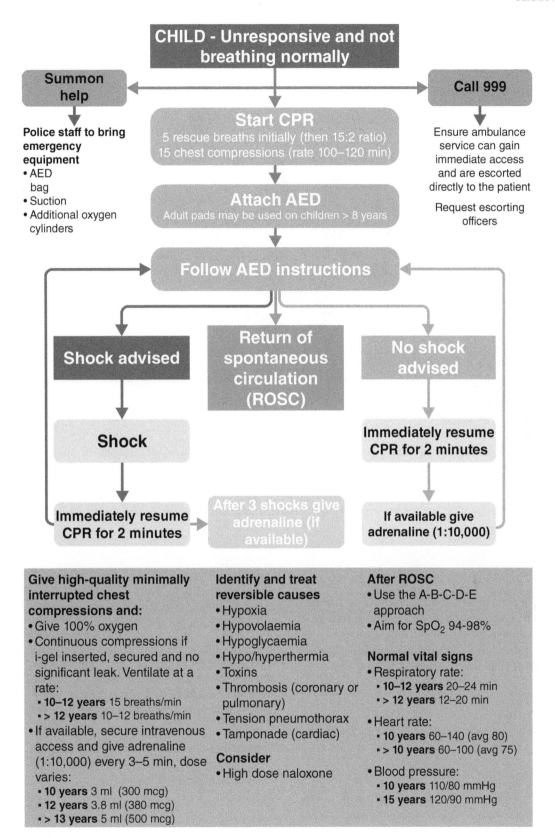

FIGURE 19.2 Child cardiac arrest algorithm. *Source:* Based on Resuscitation Council (UK) Paediatric Advanced Life Support Algorithm.

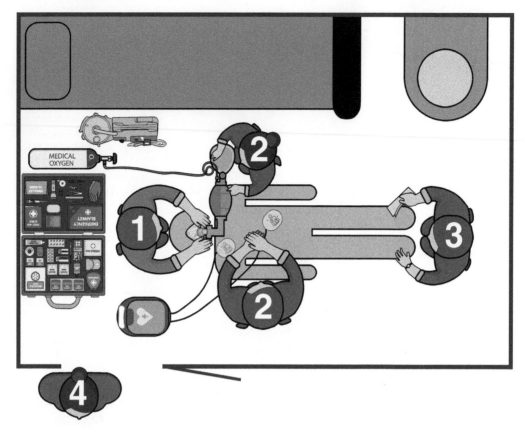

FIGURE 19.3 Resuscitation pit crew approach. 1 – HCP: The HCP bases themselves at the head, taking control of the airway, defibrillation and overseeing ventilation. Equipment should be within arm's reach. In the absence of another HCP, they lead the resuscitation. 2 – CPR operators (police staff): Two individuals rotated every two minutes. When not delivering chest compressions, operate bag-mask. 3 – Timekeeper (police staff) / Resus lead (if second HCP): Ensures CPR operators rotate every two minutes and make notes as directed by the HCP. If a second HCP, they lead the resuscitation. 4 – Runner (police staff): Prevents unnecessary crowding. Arrange additional equipment or staff and liaises with others as needed.

A-B-C-D-E APPROACH

The A-B-C-D-E approach is a systematic method for assessing and managing emergencies by focusing on Airway, Breathing, Circulation, Disability and Exposure. It is a framework to prioritise care, allowing for rapid and accurate identification of life-threatening conditions and timely interventions.

AIRWAY

The airway is always the first concern, assuming no catastrophic haemorrhage.

Assessment

Begin by looking and listening, someone sitting up talking is reassuring. However, someone unresponsive and making snoring noises requires immediate intervention.

Management

Take a stepwise approach, initially using basic manoeuvres like jaw thrust or head-tilt-chin-lift, followed by adjuncts like the nasopharyngeal (NPA) or oropharyngeal (OPA) airway, if necessary, see Figure 19.4. The most definitive airway device in custody will be an i-gel. Suction may be needed to clear fluid or vomit in the airway.

Nasopharyngeal airway The NPA can be used with semiconscious and unconscious individuals and is useful where the teeth are clenched. Typically, a 6–7 mm NPA is suitable for adults. In children, measure from the nostril to the tragus.

Oropharyngeal airway The OPA can be used with unconscious individuals. To size, measure from the middle of the incisors to the angle of the jaw.

i-gel Individuals deeply unconscious or in cardiac arrest will tolerate an i-gel, a second-generation supraglottic airway. I-gels allow for improved ventilation with a reduced risk of aspiration. They are relatively straightforward to insert and are sized according to weight, with three different adult weight options available.

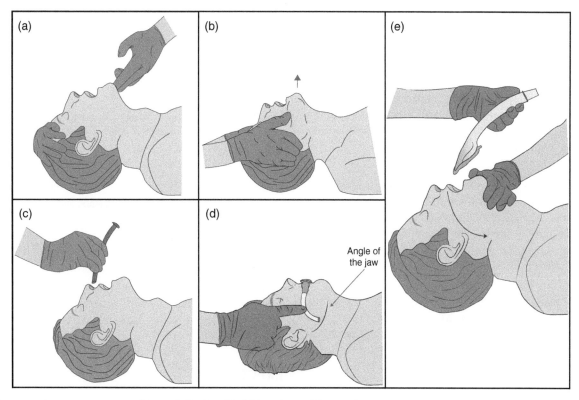

FIGURE 19.4 Airway management. (a) Head-tilt-chin-lift, (b) jaw thrust, (c) nasopharyngeal airway, (d) oropharyngeal airway and (e) i-gel.

BREATHING

Once the airway is safe, assess and manage breathing.

Assessment

Box 19.3 outlines the approach to a rapid breathing assessment.

BOX 19.3	RAPID BREATHING ASSESSMENT
Look	• Respiratory rate?
	• Equal chest movement?
	• Cyanosis?
	• Accessory muscle use?
	• Patient's position?
	• Oxygen saturations?
Listen	• Talking (full sentences or single words)?
	• Audibles wheeze or crackles?
Feel	• Is the trachea deviated?

Management

Management focuses on improving oxygenation and ventilation (breathing), including positioning to promote effective breathing.

Oxygen Unwell individuals breathing spontaneously with SpO$_2$ <94% should receive oxygen via a simple facemask or high-concentration facemask titrated to SpO$_2$ 94–98%. Simple facemasks should be started at 5 l/min, and high-concentration facemasks 10 l/min; ensure the reservoir bag is filled before applying.

Ventilation The bag-mask is a self-inflating bag used to manually ventilate in the event of critical hypoxia, inadequate respiratory effort or respiratory/cardiac arrest. Ventilation using the bag-mask is a two-person procedure. One maintains the airway using jaw thrust (or head-tilt-chin-lift) and creates a seal between the mask and the mouth and nose; another squeezes the bag to see the chest rise. Ventilate adults at a rate of 10 per minute and children 10–15 per minute unless in cardiac arrest (see Cardiac arrest).

CIRCULATION

Once breathing is optimised, move to circulation.

Assessment

Box 19.4 outlines a rapid circulation assessment.

Management

Management will depend on the complaint. For example, if there is heavy bleeding, the focus will be on controlling the bleeding. If chest pain, the management will focus on aspirin, nitrates and oxygen.

Intravenous access If able and competent, secure IV access if critically ill, at risk of cardiac arrest, or requiring IV medication or fluids. Alternatively, intraosseous may offer a quick and reliable route. It is easier to learn and maintain than IV cannulation, which is important when HCPs will only rarely have to perform (Petitpas et al. 2016).

Fluid resuscitation Acutely unwell, hypovolaemic (systolic blood pressure <100 mmHg, heart rate >90 bpm or delayed capillary refill time) individuals may require fluid resuscitation. If available, adults should receive 500 ml of normal saline over 15 minutes, repeated if necessary.

DISABILITY

Once satisfied with circulation, assess disability.

Assessment

Box 19.5 outlines a rapid disability assessment.

BOX 19.4	RAPID CIRCULATION ASSESSMENT
Look	• Colour (pale, cyanosed)?
	• Sweaty?
	• Bleeding?
	• Capillary refill time?
Listen	• Confused?
	• Chest pain?
	• Palpitations?
	• Blood pressure
Feel	• Pulse (radial, femoral or carotid)?
	• Bounding, thready and irregular?
	• Cold?
	• Clammy?

BOX 19.5	RAPID DISABILITY ASSESSMENT
Look	• Pupils
	• Blood glucose level
	• ACVPU (alert, new confusion, responds to voice, pain or unresponsive)
Listen	• Get a summary of the police risk assessment, custody record and recent checks
	• Speech normal? Slurred? Confused?
Feel	• Are they moving all limbs and head?

Management

Unconscious individuals should be placed in the recovery position. Further management will depend on the complaint but may include correcting hypoglycaemia or reversing opioids with naloxone.

EXPOSURE

Once disability is optimised, move to exposure.

Assessment

Box 19.6 outlines a rapid exposure assessment.

Management

Management will depend on the assessment. Efforts should be made to keep individuals warm and dignity maintained.

Early Warning Scores

HCPs are encouraged to measure vital signs against the National Early Warning Score (version 2) (NEWS2) (see Figure 19.5). A Custody Early Warning Score (CEWS) was developed by Border Force and adopted by other forces for use by custody staff (not HCPs). Miles et al. (2020) studied the NEWS2 and CEWS in custody and found a small correlation between increased scores and hospital referrals. However, they also noted high-risk conditions like chest pain or concealing drugs, were associated with low scores, which may be

BOX 19.6	RAPID EXPOSURE ASSESSMENT
Look	• Examine head-to-toe for any wounds or injuries
	• Check a temperature
Listen	• Do they have any complaints? Pain?
Feel	• Are they warm? Cold? Clammy

Physiological parameter	Score						
	3	2	1	0	1	2	3
Respiratory rate (per minute)	≤8		9–11	12–20		21–24	≥25
SpO₂ Scale 1 (%)	≤91	92–93	94–95	≥96			
SpO₂ Scale 2 (%)	≤83	84–85	86–87	88–92 ≥93 on air	93–94 on oxygen	95–96 on oxygen	≥97 on oxygen
Air or oxygen?		Oxygen		Air			
Systolic blood pressure (mmHg)	≤90	91–100	101–110	111–219			≥220
Pulse (per minute)	≤40		41–50	51–90	91–110	111–130	≥131
Consciousness				Alert			CVPU
Temperature (°C)	≤35.0		35.1–36.0	36.1–38.0	38.1–39.0	≥39.1	

FIGURE 19.5 National early warning score 2. *Source:* Adapted from Royal College of Physicians, 2017.

falsely reassuring. However, the study relied on a single score recorded on arrival and not as the NEWS2 is intended, monitoring repeated measurements over time.

Additionally, NEWS2 is an established tool used across Ambulance services and Acute Hospital Trusts, providing a standard language for communicating the severity of acute illness. However, there are some limitations. The tool relies on measuring all vital signs to prevent under-calculating the patient's true condition. In the context of police custody healthcare, it is noteworthy that sedatives, including methadone and buprenorphine, can depress blood pressure and pulse, rendering NEWS2 less reliable as an indicator of deterioration or acute illness. Thus, HCPs should not solely rely on NEWS2 but also on their clinical intuition. If a patient appears unwell, immediate action is warranted, regardless of their NEWS2. Conversely, it is equally important to comprehensively assess patients who may have high NEWS2 scores but appear well to ensure no underlying conditions are missed.

ACUTE BEHAVIOURAL DISTURBANCE

Acute behavioural disturbance (ABD) is an emergency characterised by extreme agitation, hyperthermia, hostility and exceptional strength without fatigue. It is most common among overweight men in their mid-thirties who frequently misuse stimulants. It is not a diagnosis but a spectrum of agitation. Complications include rhabdomyolysis, hyperkalaemia,

disseminated intravascular coagulation, metabolic acidosis, death and injury.

PATHOPHYSIOLOGY

The pathophysiology is unclear but likely a mixed physiological and psychological condition involving excessive adrenaline, noradrenaline and dopamine – increasing heart rate, blood pressure and respiratory rate, which contributes to their strength and near-constant activity. As a result, some develop metabolic acidosis, generating a strong drive to hyperventilate, reducing carbon dioxide and improving blood pH. However, restraint may impede hyperventilating, preventing carbon dioxide's 'blow off', which in severe metabolic acidosis may precipitate cardiac arrest. This may explain why some individuals report being unable to breathe when they are observed breathing hard and fast. Rather, individuals may be expressing their inability to hyperventilate and worsening acidosis.

SIGNS AND SYMPTOMS

Recognising ABD is essential to initiate appropriate management. Signs and symptoms vary and are non-specific. ABD should be considered where individuals present with two or more consensus features (Humphries et al. 2024), Box 19.7. However, the greater the number of signs and symptoms, the greater the severity.

| BOX 19.7 | ABD CONSENSUS FEATURES |

- Bizarre behaviour
- Extreme aggression
- Extreme agitation
- Near-constant physical activity
- Appears disorientated
- Exceptional strength
- Raised heart rate
- Hot to touch
- Sweating profusely
- Restrained for 15 minutes without de-escalation
- Unable to sit or stand still
- Presentation of aggression or hostility appears atypical
- Does not respond to other people being present
- Fails to improve with verbal de-escalation
- The behaviour is not explained by other factors

MANAGEMENT

Management is challenging, with the focus being de-escalation, containment, pre-rapid tranquillisation and transfer to the hospital (if necessary). Although there are differences in approaches, those with symptoms or unresponsive to oral lorazepam are unfit to detain.

De-escalation

Identify and mitigate any ongoing causes of agitation, such as loosening restraints. Communicate calmly, compassionately and respectfully while maintaining non-threatening body language. HCPs have an important role in de-escalating the individual and the police, who may also be highly charged.

Containment

Containment rather than restraint is essential, minimising risk to the individual and police. It allows individuals an opportunity to settle, de-escalating the situation. Restraint should be reserved for specific purposes, such as moving to a cell or preventing serious harm and undertaken for the minimum time necessary. Avoid restraint solely to prevent violence when containment is available. Custody officers may worry about the increased risk of self-harm. However, it must be stressed restraint is dangerous and carries significant risks. Cells provide an ideal environment for containment without stimuli, dimmed lights and monitored remotely via CCTV. If individuals are hot, cells should be cooled or moved to an exercise yard.

Pre-rapid Tranquilisation

If de-escalation and containment fail, the Faculty of Forensic & Legal Medicine (2019) recommends 1–2 mg oral lorazepam. However, those at the extreme end of the spectrum may not accept or respond sufficiently. More recently, ABD has been recognised by ambulance services as an emergency, with some specialist paramedics able to administer parental sedation in such circumstances.

Transfer to Hospital (If Necessary)

Ideally, transport to the hospital via ambulance. However, where the individual remains highly aggressive, a police van may be preferable, with the ambulance following.

| SCENARIO 19.3 | Acute behavioural disturbance |

You are asked to see someone in the holding cell. The custody officer is concerned because he appears very aggressive and is fighting restraints and they are worried it is ABD. In the holding cell, you see a large adult male being restrained by six officers, who look stressed, tired and sweaty. The male is making loud noises; it is possible to make out the odd word. He is very sweaty and feels warm. You cannot get any vital signs from him. The officer reports he has been like this for about 45 minutes.

1. *Outline your approach to this assessment.*

2. *Outline the risk(s) to:*
   b. *The individual.*
   c. *The police.*

3. *What are your prioritises?*

4. *Outline your management of this scenario.*

ALCOHOLIC KETOACIDOSIS

Alcoholic ketoacidosis is a serious metabolic complication that can occur following a binge of alcohol. It is characterised by increased ketones (ketosis) and decreased blood pH (acidosis). Alcoholic ketoacidosis can be a life-threatening condition if not properly recognised and treated.

SIGNS AND SYMPTOMS

Alcoholic ketoacidosis can present with a wide range of symptoms:

- Nausea and vomiting
- Abdominal pain

- Dehydration

- Rapid and deep breathing

- Confusion

- Fatigue and weakness

- Capillary ketones ≥ 0.6 mmol/l or urinary ketones ++/+++/++++

Devices designed for measuring ketones in diabetes can be used to measure ketones in suspected alcoholic ketoacidosis. Diagnosis is based on a combination of history, examination, and raised ketones. Capillary ketones ≥ 0.6 mmol/l indicate some degree of ketosis, while levels ≥ 1.5 mmol/l suggest a more severe state of ketosis. Similarly, the greater the presence of urinary ketones, the greater the degree of ketosis.

MANAGEMENT

Treatment typically involves IV fluids and electrolyte replacement in a hospital setting. Therefore, individuals are unfit to be detained in custody.

ANAPHYLAXIS

Anaphylaxis is a life-threatening allergic reaction, with a rapid onset of airway constriction, difficulty breathing, circulation problems such as hypotension and tachycardia and skin changes such as a rash, angioedema and itchy skin. Prompt recognition and treatment with intramuscular adrenaline and airway and breathing management, are priorities to save lives. Common triggers include food and insect stings/venom. However, in 30% of cases, the trigger is unknown (Resuscitation Council UK 2021).

If anaphylaxis is suspected, call **999**, stating 'Anaphylaxis' triggering a category one response from the ambulance service.

SIGNS AND SYMPTOMS

Anaphylaxis should be suspected with any of the following (Resuscitation Council UK 2021):

- Rapid onset and progression of symptoms (see Box 19.8)

- Life-threatening airway, breathing or circulatory concern

- Sudden onset of skin changes such as rash, flushing, urticaria and swelling (angioedema)

- Signs of shock

MANAGEMENT

See Figure 19.6 for the management of anaphylaxis. The priority is early intramuscular adrenaline. Some individuals may carry adrenaline auto-injectors (i.e. EpiPen®, Emerade® or Jext®); these should only be used if no other suitable

BOX 19.8	ANAPHYLAXIS SYMPTOMS
Airway	• Tongue or throat swelling
	• Difficulty swallowing
	• Hoarse voice
	• Stridor
Breathing	• Shortness of breath
	• Difficulty breathing or tachypnoea
	• Stridor, wheeze or bronchospasm
	• SpO₂ < 92%
	• Cyanosis
	• Confusion/ agitation secondary to hypoxia
	• Respiratory fatigue or arrest
Circulatory	• Pale and clammy presentation
	• Hypotension
	• Tachycardia
	• Feeling faint/dizzy
	• Decreased level of consciousness
	• Bradycardia (late-onset symptom)
	• Cardiac arrest
Other	• Vomiting or diarrhoea
	• Abdominal cramps or pains
	• Rash – urticarial or hives
	• Swelling or angioedema
	• Itchy skin
	• Anxiety

adrenaline preparation is available.[1] Serial observations and cardiorespiratory assessment must be taken throughout. All cases of suspected anaphylaxis will need to be referred to the hospital.

Avoid rapid changes in posture; the patient should remain in a semi-recumbent position during treatment. If the patient feels faint, advise them not to move position; any sudden movements can lead to cardiac arrest.

Salbutamol

Administer nebulised 5 mg salbutamol,[2] oxygen-driven,[3] if wheeze, bronchospasm or respiratory distress noted, if available (Resuscitation Council UK 2021).

---

[1] Auto-injectors only deliver 300 mcg adrenaline, with some devices prone to administration failures.
[2] For adults and children over 5-years-old.
[3] A flow rate of 6 l/min is needed to drive most nebulisers.

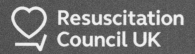

Anaphylaxis

Anaphylaxis?

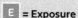

| A = Airway | B = Breathing | C = Circulation | D = Disability | E = Exposure |

Diagnosis – look for:

- Sudden onset of Airway and/or Breathing and/or Circulation problems[1]
- And usually skin changes (e.g. itchy rash)

Call for HELP
Call resuscitation team or ambulance

- Remove trigger if possible (e.g. stop any infusion)
- Lie patient flat (with or without legs elevated)
  - A sitting position may make breathing easier
  - If pregnant, lie on left side

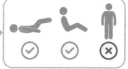

Give intramuscular (IM) adrenaline[2]

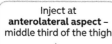
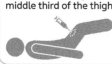

Inject at **anterolateral aspect – middle third of the thigh**

- Establish airway
- Give high flow oxygen
- Apply monitoring: pulse oximetry, ECG, blood pressure

If no response:
- Repeat IM adrenaline after 5 minutes
- IV fluid bolus[3]

If no improvement in Breathing or Circulation problems[1] despite TWO doses of IM adrenaline:
- Confirm resuscitation team or ambulance has been called
- Follow REFRACTORY ANAPHYLAXIS ALGORITHM

1. Life-threatening problems

Airway
Hoarse voice, stridor

Breathing
↑work of breathing, wheeze, fatigue, cyanosis, SpO$_2$ <94%

Circulation
Low blood pressure, signs of shock, confusion, reduced consciousness

2. Intramuscular (IM) adrenaline
Use adrenaline at 1 mg/mL (1:1000) concentration

Adult and child >12 years:	500 micrograms IM (0.5 mL)
Child 6–12 years:	300 micrograms IM (0.3 mL)
Child 6 months to 6 years:	150 micrograms IM (0.15 mL)
Child <6 months:	100–150 micrograms IM (0.1–0.15 mL)

The above doses are for IM injection **only**.
Intravenous adrenaline for anaphylaxis to be given **only by experienced specialists** in an appropriate setting.

3. IV fluid challenge
Use crystalloid

Adults:	500–1000 mL
Children:	10 mL/kg

FIGURE 19.6 Anaphylaxis management. *Source:* Reproduced from Emergency treatment of anaphylaxis; Guidelines for healthcare providers, 2021 / with permission of Resuscitation Council (UK).

ASTHMA (ACUTE EXACERBATION)

Asthma exacerbations can present as shortness of breath, wheezing, coughing and chest tightness (Scottish Intercollegiate Guidelines Network and British Thoracic Society 2019).

A full assessment should be undertaken, including peak expiratory flow (PEF), subjective and objective symptoms of respiratory distress and auscultation of lung fields (if able). Clinical assessment should identify the severity of the episode and guide management.

MILD ASTHMA

Mild asthma presents with none of the features of moderate, severe or life-threatening asthma.

Management

- Move to a quiet and calm environment.
- Two puffs (100 mcg) salbutamol inhaler.
- If fails to improve treat as 'moderate'.

MODERATE, SEVERE AND LIFE-THREATENING ASTHMA

See Figures 19.7 and 19.8 for the management of adults and children with moderate, severe or life-threatening asthma. While adults with severe asthma responding to treatment may remain fit to detain,[4] children should be referred to a hospital. All cases of life-threatening asthma will require an emergency ambulance and referral to the hospital.

CARDIAC CHEST PAIN

Cardiac chest pain can be broadly characterised as either stable angina, which may be managed in custody (see Chapter 8 – Minor Illness) or an acute coronary syndrome (ACS), which cannot. ACS includes myocardial infarction (heart attack) and unstable angina caused by a partial or total occlusion of the coronary arteries, usually by a thrombus.[5] Suspected ACS requires rapid transport to the hospital by ambulance.

SIGNS AND SYMPTOMS

ACS can present with a range of symptoms and not the typically described chest pain radiating in the left arm and jaw (see Box 19.9). Females and those with diabetes may present with vague or atypical signs. For this reason, HCPs should have a high index of suspicion for ACS in any unexplained chest pain or breathing difficulty.

MANAGEMENT

Management is primarily supportive whilst awaiting the ambulance, see Figure 19.9. Keep the individual calm and seated or semi-recumbent to avoid stress or exertion. Because of the risk of cardiac arrest, have the AED collected. Other treatment options may include oxygen, aspirin and glyceryl trinitrate.

DELIRIUM TREMENS

Delirium tremens is an emergency with mortality up to 35% if left untreated. It occurs during alcohol withdrawal and represents the most extreme form of the condition.

SIGNS AND SYMPTOMS

Symptoms start 48–96 hours following the last alcoholic drink. In addition to the typical alcohol withdrawal signs and symptoms, individuals may present with the following:

- Confusion
- Disorientation
- Fever
- Hallucinations (typically tactile or visual)
- Hyperreflexia (over responsive reflexes)
- Hypertension (later stages may develop hypotension)
- Sinister delusions

MANAGEMENT

Delirium tremens can only be safely managed in a hospital and individuals should be urgently referred.

HYPO/HYPERGLYCAEMIA

Complications associated with blood glucose levels outside accepted levels can give rise to emergencies in custody.

HYPOGLYCAEMIA

Hypoglycaemia is a BGL < 4.0 mmol/l. Mild hypoglycaemia is an episode in which individuals self-treat (able to swallow) and severe hypoglycaemia when requiring third-party intervention (unable to swallow).

Signs and Symptoms

Box 19.10 outlines the signs any symptoms of hypoglycaemia.

---

[4] The exception being pregnancy. All pregnant patients with severe asthma should be referred to the hospital immediately.
[5] Cocaine can cause coronary artery spasm and occlusion.

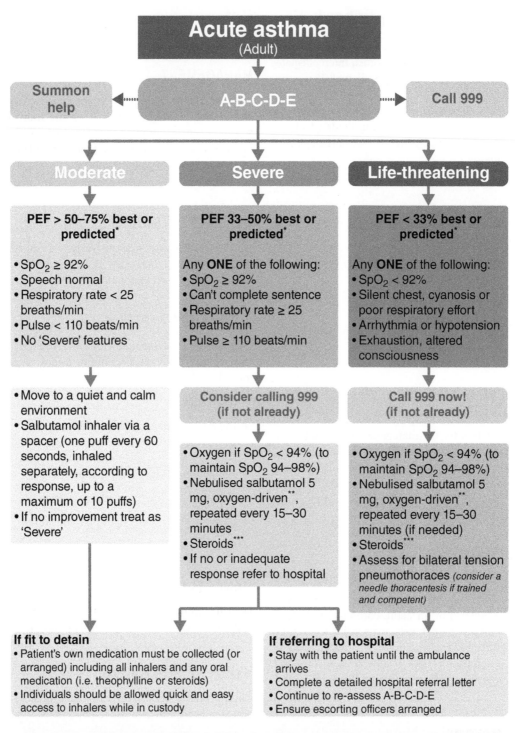

FIGURE 19.7 Asthma management (adult). *Source:* Adapted from Scottish Intercollegiate Guidelines Network and British Thoracic Society (2019).

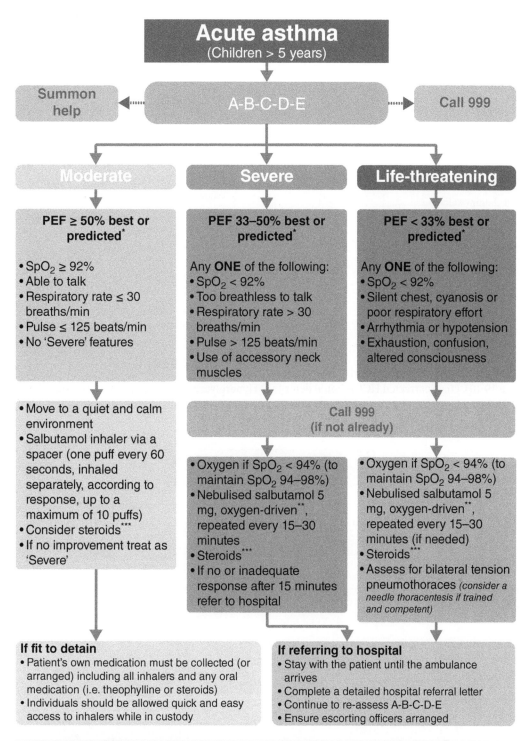

FIGURE 19.8 Asthma management (child). *Source:* Adapted from Scottish Intercollegiate Guidelines Network and British Thoracic Society (2019).

BOX 19.9	ACUTE CORONARY SYNDROME SIGNS AND SYMPTOMS

- Central chest pain
  - Dull, aching, pressure or crushing
  - Radiating arm(s), back, neck or jaw
  - Gradual onset over several minutes
  - Unaffected by inhalation/exhalation
- Pale, cold and clammy skin
- Nausea and vomiting
- Breathing difficulties
- Palpitations
- A sense of impending doom

BOX 19.10	SYMPTOMS OF HYPOGLYCAEMIA

Adrenergic	Neuroglycopenic
• Sweating	• Confusion
• Palpitations	• Drowsiness leading to coma
• Tremor	• Altered behaviour
• Anxiety	• Aggression
• Numbness	• Difficulty speaking
• Headache	• Unsteady on feet
• Nausea	

Management

The primary focus after A-B-C-D-E is correcting the blood glucose (see Figure 19.10). Once corrected HCPs should determine the reason for hypoglycaemia and the need for hospital or further monitoring, see Box 19.11 for an example of hyperglycaemia managment.

HYPERGLYCAEMIA

Hyperglycaemia is a BGL above 14.0 mmol/l. Hyperglycaemic type 1 diabetics are at risk of developing Diabetic Ketoacidosis

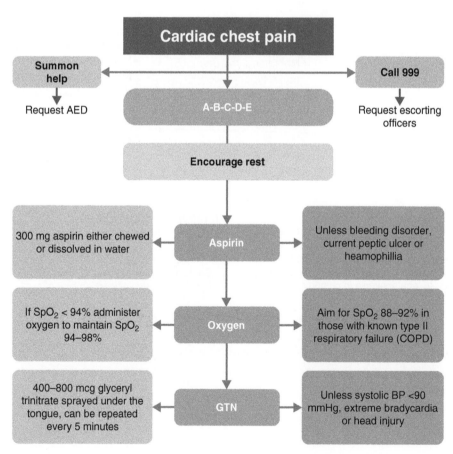

FIGURE 19.9 ACS management.

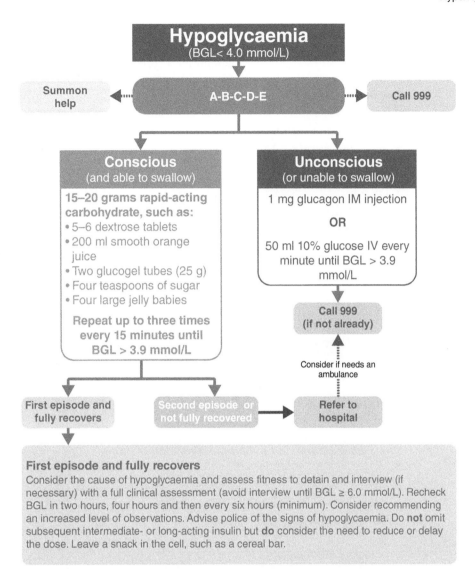

FIGURE 19.10 Hypoglycaemia management.

BOX 19.11	HYPOGYLCAEMIA RISK FACTORS

- Earlier hypoglycaemia
- Impaired hypoglycaemia awareness
- Infection/sepsis
- Increased exercise
- Alcohol
- Vomiting or diarrhoea
- Missed or late meals
- Less carbohydrate than normal
- No access to snacks between meals

(DKA) and type 2 diabetics are at risk of both DKA and hyperosmolar hyperglycaemic state (HHS).

Signs and Symptoms

The signs and symptoms associated with DKA and HHS are listed in Box 19.12.

Management

Management depends on the type of diabetes, the BGL and the presence of any red flags, see Figure 19.11. Individuals with evidence of DKA or HHS, should be referred to hospital. Capillary blood ketone meters may be helpful in differentiating between simple hyperglycaemia and DKA, providing a more accurate reflection of ketones than urinary ketones.

For simple hyperglycaemia without raised ketones or red flags, the priority should be correcting their BGL. This will

BOX 19.12	SIGNS AND SYMPTOMS DKA AND HHS

Diabetic ketoacidosis	Hyperosmolar hyperglycaemic state
• Thirsty	• Thirsty
• Increased urination	• Increased urination
• Abdominal pain	• Nausea
• Nausea or vomiting	• Dry skin
• Diarrhoea	• Disorientation leading to loss of consciousness
• Increased respiratory rate/depth	
• Blurred vision	
• Acetone breath	

depend on their type of diabetes and current medication regimen. Individuals prescribed a rapid-acting insulin may administer a correction dose. There are numerous formulas for calculating correction doses and individuals may have their own formula. One formula calculates doses based on an individual's daily insulin dose, see Box 19.13.

OVERDOSE

Drug overdoses are, sadly, a common occurrence in custody. Many of those we see have drug problems, obtaining illicit drugs from various sources with inconsistent potency and contents. Additionally, any time spent in prison often leads to a reduction in an individual's tolerance to drugs. Suspected overdoses may become apparent shortly after detention, or may occur several hours later. HCPs should consider drug overdose as a possible cause for all cases of reduced consciousness.

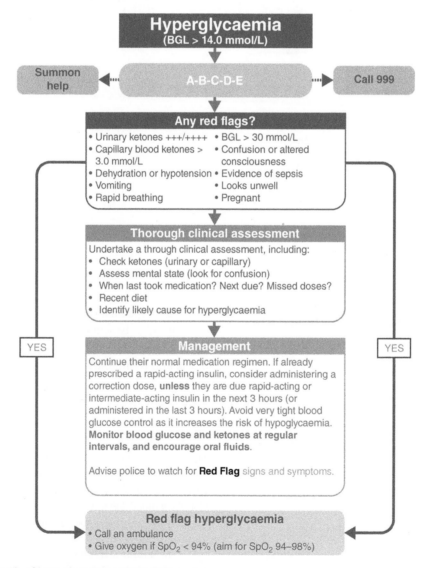

FIGURE 19.11   An example of hyperglycaemia management.

<table>
<tr><td>**BOX 19.13**</td><td>**CALCULATING CORRECTION DOSE**</td></tr>
</table>

Insulin total daily dose = Total number of insulin units daily (long and rapid acting)

Correction factor = 100 ÷ insulin total daily dose

<u>Worked example</u>
Insulin total daily dose = Lantus 24 units + Novorapid 16 units = 40 units
Correction factor = 100 ÷ 40 = 2.5
1 unit rapid-acting insulin will reduce BGL 2.5 mmol/L

BGL 19 mmol/L (target 10 mmol/L)
19.0 − 10.0 = 9 ÷ 2.5 = 3.6
Round to nearest whole number = 4 units rapid-acting insulin

Source: Adapted from NHS Tayside (2023).

ASSESSMENT

All overdoses should be assessed using the A-B-C-D-E approach. Pay particular attention to the pupils, which may point towards a drug type. There are different toxidromes specific to certain drug types (see Box 19.14). However, because of poly-drug use or 'mixing' of drugs, an individual may not present with one single toxidrome.

MANAGEMENT

Management is mostly supportive of using the A-B-C-D-E approach. All drug overdoses should be transferred to hospital.

Opioid Overdose

Opioid overdoses are common and easily reversible with naloxone, an opioid antagonist, see Figure 19.12. The half-life of naloxone is shorter than most opioids, so repeated doses may be necessary. All opioid overdoses require 999 ambulance transport to hospital for a period of observation.

SEIZURES

Seizures are a disturbance in the brain's electrical activity resulting in temporary changes in muscle activity, behaviours, sensations or state of awareness. They can present in several different ways, ranging from periods of apparent inattention (absences) to focal seizures where only part of the body is affected to generalised seizures involving the whole body and a loss of responsiveness and awareness.

Seizures can be caused by:

- Epilepsy
- Drug side effects or overdose
- Head trauma
- Stroke

<table>
<tr><td>**BOX 19.14**</td><td>**TOXIDROMES**</td></tr>
</table>

Toxidrome *(and drug examples)*	Vital signs (Temp, HR, RR, BP)	Pupils	Other symptoms
Sympathomimetic *(cocaine, amphetamine, ephedrine, pseudoephedrine)*	↑	Dilated	Hyperalert, agitated, hallucinations, sweating, tremors, hyperreflexia, seizures
Anticholinergic *(antihistamines, tricyclics, anti-Parkinson drugs, antispasmodics, phenothiazines)*	↑	Dilated	Hypervigilant, agitated, hallucinations, coma, dry mucous membranes, urinary retention, myoclonus, seizures
Hallucinogenic *(MDMA, ecstasy, LSD, phencyclidine)*	↑	Dilated	Hallucinations, agitated, nystagmus
Serotonin syndrome *(MAOIs, SSRI, tricyclic antidepressants, L-tryptophan)*	↑	Dilated	Tremor, myoclonus, hyperreflexia, clonus, sweating, flushed skin, muscle rigidity, diarrhoea
Opioid *(codeine, heroin, morphine, oxycodone)*	↓	Small or pinpoint	Reduced level of consciousness, coma
Sedative/hypnotic *(benzodiazepines, barbiturates, alcohol)*	↓	Dilated	Reduced level of consciousness, coma, confusion
Cholinergic *(organophosphate insecticides, nerve agents, nicotine)*	↓	Small	Confusion, coma, salivation, incontinence, diarrhoea, vomiting, sweating, weakness, seizures

- Alcohol withdrawal

- Meningitis/encephalitis

- Hypo/hyperglycaemia

Fortunately, most seizures are short-lived (less than one minute) and self-terminate. Seizures in those with no history of epilepsy are a red flag and require immediate hospital referral (see Box 19.15). In epilepsy, the greatest risk is usually from the effects such as, injuries sustained in a fall from standing or aspiration of vomit. However, prolonged seizures can cause hypoxia due to trismus and ineffective respiratory muscle control.

BOX 19.15   SEIZURE RED FLAGS

Red flags

Refer to the hospital

- No history of epilepsy

- Significant injury

- Prolonged seizure (5 minutes)

- Second seizure with no recovery between

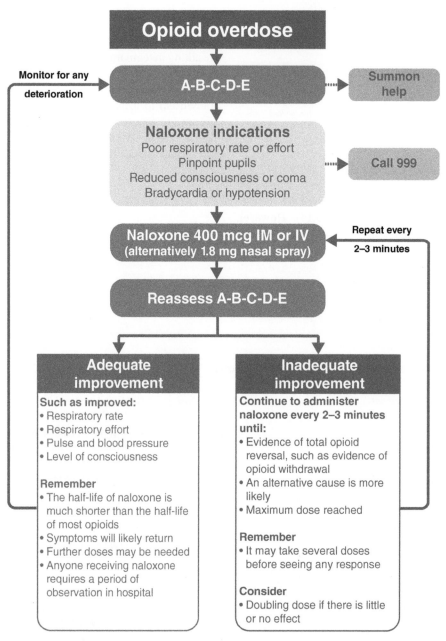

FIGURE 19.12   Opioid overdose management.

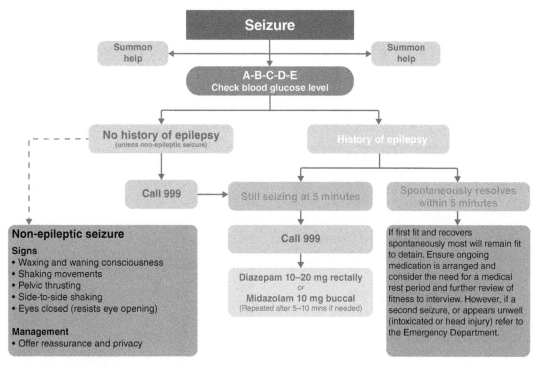

FIGURE 19.13   Seizure management.

ASSESSMENT

Use the A-B-C-D-E approach. Establish the time seizure activity was noted and the likely cause (i.e. epileptic or alcohol withdrawal).

MANAGEMENT

Make the immediate area safe by removing harmful objects and placing something soft under their head. Figure 19.13 outlines the further management of seizures. Consider supplemental oxygen. If a known epileptic has a seizure in keeping with their normal pattern and recovers fully with no injuries, then there is no need to be sent to hospital. They may, however, be unfit for an interview for some time post-seizure.

Prolonged seizures (over 5 minutes) require an anticonvulsant such as diazepam or midazolam.

NON-EPILEPTIC SEIZURES

There is a category of seizures known as non-epileptic seizures.[6] These are episodes that may mimic seizures but do not originate from aberrant electrical activity in the brain. Instead, they are a psychological condition rather than a physiological one, in response to triggers perceived as threatening or challenging. They may be indistinguishable from true seizures or may present atypically. In recent years, it has been recognised non-epileptic seizures are not under conscious control and are not fabricated.

Management

The priority is making the immediate area safe by removing harmful objects and placing something soft under their head. Provide reassurance and privacy. Anticonvulsants are not indicated, even if events last over five minutes, as non-epileptic seizures do not cause any damage to the brain.

SEPSIS

Sepsis is a life-threatening response to an infection, usually respiratory, urinary, gastrointestinal or wound infections. Those at higher risk of sepsis include:

- Women post-delivery, miscarriage or termination
- Over 75
- Immunosuppressed[7]
- Diabetes
- Recent surgery or serious illness

SIGNS AND SYMPTOMS

Sepsis may present with a variety of signs and symptoms. For this reason, screen for sepsis those appearing clinically unwell or have a NEWS2 of 5 or above (see Figure 19.14).

---

[6] Also known as psychogenic non-epileptic seizure, psychogenic seizure, pseudo seizure, non-epileptic attack (disorder).

[7] Cancer treatment, organ or bone marrow transplant, HIV or AIDS, kidney failure or some medications (i.e. steroids, methotrexate or azathioprine).

SEPSIS SCREENING TOOL COMMUNITY CARE

AGE 16+

01 START THIS CHART IF THE PATIENT LOOKS UNWELL OR HAS ABNORMAL PHYSIOLOGY

RISK FACTORS FOR SEPSIS INCLUDE:

☐ Age > 75
☐ Impaired immunity (e.g. diabetes, steroids, chemotherapy)

CONSIDER ANY ADVANCE DIRECTIVE/ CARE PLAN

☐ Recent trauma / surgery / invasive procedure
☐ Indwelling lines / IVDU / broken skin

02 COULD THIS BE DUE TO AN INFECTION?

YES

LIKELY SOURCE:

☐ Respiratory ☐ Urine ☐ Skin / joint / wound ☐ Indwelling device
☐ Brain ☐ Surgical ☐ Other

NO → SEPSIS UNLIKELY, CONSIDER OTHER DIAGNOSIS

03 ANY RED FLAG PRESENT?

YES

☐ Objective evidence of new or altered mental state
☐ Respiratory rate ≥ 25 per minute
☐ Needs O2 (40% +) to keep SpO2 ≥ 92% (≥88% in COPD)
☐ Systolic BP ≤ 90 mmHg (or drop of >40 from normal)
☐ Heart rate ≥ 130 per minute
☐ Not passed urine in 18 hours (<0.5ml/kg/hr if catheterised)
☐ Non-blanching rash / mottled / ashen / cyanotic

YES →

RED FLAG SEPSIS
START BUNDLE

04 ANY AMBER FLAG PRESENT?

NO

☐ Family report abnormal behaviour or mental state
☐ Reduced functional ability
☐ Respiratory rate 21-24
☐ Systolic BP 91-100 mmHg
☐ Heart rate 91-129 or new dysrhythmia
☐ SpO2 ≤ 92% or increased O2 requirement
☐ Not passed urine in 12-18 h (<0.5ml/kg/hr if catheterised)
☐ Immunocompromised
☐ Signs of infection including wound infection
☐ Temperature <36°C

1 SAME DAY ASSESSMENT BY GP / TEAM LEADER

2 IS URGENT REFERRAL TO HOSPITAL REQUIRED?

YES →

3 AGREE AND DOCUMENT ONGOING MANAGEMENT PLAN (INCLUDING OBSERVATION FREQUENCY AND PLANNED SECOND REVIEW)

NO AMBER FLAGS: ROUTINE CARE AND GIVE SAFETY-NETTING ADVICE:

CALL 111 IF CONDITION CHANGES OR DETERIORATES. SIGNPOST TO AVAILABLE RESOURCES AS APPROPRIATE

CALL 999 IF ANY OF: →
Slurred speech or confusion
Extreme shivering or muscle pain
Passing no urine (in a day)
Severe breathlessness
'I feel I might die'
Skin mottled, ashen, blue or very pale

RED FLAG BUNDLE:

DIAL 999 AND ARRANGE BLUE LIGHT TRANSFER
IF PRESCRIBER AVAILABLE & TRANSIT TIME >1H GIVE IV ANTIBIOTICS

Ensure communication of 'Red Flag Sepsis' to crew. Advise crew to pre-alert as 'Red Flag Sepsis'. Where possible a written handover is recommended including observations and antibiotic allergies.

The controlled copy of this document is maintained by The UK Sepsis Trust. Any copies of this document held outside of that area, in whatever format (e.g. paper, email attachment) are considered to have passed out of control and should be checked for currency and validity.

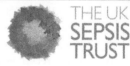

THE UK SEPSIS TRUST

UKST 2024 1.0 PAGE 1 OF 1

The UK Sepsis Trust registered charity number (England & Wales) 1158843 (Scotland) SC050277. Company registration number 8644039. Sepsis Enterprises Ltd. company number 9583335. VAT reg. number 293133408.

FIGURE 19.14 Sepsis screening tool community. *Source:* Reproduced with permission of The UK Sepsis Trust.

MANAGEMENT

Any suspected sepsis must be transported to hospital, including amber flag sepsis. Those with Red Flag Sepsis will require 999 ambulance transport and:

- Assessment and management of A-B-C-D-E
- If necessary, administer oxygen to maintain SpO_2 of ≥94% (88% in COPD)
- Depending on skillset and equipment, consider IV fluid bolus for hypotension

WERNICKE'S ENCEPHALOPATHY

Wernicke's encephalopathy is a severe neurological disorder caused by a thiamine deficiency. It can present acutely, developing rapidly over hours to days. It is essential to recognise as delays in treatment can lead to irreversible brain damage or death.

SIGNS AND SYMPTOMS

The classical features are confusion, ataxia and ophthalmoplegia.[8] Individuals may present with confusion, disorientation and agitation before progressing to coma. Ataxia is impaired motor coordination, including a wide-based unsteady gait, speech difficulties and poor fine motor skills. Ophthalmoplegia is abnormal eye movements or paralysis, resulting in difficulty moving an eye or both eyes in all directions. However, not all individuals will present with the complete triad of symptoms.

MANAGEMENT

Individuals with suspected Wernicke's encephalopathy should be transferred immediately to hospital for high-dose intravenous thiamine.

DEATHS IN CUSTODY

Death in custody includes any death in custody or at hospital following transfer. Any death is a tragedy and deeply upsetting for the deceased's family and friends. However, deaths can also have a profound impact on HCPs. Such incidents receive intense scrutiny, media attention and ultimately an inquest (coronal or fatal accident inquiry). All deaths are referred for investigation by the Independent Office for Police Conduct (or equivalent).

HCPs should have guidelines following a death in custody, outlining the immediate and short-term actions and responsibilities, including a de-brief of the HCPs involved and a review and completion of incident reporting systems. Priority should be the welfare and support of the HCPs involved, allocating resources to meet the ongoing needs of others detained in the suite and responding to any immediate risks identified (for example, if drug-related other individuals may have been exposed) and replenishing of stock and completion of medical records, usually completed retrospectively if managing an acute emergency.

Following a death in custody, police may implement local post-incident procedures, including preserving the scene (i.e. cell). They will likely initiate Post-Incident Management, often called the 'PIM', to facilitate the investigation process. The PIM involves documenting all relevant information and decisions, including identifying witnesses and key police witnesses who can give direct evidence relating to the death. HCPs may be considered key police witnesses. HCPs should have well-documented guidelines or procedures following a death in custody concerning their organisational response and engagement with the PIM.

CONCLUSION

In conclusion, this chapter provides a comprehensive and detailed exploration of managing various emergencies, emphasising the A-B-C-D-E approach. The chapter equips HCPs with the necessary knowledge and skills to effectively handle medical, psychiatric, and substance-related emergencies, ensuring timely and appropriate care. The inclusion of specific equipment and management strategies, alongside the consideration of ambulance transport and the complexities of decision-making in critical situations, reflects the real-world challenges faced by HCPs. The chapter also underscores the significance of continuous learning and adherence to guidelines, ensuring HCPs are always prepared to provide the best possible care in emergencies.

| LEARNING |
| ACTIVITIES |

1. Using the equipment and resources (including police staff) available in your setting, practice responding to various stimulated emergencies in the cells. Be sure to include acute behavioural disturbance.

2. Write a reflection of a situation where you dealt with an emergency in custody. Consider what went well or not so well and how you manage the pressure of being the only HCP present.

3. In a scenario where multiple individuals require urgent medical attention simultaneously, explain how you would prioritise care. What factors would influence your decisions, and how would you manage limited resources while ensuring effective treatment for all individuals?

---

[8] A paralysis or weakness of eye muscles, leading to uncontrolled, jerky eye movements (nystagmus) or the inability to move eyes in all directions.

RESOURCES

Online

- College of Policing | Post-incident procedures following death or serious injury | https://www.college.police.uk/app/post-incident-procedures-following-death-or-serious-injury/post-incident-procedures-following-death-or-serious-injury

- Faculty of Forensic & Legal Medicine | Acute behavioural disturbance: Guidelines on management in police custody | https://fflm.ac.uk/resources/publications/acute-behavioural-disturbance-abdguidelines-on-management-in-police-custody/

Organisations

- Resuscitation Council UK | www.resus.org.uk

- TOXBASE | www.toxbase.org

- The UK Sepsis Trust | www.sepsistrust.org

REFERENCES

Faculty of Forensic & Legal Medicine (2019). *Acute Behavioural Disturbance (ABD): Guidelines on Management in Police Custody*. London: Faculty of Forensic and Legal medicine https://fflm.ac.uk/wp-content/uploads/2019/05/AcuteBehaveDisturbance_Apr19-FFLM-RCEM.pdf (accessed 23 September 2021).

Humphries, C., Kelly, A., Sadik, A. et al. (2024). Consensus on acute behavioural disturbance in the UK: a multidisciplinary modified Delphi study to determine what it is and how it should be managed. *Emergency Medicine Journal* 41: 4–12.

Miles, T., Webb, V., Kevern, P. et al. (2020). Custody early warning scores; do they predict patient deterioration in police custody? *Journal of Forensic and Legal Medicine* 76: 102069.

NHS Tayside (2023). Adjusting insulin. https://www.nhstayside.scot.nhs.uk/OurServicesA-Z/DiabetesOutThereDOTTayside/PROD_263751/index.htm (accessed 11 July 2023).

Petitpas, F., Guenezan, J., Vendeuvre, T. et al. (2016). Use of intra-osseous access in adults: a systematic review. *Critical Care* 20: 102.

Resuscitation Council UK (2021). *Emergency Treatment of Anaphylaxis; Guidelines for Healthcare Providers*. London: Resuscitation Council UK https://www.resus.org.uk/sites/default/files/2021-05/Emergency%20Treatment%20of%20Anaphylaxis%20May%202021_0.pdf (accessed 08 October 2023).

Scottish Intercollegiate Guidelines Network and British Thoracic Society (2019). [SIGN158] British guideline on the management of asthma. Healthcare Improvement Scotland. https://www.brit-thoracic.org.uk/document-library/guidelines/asthma/bts-sign-asthma-guideline-2014/ (accessed 10 October 2023).

FURTHER READING

Association of Ambulance Chief Executives and NHS England | National Framework for healthcare professional ambulance responses | https://www.england.nhs.uk/wp-content/uploads/2019/07/C1172-aace-national-framework-for-hcp-ambulance-responses.pdf

Peel, M. (2022) Acute behavioural disturbance: recognition, assessment and management. *Emergency Nurse* 32 (3): 35357781. doi: 10.7748/en.2022.e2126

TREND-UK | Hypoglycaemia in adults in the community: recognition, management and prevention | https://www.mytype1diabetes.nhs.uk/media/1167/hcp_hypo_trend_final.pdf

Index

Note: Page numbers following *f* refer to figure

Police Custody Healthcare for Nurses and Paramedics, First Edition. Edited by Matthew Peel, Jennie Smith, Vanessa Webb, and Margaret Bannerman.
© 2025 John Wiley & Sons Ltd. Published 2025 by John Wiley & Sons Ltd.
Companion website: www.wiley.com/go/policecustodyhealthcare